Changing Paradigms in the Management of Breast Cancer

Marissa Howard-McNatt
Editor

Changing Paradigms in the Management of Breast Cancer

Springer

Editor
Marissa Howard-McNatt, MD
Associate Professor of Surgery
Director Breast Care Center
Wake Forest School of Medicine
Winston-Salem, NC, USA

ISBN 978-3-319-60335-3 ISBN 978-3-319-60336-0 (eBook)
DOI 10.1007/978-3-319-60336-0

Library of Congress Control Number: 2017947154

Printed on acid-free paper

This Springer imprint is published by Springer Nature
The registered company is Springer International Publishing AG
The registered company address is: Gewerbestrasse 11, 6330 Cham, Switzerland

To my husband, Stephen,
our three beautiful daughters,
and my beloved parents.

Preface

This is the first edition of *Changing Paradigms in the Management of Breast Cancer*. Breast cancer treatment has evolved over the past 20 years. Breast conservation and mastectomy have been the mainstay of treatment; however, sentinel lymph node biopsy has become the standard of care. Surgically, we have had debates on, and now hopefully resolution of, margin status, and we have witnessed the rise of contralateral prophylactic mastectomy. On the systemic side, there has been an increase in targeted therapy especially with Her2 agents. The use of genomic profiling has also spurred an era of new management of breast cancer patients. Many aspects of breast cancer care continue to evolve.

This text is designed to present a comprehensive and state-of the-art approach to the management of breast cancer within the fields of surgery, medical oncology, and radiation oncology. Sections will address changes in these fields. We will start with examining new techniques in breast imaging. This will be followed by surgical issues including the management of the axilla, surgical margins, and nipple-sparing and contralateral mastectomies as well as current trends in breast reconstruction. Atypical lesions of the breast will be highlighted. Subsequent chapters will focus on issues in medical oncology including triple-negative breast cancer and metastatic disease. New paradigms in radiation oncology treatment will be explored. Breast cancer treatment in the elderly and in the young and genetic risk in breast cancer management will also be discussed. Written by a diverse and distinguished group of experts in their field, each of these sections will address advances and changes in the field. A brief review of the existing literature addressing the particular topic will be included in each section. Finally, I would like to thank Maureen Alexander for helping in the preparation of the manuscript.

Access to a comprehensive multidisciplinary resource for breast cancer patients is currently limited in the literature. As such, there is no single source to provide information on advances and outcomes for physicians, fellows, residents, nurse practitioners, and physician assistants caring for breast cancer patients in a multidisciplinary setting. We hope that *Changing Paradigms in the Management of Breast Cancer* becomes a useful resource for clinicians and adds to the knowledge necessary to provide up-to-date care for our patients with breast cancer.

Winston-Salem, NC, USA Marissa Howard-McNatt, MD

Contents

1 **Breast Imaging: Tomosynthesis, Elastography, Breast MRI and Emerging Techniques** 1
Nancy A. Resteghini, Michael D.C. Fishman, and Priscilla J. Slanetz

2 **Nipple-Sparing Mastectomy** 17
Suzanne B. Coopey and Barbara L. Smith

3 **Contralateral Prophylactic Mastectomy: Current Perspectives** 33
Katharine Yao

4 **Management of the Axilla in Breast Cancer** 47
Toan T. Nguyen and Judy C. Boughey

5 **Margins and Breast Cancer** 59
Anees B. Chagpar

6 **Percutaneous Ablation in the Treatment of Breast Cancer** 71
Vivian J. Bea, Dalliah Black, and Kelly Hunt

7 **New Technology and Techniques in Breast Reconstruction** 85
Christine Velázquez and Ivo Alexander Pestana

8 **New Thoughts on Atypias of the Breast: Flat Epithelial Atypia, Atypical Ductal Hyperplasia, and Lobular Neoplasia** 117
Megan E. Sullivan

9 **New Techniques in Radiation Oncology** 127
Ryan T. Hughes and Doris R. Brown

10 **Radiotherapy and Regional Nodes** 139
Andrew Zhang, Bruce G. Haffty, and Sharad Goyal

11 **Triple-Negative Breast Cancer** 155
Tiffany P. Avery

12 New Treatments for Metastatic Breast Cancer 167
Ana Christina Garrido-Castro and Beth Overmoyer

13 Breast Cancer Treatment in Elderly Patients. 199
Akiko Chiba and Marissa Howard-McNatt

14 Breast Cancer Treatment in Young Women. 209
Susan K. Boolbol and Sarah Cate

15 Genetic Risk Prediction in Breast Cancer 217
Anvy Nguyen, Jennifer K. Plichta, Jessica Cintolo-Gonzalez,
Kinyas Kartal, Molly Elizabeth Griffin, and Kevin Hughes

Correction to: Percutaneous Ablation in the Treatment of Breast Cancer C1

Index. 233

Contributors

Tiffany P. Avery, MD Department of Hematology and Oncology, Wake Forest Baptist Health, Winston-Salem, NC, USA

Vivian J. Bea, MD Department of Breast Surgical Oncology, University of Texas MD Anderson Cancer Center, Houston, TX, USA

Dalliah Black, MD Department of Breast Surgical Oncology, University of Texas MD Anderson Cancer Center, Houston, TX, USA

Susan K. Boolbol, MD Mount Sinai Beth Israel Hospital, New York, NY, USA

Judy C. Boughey, MD Department of Surgery, Mayo Clinic, Rochester, MN, USA

Doris R. Brown, MD, PhD Department of Radiation Oncology, Wake Forest Baptist Health, Winston-Salem, NC, USA

Sarah Cate, MD Mount Sinai Beth Israel Hospital, New York, NY, USA

Anees B. Chagpar, MD, MSc, MA, MPH, MBA Department of Surgery, Yale University School of Medicine, New Haven, CT, USA

Akiko Chiba, MD Department of Surgical Oncology, Wake Forest Baptist Health, Winston-Salem, NC, USA

Jessica Cintolo-Gonzalez, MD Brigham and Women's Hospital, Boston, MA, USA

Suzanne B. Coopey, MD Division of Surgical Oncology, Massachusetts General Hospital, Boston, MA, USA

Michael D. C. Fishman, MD Department of Radiology, Harvard Medical School, Beth Israel Deaconess Medical Center, Boston, MA, USA

Ana Christina Garrido-Castro, MD Department of Medical Oncology, Harvard Medical School, Dana-Farber Cancer Institute, Susan F. Smith Center for Women's Cancer, Boston, MA, USA

Sharad Goyal, MD, MS Department of Radiation Oncology, Rutgers Cancer Institute of New Jersey and Rutgers Robert Wood Johnson Medical School, New Brunswick, NJ, USA

Molly Elizabeth Griffin, BA Division of Surgical Oncology, Massachusetts General Hospital, Boston, MA, USA

Bruce G. Haffty, MD Department of Radiation Oncology, Rutgers Cancer Institute of New Jersey and Rutgers Robert Wood Johnson Medical School, New Brunswick, NJ, USA

Marissa Howard-McNatt, MD Department of Surgery, Wake Forest Baptist Health, Winston-Salem, NC, USA

Kevin Hughes, MD Division of Surgical Oncology, Massachusetts General Hospital, Boston, MA, USA

Ryan T. Hughes, MD Department of Radiation Oncology, Wake Forest Baptist Health, Winston-Salem, NC, USA

Kelly Hunt, MD, FACS, BSC Department of Breast Surgical Oncology, University of Texas MD Anderson Cancer Center, Houston, TX, USA

Kinyas Kartal, MD Division of Surgical Oncology, Massachusetts General Hospital, Boston, MA, USA

Anvy Nguyen, MD Department of Breast Oncology, Susan F. Smith Center for Women's Cancers, Dana-Farber Cancer Institute, Boston, MA, USA

Toan T. Nguyen, MD Department of Surgery, Mayo Clinic, Rochester, MN, USA

Beth Overmoyer, MD, FACP Department of Medical Oncology, Harvard Medical School, Dana-Farber Cancer Institute, Susan F. Smith Center for Women's Cancer, Boston, MA, USA

Ivo Alexander Pestana, MD, FACS Department of Plastic and Reconstructive Surgery, Wake Forest University Baptist Medical Center, Winston-Salem, NC, USA

Jennifer K. Plichta, MD, MS Department of Surgery, Duke University Medical Center, Durham, NC, USA

Nancy A. Resteghini, DO, MS Department of Radiology, Beth Israel Deaconess Medical Center, Boston, MA, USA

Priscilla J. Slanetz, MD, MPH Department of Radiology, Harvard Medical School, Beth Israel Deaconess Medical Center, Boston, MA, USA

Barbara L. Smith, MD, PhD Division of Surgical Oncology, Massachusetts General Hospital, Boston, MA, USA

Megan E. Sullivan, MD Department of Pathology and Laboratory Medicine, Evanston Hospital, North Shore University Health System, Evanston, IL, USA

Christine Velázquez, MD Department of General Surgery, Wake Forest University Baptist Medical Center, Winston-Salem, NC, USA

Katharine Yao, MD Division of Surgical Oncology, Department of Surgery, NorthShore University HealthSystem, Evanston, IL, USA

Pritzker School of Medicine, University of Chicago, Evanston, IL, USA

Andrew Zhang, MD Department of Radiation Oncology, Rutgers Cancer Institute of New Jersey and Rutgers Robert Wood Johnson Medical School, New Brunswick, NJ, USA

Breast Imaging: Tomosynthesis, Elastography, Breast MRI and Emerging Techniques

1

Nancy A. Resteghini, Michael D.C. Fishman, and Priscilla J. Slanetz

Breast imaging plays a critical role in the detection, diagnosis, and management of women diagnosed with breast cancer. Although there are a multitude of risk factors associated with breast cancer, such as female gender, increasing age, and family history, the density of breast tissue as evident on mammography has more recently been identified as an independent risk factor [1]. Although some studies suggest that the lifetime risk increases by four to six times for women with dense breast tissue, this is misleading as this compares women with extremely dense tissue to women with predominantly fatty breasts, both of which represent a minority of the population [2]. More realistically, the lifetime risk is only increased by 1.2–2.1 times in a woman with heterogeneously dense or extremely dense breasts, respectively, when compared to the average woman who has scattered fibroglandular tissue [1, 3, 4]. However, as breast density is known to lower the sensitivity of mammography due to "masking" of cancers, the integration of newer modalities for the management of newly diagnosed breast cancer, such as digital breast tomosynthesis, ultrasound, and magnetic resonance imaging (MRI), continues to evolve. In addition, recent legislative efforts that mandate direct patient notification of breast density exist in

N.A. Resteghini, DO, MS (✉)
Department of Radiology, Beth Israel Deaconess Medical Center, 330 Brookline Avenue, Boston, MA 02215, USA
e-mail: nrestegh@bidmc.harvard.edu

M.D.C. Fishman, MD
Department of Radiology, Harvard Medical School, Beth Israel Deaconess Medical Center, 330 Brookline Avenue, Shapiro 460, Boston, MA 02115, USA
e-mail: mfishma1@bidmc.harvard.edu

P.J. Slanetz, MD, MPH
Department of Radiology, Harvard Medical School, Beth Israel Deaconess Medical Center, 330 Brookline Avenue, Boston, MA 02478, USA
e-mail: pslanetz@bidmc.harvard.edu

M. Howard-McNatt (ed.), *Changing Paradigms in the Management of Breast Cancer*, DOI 10.1007/978-3-319-60336-0_1

nearly 50% of states in the USA. Consequently, there is a growing research on developing more sensitive and specific tools to "see through" the dense tissue and therefore permit earlier cancer detection, which should translate into improved outcomes.

In this chapter, we review the current role of digital mammography, digital breast tomosynthesis, ultrasound, and magnetic resonance imaging (MRI) for routine and supplemental screening of breast cancer and review the role of these modalities in the management of breast cancer. We also will discuss the role of two emerging modalities – contrast-enhanced mammography and abbreviated MRI. By providing insight into the advantages and disadvantages of the currently available imaging modalities, providers should be able to optimize the imaging evaluation of women with suspected and newly diagnosed breast cancer.

Digital Mammography and Breast Tomosynthesis

Mammography consists of two-dimensional (2D) images of a three-dimensional (3D) breast. For screening of asymptomatic women, mediolateral oblique (MLO) and craniocaudal (CC) projections of each breast are acquired [5]. In all centers accredited by the American College of Radiology (ACR), an MQSA-certified breast radiologist interprets the screening examination and will recall the patient for additional diagnostic imaging if a finding is deemed to warrant further evaluation. In most practices, approximately 10% of asymptomatic women in the screening population are recalled for diagnostic evaluation. When the woman returns, she may undergo additional diagnostic mammographic views or ultrasound. Any woman who has a focal symptom or findings concerning for breast cancer on clinical examination undergoes diagnostic mammography, which typically entails the standard CC and MLO views, additional spot compression imaging, and usually ultrasound. Based on the diagnostic work-up, the patient may return to routine screening or be asked to undergo either follow-up imaging or image-guided biopsy. Interpretation of mammography is standardized using the Breast Imaging Reporting and Data System (BIRADS) lexicon [5]. In addition to describing any finding (such as asymmetry, mass, calcifications, or architectural distortion) using standardized terminology, the breast density (i.e., the relative amount of glandular tissue to fat in the breast) is also reported according to four categories: predominantly fatty, scattered fibroglandular, heterogeneously dense, or extremely dense (Fig. 1.1) [5]. Finally, a final assessment category between 0 and 6 is added to the breast imaging report as a standardized way to summarize the clinical significance of the imaging findings.

At present, although controversy persists surrounding the optimal screening interval, mammography remains the only modality that has been proven to reduce mortality from breast cancer by up to 30% [6]. The controversy surrounding screening stems from concerns over the number of false positives, especially in younger women with dense tissue, and the potential of overdiagnosis of ductal carcinoma in situ (DCIS). Both of these concerns do warrant an informed discussion with every woman, but given that there is no other proven test for early detection of breast cancer, nearly all women still opt to participate in screening. In addition, given the

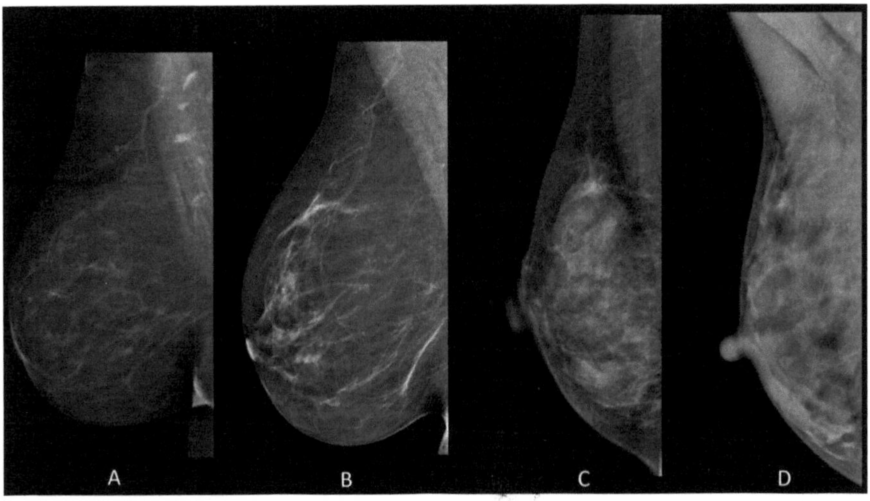

Fig. 1.1 Breast tissue patterns according to the fifth edition of the BIRADS lexicon. (**a**) Predominantly fatty, (**b**) scattered fibroglandular, (**c**) heterogeneously dense, and (**d**) extremely dense

mortality benefit, many major medical organizations continue to recommend annual screening mammography starting at the age of 40 years for the average-risk woman and earlier if the patient is deemed to be at elevated risk.

With sensitivity of approximately 90% and specificity of 89% for the average breast (scattered fibroglandular tissue), the presence of dense breast tissue (heterogeneously dense or extremely dense) lowers the sensitivity of mammography to as low as 62–68% on film-screen but this increases to approximately 83% with digital techniques [7–9]. As mammographic sensitivity is lower in women with dense breast tissue, practice is evolving on how best to screen these women, as approximately 40–50% of the US population is known to have dense breast tissue. A recent change in the BIRADS lexicon on how breast density is characterized also likely will lead to an even greater percentage of women being characterized as "dense" as the current edition recommends that any patch of dense tissue be classified as "dense" [5]. In addition, it is important to recognize that in most practices, breast density is subjectively assessed and that there is considerable inter-reader variability, especially for a majority of women (those who either have scattered fibroglandular tissue or heterogeneously dense tissue) [7, 10–12]. Breast density can also be affected by patient age, parity, hormone replacement therapy, body mass index, and genetic predisposition [13–15]. For women with dense tissue, the multicenter prospective DMIST study of 49,528 women showed that screening with digital mammography increased cancer detection by women with heterogeneously dense or extremely dense breasts on mammography (difference, 0.11; 95% confidence interval, 0.04–0.18; $P = 0.003$) [16] (Fig. 1.2). Consequently, women with dense tissue ideally should be imaged using digital equipment whenever possible. Fortunately, in 2016, greater than 95% of accredited imaging facilities have digital technology [17].

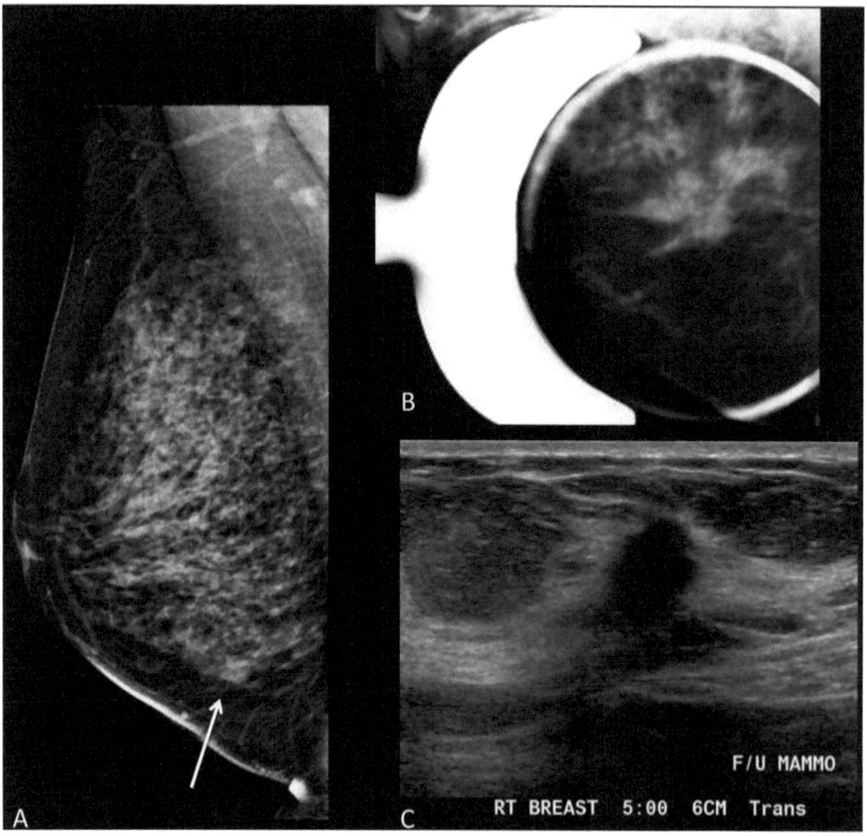

Fig. 1.2 Forty-six-year-old woman with 2 cm mass in the lower inner right breast on screening mammography. (**a**) MLO view shows an asymmetry inferiorly. (**b**) Spot compression MLO view confirms an irregular mass with distortion. (**c**) Ultrasound shows an irregular hypoechoic shadowing mass. Biopsy revealed grade 2 invasive lobular carcinoma

However, mammography has other limitations. Given that up to 10% of women may be recalled for additional imaging for a majority of findings that ultimately are dismissed or are benign, there is a continued need to improve this technology, that is, increase cancer detection while decrease the recall rate from screening. At present, with conventional mammographic imaging, superimposed or overlapping breast tissue on one of the 2D images is the leading cause for recall from screening, which is more common in women with dense breasts [18, 19].

Digital breast tomosynthesis (DBT) is a newer modality that can overcome some of the current limitations of conventional digital mammography [19]. First approved by the Food and Drug Administration (FDA) in 2011, this technology acquires both an arc of projection images that are reconstructed into a pseudo-3D dataset and conventional images (either as a separate acquisition or reconstructed from the 3D dataset). When acquired as a separate acquisition, combining DBT with conventional digital mammography comes with at least two times the radiation dose to the patient as compared to digital mammography alone. However, DBT has substantial advantages as the interpreting radiologist can scroll through the 3D dataset almost entirely eliminating overlapping breast tissue [20–22]. In addition, in several recent studies, when combined with digital mammography, digital breast tomosynthesis has been shown to decrease recall rates and improve detection of invasive breast cancers as compared to digital mammography alone (Fig. 1.3) [23–26]. A recent observational study by Rose et al. where DBT was integrated into a screening practice resulted in significant decreases in recall rates from 8.7 to 5.5% ($p < 0.001$) with increase in detection of invasive cancer from 2.8 to 4.3 per 1000 screening examinations and an increase in the positive predictive value for recalls from 4.7 to 10.1% ($p < 0.001$) [24]. Sharpe et al. evaluated 85,852 patients in a prospective study and demonstrated that DBT was associated with a 54.3% increase in the cancer detection rate compared with 2D mammography (3.5–5.4 per 1000; absolute change, +1.9 per 1000; relative change, +54.3%; $P < 0.018$) [18].

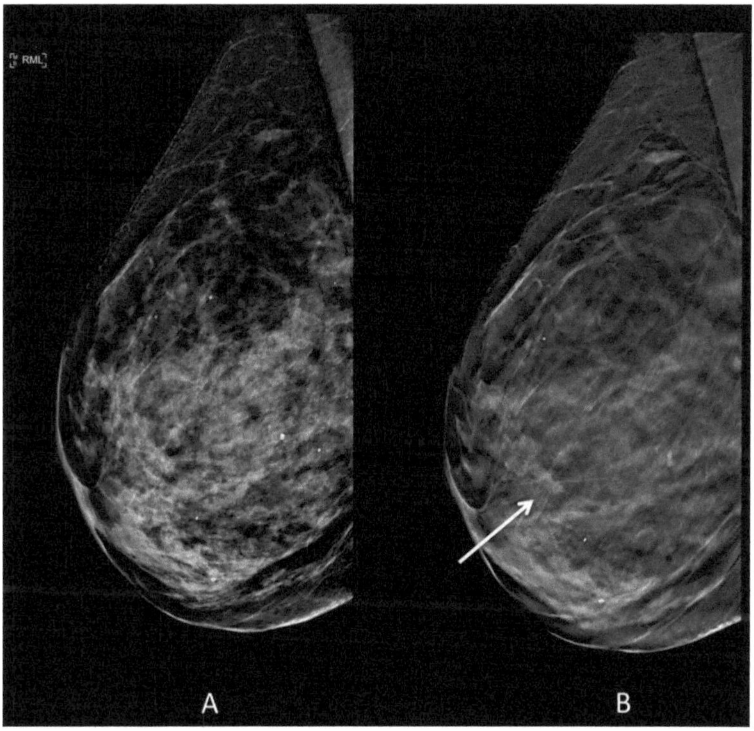

Fig. 1.3 Seventy-six-year-old woman with dense breast parenchyma for annual full-field digital mammogram with digital breast tomosynthesis (DBT). (**a**) Conventional 2D lateral view is negative for malignancy. (**b**) Architectural distortion (*arrow*) is identified only on DBT image. A mass was seen on subsequent ultrasound (not shown) with subsequent biopsy pathology of grade 1 invasive ductal carcinoma

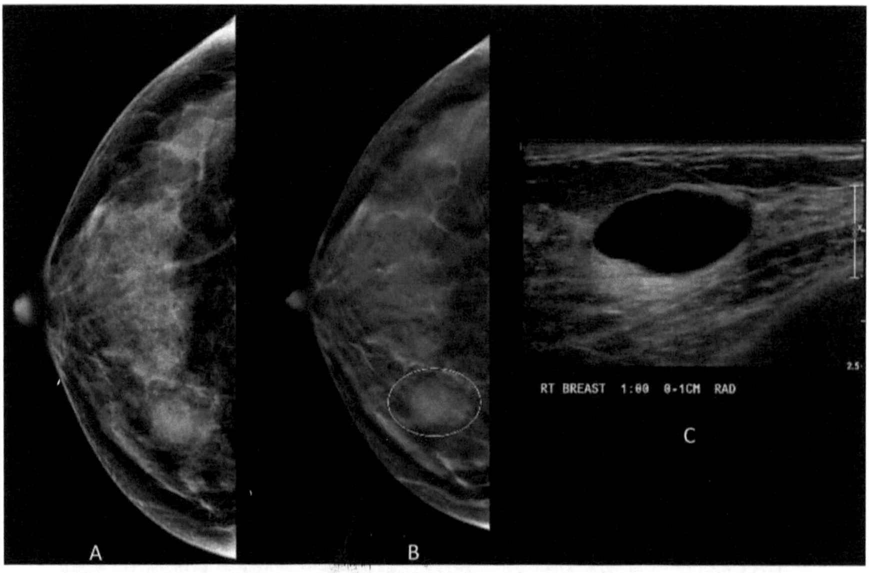

Fig. 1.4 Forty-three-year-old woman with obscured mass in the inner right breast on conventional MLO view (**a**) Tomosynthesis reveals circumscribed margins (**b**) Instead of additional diagnostic mammographic views to better characterize the margins, the patient was recalled to undergo ultrasound that revealed a simple cyst (**c**)

Although DBT clearly adds value in the screening setting, it also is helpful in the diagnostic work-up of patients with suspicious findings on clinical exam or those recalled from screening. This is particularly true in women with scattered fibroglandular tissue or heterogeneously dense breast tissue, as DBT can detect additional suspicious areas in women with newly diagnosed cancer or provide reassurance that the area of concern is benign or not clinically significant, resulting in fewer biopsies and specifically, fewer false-positive biopsies [27–30]. Digital breast tomosynthesis is particularly useful in characterizing margins of masses that are otherwise obscured by overlapping breast tissue on conventional imaging [31, 32]. Consequently, imaging protocols continue to evolve. For example, in most centers where a majority of women undergo screening using both digital mammography and DBT, if a circumscribed mass is seen on DBT, the patient is recalled for ultrasound only, thereby frequently avoiding any further diagnostic mammographic views and associated radiation (Fig. 1.4). While DBT considerably improves cancer detection and lowers recall rates, it remains an imperfect modality, particularly for women with extremely dense tissue. In order to detect malignancy, DBT relies on interfaces between the glandular tissue and fat, which is essentially non-existent in this subgroup of women [12].

Ultrasound and Elastography

Ultrasound uses sound waves to image the breast tissue and therefore comes with no radiation exposure to the patient. In most circumstances, breast ultrasound serves to complement mammography as a diagnostic tool for characterization of breast findings on both clinical exam and imaging. Breast ultrasound is mainly used to differentiate cystic from solid masses and can often classify benign from malignant masses for some women [33]. Ultrasound guidance for percutaneous core needle biopsy expedites the diagnosis of breast malignancy or confirms a benign diagnosis. In addition, image-guided biopsy streamlines the management of women eventually diagnosed with breast cancer by providing improved preoperative planning with diagnostic accuracy comparable to an open surgical biopsy [34].

One limitation of breast ultrasound, however, is the inconsistent differentiation of benign from malignant lesions. While not widely available, some breast imaging practices are beginning to incorporate breast elastography into diagnostic imaging. This technique can be performed at the time of the diagnostic breast ultrasound and provides information about tissue stiffness [35–37]. Typically, invasive cancers are "stiffer" or less elastic than normal breast tissue or even benign breast lesions [36, 38]. By incorporating this technique into diagnostic imaging, it has the potential to improve ultrasound specificity and decrease the number of benign breast biopsies (Fig. 1.5) [37–39].

More recent studies suggest that ultrasound of the whole breast can be performed to screen high-risk women and women with dense breast tissue with several studies showing that ultrasound can detect mammographically occult malignancy [40–42]. A study of 13,547 women undergoing screening mammography and ultrasound showed that with the addition of screening ultrasound, for all women, sensitivity for breast cancer detection increased from 74.7 to 97.3%, and in the cohort of women with extremely

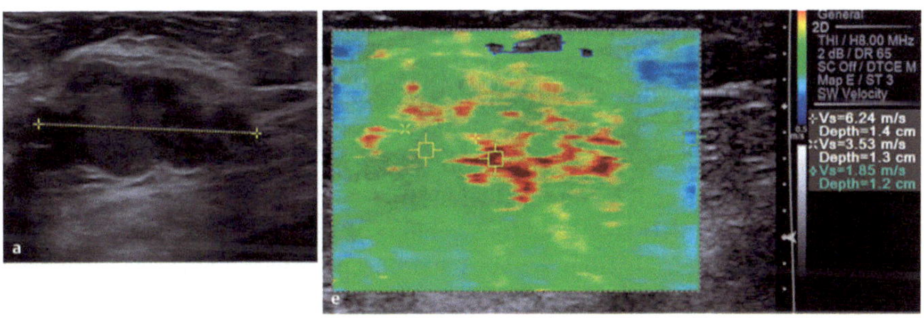

Fig. 1.5 Elastography showing that the solid macrolobulated mass seen on gray-scale ultrasound (*left image*) has high velocities highly suspicious for malignancy (*right image*). Biopsy confirmed invasive ductal carcinoma (Reprinted with permission from Ref. [80], Richard G. Barr, Breast Elastography. Thieme Publishers Inc. 2014)

dense breast tissue, the sensitivity increased from 47.6 to 76.1% [8]. As a result of this data, some advocate for supplemental ultrasound screening of all women with dense breast tissue. However, the incremental cancer detection is 0.3–14.0 cancers/1000 women screened depending on the patient's risk status (being closer to 4–7/1000 if high risk and closer to 2/1000 if low or average risk) [43]. In addition, supplemental screening with ultrasound leads to substantial false positives with positive biopsy rates less than 10% [41–44]. Therefore, not all clinicians advocate for screening with this modality. In fact, based on current evidence and weighing the risks and benefits of the various available modalities, if a patient is considered high risk, MRI is the preferred supplemental screening modality (discussed in further detail below), whereas if the patient is low or average risk, digital mammography with DBT is advisable [45].

Breast Magnetic Resonance Imaging

Magnetic resonance imaging of the breast is an imaging technique that uses a high-field magnet to image the breast tissue and demonstrates high sensitivity and specificity for breast cancer [46]. During the study, which is most commonly performed on a 1.5-Tesla magnet, the patient lies prone with the breasts pendent within a dedicated imaging coil. After acquiring some non-contrast images, intravenous contrast is administered (unless the study is only being performed to assess silicone implant integrity) to highlight the neo-vascularity of the tissue, and dynamic imaging is done for approximately 5–6 min after contrast injection. Since MRI highlights contrast enhancement, breast tissue density is less relevant in limiting sensitivity, as compared to mammography. In order to minimize background parenchymal enhancement (marked background enhancement does lower detection of DCIS and invasive lobular cancers) and minimize false positives (highest in perimenopausal women), the ideal time for breast MRI is between days 5 and 15 of the menstrual cycle, as the uptake of intravenous contrast is affected by hormonal fluctuations. However, in newly diagnosed cancer patients, it is not always possible to time the study accordingly. Therefore, when patients are imaged outside of this window, there is a greater chance of a false positive. Given that MRI does carry the risk of false positives, it is important to obtain histopathologic confirmation via MRI-guided breast biopsy for any finding prior to finalizing management recommendations.

Currently, breast MRI is utilized for screening as well as breast cancer diagnosis and staging. Clinical trials from the USA and Europe have demonstrated that MRI can significantly improve cancer detection that is otherwise clinically, mammographically, and sonographically occult [42, 47, 48], particularly in women at elevated lifetime risk for breast cancer. According to the American College of Radiology (ACR) Appropriateness Criteria, current indications for breast MRI include evaluation of silicone implant integrity, screening of high-risk patients (defined as women with greater than 20% lifetime risk), defining extent of disease in women with newly diagnosed breast cancer or women undergoing neoadjuvant chemotherapy, evaluation for recurrence, identification of an unknown primary in woman with metastatic disease, and problem solving of incompletely characterized imaging findings on other modalities [49].

Several studies, primarily in high-risk populations, have demonstrated that MRI detects an additional 3.5–28.6 cancers/1000 screened as compared to screening mammography alone [42, 50–59]. One of the larger studies, ACRIN 6666, which included women who were of intermediate to high risk and some of whom had dense breast tissue yielded 14.7 additional cancers per 1000 women screened [42].

Breast MRI can also be useful in defining extent of disease, including the presence of multifocal and multicentric disease in patients with known malignancy, especially in those with dense tissue. Multiple clinical studies have shown that on average, MRI reveals occult disease in the ipsilateral breast in approximately 15% (range 12–27%) and disease in the contralateral breast in 4% (range 3–24%) [60, 61]. MRI has also been shown to be particularly useful in determining the extent of disease in women with invasive lobular cancer, as this subtype is often underestimated by mammography and physical examination [62, 63]. Finally, as breast MRI visualizes the chest wall, surrounding tissues, and axilla, it also can assess chest wall invasion and axillary nodal involvement [60, 61].

Another potential indication for breast MRI is in the evaluation of residual disease in patients who have close or positive pathologic margins prior to re-excision. In patients with locally advanced breast cancer who undergo neoadjuvant chemotherapy prior to definitive surgical treatment, MRI can assist with assessing response to therapy and at times can help guide the choice of chemotherapeutic regimen (Fig. 1.6) [61, 64]. Multiple studies have shown that MR is more accurate than

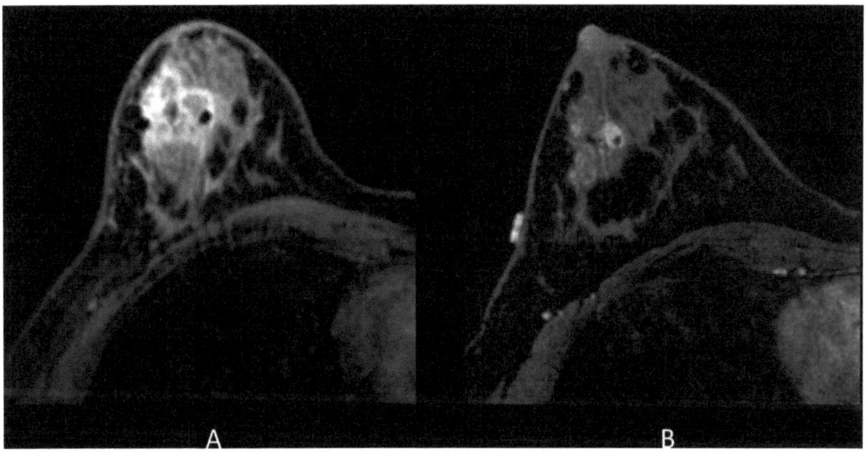

Fig. 1.6 Thirty-one-year-old woman who presented with right breast 3 cm palpable lump. Ultrasound guided biopsy confirmed grade 3 invasive ductal carcinoma. At the time of biopsy, a suspicious axillary node was identified and a fine needle aspiration confirmed metastatic disease. The patient subsequently underwent breast MRI to determine the extent of disease. (**a**) Pretreatment MRI confirmed extensive disease in the right breast and several suspicious right axillary lymph nodes. The patient then underwent neoadjuvant chemotherapy. (**b**) Posttreatment MRI showed partial response to therapy

mammography, ultrasound, or physical examination in determining residual disease after therapy [64]. However, if utilized for this indication, it is critical that MRI be performed prior to the start of chemotherapy and subsequent to therapy, either after completion of part or the entire regimen.

In an effort to better differentiate benign from malignant lesions on MRI, some centers now routinely utilize diffusion-weighted imaging (DWI), a specialized MR sequence that assesses alterations in water movement across cell membranes [65]. Using this acquisition, a quantitative map of water diffusion can be created (apparent diffusion coefficient (ADC) map) which can be used to help classify an enhancing lesion as more likely benign (high ADC value) or malignant (low ADC value) (Fig. 1.7). Smaller-range region of interest focused on highest signal is optimal for measurements. In recent studies, the threshold range for discriminating benign from malignant is approximately 1.1–1.2 × 10^{-3} mm^2/s with associate sensitivity of 82.8–92.8% and specificity of 80.2–90% [66, 67]. In addition to characterizing focal lesions, the change in ADC value has been shown to correlate with tumor response from neoadjuvant chemotherapy and therefore may aid in guiding therapy [68, 69].

Finally, as MR technology continues to advance, it is now possible to perform an ultrafast MR acquisition, which is comprised of high-temporal-resolution and 3D whole-breast images. Performed on a 3-Tesla magnet (not widely available in the USA), this dynamic contrast-enhanced MR protocol consists of standard and contrast-enhanced ultrafast images. A retrospective study of 60 patients with 33 malignancies using this technique revealed statistically significant difference in enhancement rate

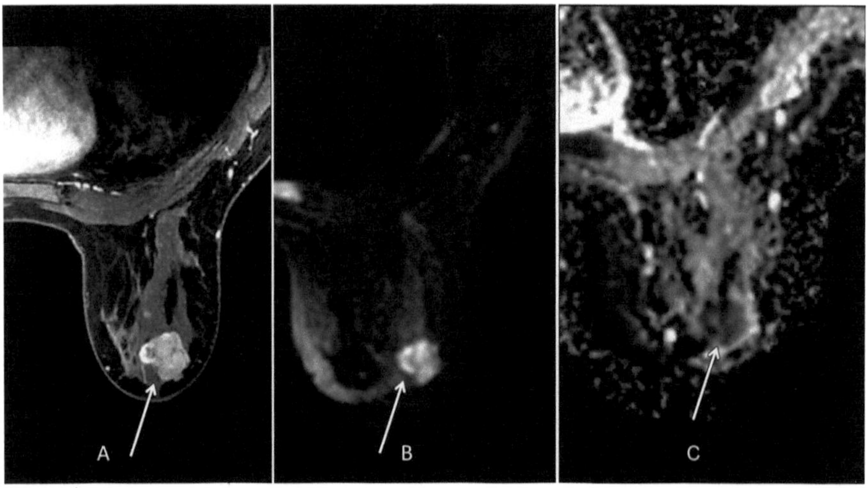

Fig. 1.7 Thirty-nine-year-old woman with biopsy proven right breast retroareolar triple-negative grade 3 invasive ductal carcinoma who underwent MRI to evaluate extent of disease. (**a**) Post-contrast VIBRANT sequence demonstrates 2.6-cm-irregular-enhancing mass corresponding to known malignancy. (**b**) Hyperintense signal in mass on diffusion-weighted imaging (DWI). (**c**) Hypointense signal in mass on apparent diffusion coefficient (ADC) represents restricted diffusion with ADC average of 0.765 × 10^{-3} mm^2/s (less than 1.1–1.2 × 10^{-3} mm^2/s suspicious for malignancy)

and kinetic features between benign and malignant lesions [70]. Therefore, this technique has the potential to decrease the false positives of breast MRI thereby reducing the number of benign biopsies in women being imaged with MRI.

Emerging Technologies: Contrast-Enhanced Mammography

Contrast-enhanced mammography (CEM) is a promising tool currently FDA-approved for diagnostic imaging. At a radiation dose similar to a conventional mammogram, this technology acquires a low-energy and high-energy mammographic image centered at the k-edge of iodine following intravenous administration of an iodinated contrast agent. The low-energy acquisition is comparable to a conventional mammogram and subtraction of the two acquisitions highlights tumor neo-vascularity. Early studies in the diagnostic setting have shown that CEM is more sensitive than conventional mammography [71–73] and has a sensitivity of 96–100%, which is comparable to MRI [74, 75]. When used to determine extent of disease in a newly diagnosed cancer patient, CEM is slightly less sensitive than MRI but it comes with fewer false positives, that is, better specificity (Fig. 1.8) [76, 77]. Given these results, it seems reasonable to use this modality for patients with a newly diagnosed cancer who are unable to undergo MRI due to severe claustrophobia, gadolinium allergy, or presence of internal ferromagnetic material in order to

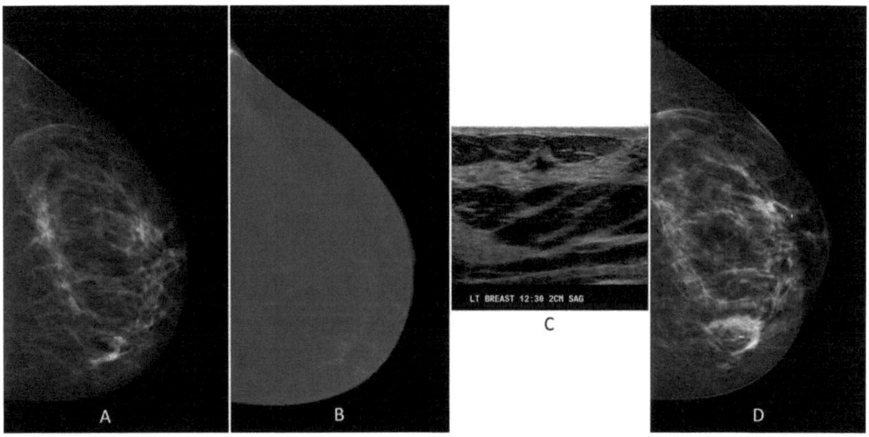

Fig. 1.8 Thirty-nine-year-old woman with indeterminate calcifications in the medial left breast on screening mammogram. (**a**) Craniocaudal (CC) view of left breast mammogram demonstrates pleomorphic calcifications in the medial left breast. (**b**) Recombined CC view from contrast-enhanced mammogram (CEM) confirms the suspicious medial calcifications with associated irregular non-mass enhancement. In addition, there is 7-mm-enhancing mass in the anterior lateral left breast. (**c**) Suspicious hypoechoic left breast mass with irregular margins identified on subsequent diagnostic ultrasound, corresponding to mass only identified on CEM. (**d**) Post-biopsy CC mammogram confirms appropriate clip placement in expected location of left breast mass and left breast calcifications, which were confirmed as grade 1 invasive ductal carcinoma and grade 3 DCIS, respectively

determine the extent of disease. In addition, based on an early study of 26 patients with mammographic or clinical findings warranting biopsy, of which 13 ultimately were proven to be invasive cancers, CEM detected all malignancies and accurately identified disease extent [78]. CEM may also have a role in problem solving of incompletely characterized findings on mammography or ultrasound, detection of mammographically occult findings, and assessment of recurrence [76].

Finally, although CEM has not been extensively studied in the screening population, as the technology can "see through" dense tissue, it may be useful in screening women with dense breast tissue, especially the extremely dense cohort where DBT has less benefit. In an unpublished study by Phillips et al. that compared MRI screening to CEM screening in high-risk women, CEM was well-tolerated and even preferred over MRI by a majority of participants [79].

Abbreviated (Fast) MRI

Having applicability in the screening setting, this technique consists of markedly shortened scan times on an existing MR clinical scanner (scan time of 5 min rather than 30 min). The interpreting radiologist is provided only a maximum intensity projection image (MIP), a pre-contrast image, a single post-contrast image acquired approximately 1 min after injection of IV contrast, and subtraction image of the pre- and post-contrast images. Using this limited information, several retrospective studies have shown that cancer detection is comparable to the full diagnostic protocol [69, 70]. Although this shortened MR screening protocol has yet to be adopted in practice, it has great promise to revolutionize how we screen women for breast cancer, particularly women of intermediate-risk and possibly even all women with dense breast tissue. More study is needed to determine which cohorts will be most cost-effective with this approach.

Conclusion

Over the past few decades, there have been major advances in the early detection and management of breast cancer. Current imaging tools include digital mammography, digital breast tomosynthesis, ultrasound, and magnetic resonance imaging. Although there continue to be advances in these modalities, other techniques, such as contrast-enhanced mammography and abbreviated MRI, have great promise to revolutionize how we care for patients in the coming years.

References

1. Yaffe M, Boyd N. Mammographic breast density and cancer risk: the radiological view. Gynecol Endocrinol. 2005;21(suppl 1):S6–S11.
2. Mandelson MT, Oestreicher N, Porter PL, White D, Finder CA, Taplin SH, White E. Breast density as a predictor of mammographic detection: comparison of interval- and screen-detected cancers. J Natl Cancer Inst. 2000;92(13):1081–7.

3. Lee CI, Bassett LW, Lehman CD. Breast density legislation and opportunities for patient-centered outcomes research. Radiology. 2012;264(3):632–6.
4. Carney PA, Miglioretti DL, Yankaskas BC, et al. Individual and combined effects of age, breast density, and hormone replacement therapy use on the accuracy of screening mammography. Ann Intern Med. 2003;138(3):168–75.
5. D'Orsi CJ, Mendelson EB, Morris EA, et al. Breast imaging reporting and data system: ACR BI-RADS. 5th ed. Reston: American College of Radiology; 2012.
6. Tabár L, Vitak B, Chen TH, et al. Swedish two-county trial: impact of mammographic screening on breast cancer mortality during 3 decades. Radiology. 2011;260(3):658–63.
7. Winkler NS, Raza S, Mackesy M, Birdwell RL. Breast density: clinical implications and assessment methods. Radiographics. 2015;35(2):316–24.
8. Kolb TM, Lichy J, Newhouse JH. Comparison of the performance of screening mammography, physical examination, and breast US and evaluation of the factors that influence them: an analysis of 27,825 patient evaluations. Radiology. 2002;225:165–75.
9. Kerlikowske K, Hubbard RA, Miglioretti DL, Geller BM, Yankaskas BC, Lehman CD, Taplin SH, Sickles EA, Breast Cancer Surveillance Consortium. Comparative effectiveness of digital versus film-screen mammography in community practice in the United States: a cohort study. Ann Intern Med. 2011;155(8):493–502.
10. McCormack VA, dos Santos Silva I. Breast density and parenchymal patterns as markers of breast cancer risk: a meta-analysis. Cancer Epidemiol Biomark Prev. 2006;15(6):1159–69.
11. Nicholson BT, LoRusso AP, Smolkin M, Bovbjerg VE, Petroni GR, Harvey JA. Accuracy of assigned BI-RADS breast density category definitions. Acad Radiol. 2006;13(9):1143–9.
12. Rafferty E, Durand M, Conant E, Copit D, et al. Breast cancer screening using tomosynthesis and digital mammography in dense and nondense breasts. JAMA. 2016;315(16):1784–6.
13. Tseng M, Sellers TA, Vierkant RA, Kushi LH, Vachon CM. Mediterranean diet and breast density in the Minnesota breast cancer family study. Nutr Cancer. 2008;60(6):703–9.
14. Sellers TA, Vachon CM, Pankratz VS, Janney CA, Fredericksen Z, Brandt KR, Huang Y, Couch FJ, Kushi LH, Cerhan JR. Association of childhood and adolescent anthropometric factors, physical activity, and diet with adult mammographic breast density. Am J Epidemiol. 2007;166(4):456–64.
15. Vachon CM, Kushi LH, Cerhan JR, Kuni CC, Sellers TA. Association of diet and mammographic breast density in the Minnesota breast cancer family cohort. Cancer Epidemiol Biomark Prev. 2000;9(2):151–60.
16. Pisano ED, Gatsonis C, Hendrick E, Yaffe M, Baum JK, Acharyya S. Digital mammographic imaging screening trial (DMIST) investigators group et al. diagnostic performance of digital versus film mammography for breast-cancer screening. N Engl J Med. 2005;353(17):1773–83.
17. http://www.fda.gov/RadiationEmittingProducts/MammographyQualityStandardsActandProgram/DocumentArchives/ucm432658.htm
18. Sharpe RE Jr, Venkataraman S, Phillips J, Dialani V, Fein-Zachary VJ, Prakash S, Slanetz PJ, Mehta TS. Increased cancer detection rate and variations in the recall rate resulting from implementation of 3D digital breast tomosynthesis into a population-based screening program. Radiology. 2016;278(3):698–706.
19. Zuckerman SP, Conant EF, Keller BM, Maidment AD, Barufaldi B, et al. Implementation of synthesized two-dimensional mammography in a population-based digital breast tomosynthesis screening program. Radiology. 2016;28:160366.
20. Niklason LT, Christian BT, Niklason LE, et al. Digital tomosynthesis in breast imaging. Radiology. 1997;205(2):399–406.
21. Good WF, Abrams GS, Catullo VJ, et al. Digital breast tomosynthesis: a pilot observer study. AJR Am J Roentgenol. 2008;190(4):865–9.
22. Nees AV. Digital breast tomosynthesis. In: Whitman GJ, Haygood TM, editors. Digital mammography: a practical approach. New York: Cambridge University Press; 2012. p. 109–24.
23. Roth RG, Maidment AD, Weinstein SP, Roth SO, Conant EF. Digital breast tomosynthesis: lessons learned from early clinical implementation. Radiographics. 2014;34(4):E89–102.
24. Rose SL, Tidwell AL, Bujnoch LJ, Kushwaha AC, Nordmann AS, Sexton R Jr. Implementation of breast tomosynthesis in a routine screening practice: an observational study. AJR Am J Roentgenol. 2013;200(6):1401–8.

25. McDonald ES, Oustimov A, Weinstein SP, et al. Effectiveness of digital breast tomosynthesis compared with digital mammography: outcomes analysis from 3 years of breast cancer screening. JAMA Oncol. 2016;2(6):737–43.
26. Margolies L, Cohen A, Sonnenblick E, et al. Digital breast tomosynthesis changes management in patients seen at a tertiary care breast center. ISRN Radiol. 2014;2014:658–929.
27. Gur D, Abrams GS, Chough DM, et al. Digital breast tomosynthesis: observer performance study. AJR Am J Roentgenol. 2009;193:586.
28. Gennaro G, Toledano A, di Maggio C, et al. Digital breast tomosynthesis versus digital mammography: a clinical performance study. Eur Radiol. 2010;20:1545.
29. Hakim CM, Chough DM, Ganott MA, et al. Digital breast tomosynthesis in the diagnostic environment: a subjective side-by-side review. AJR Am J Roentgenol. 2010;195:W172.
30. Rafferty EA, Park JM, Philpotts LE, et al. Assessing radiologist performance using combined digital mammography and breast tomosynthesis compared with digital mammography alone: results of a multicenter, multireader trial. Radiology. 2013;266:104.
31. Chan HP, Wei J, Sahiner B, et al. Computer-aided detection system for breast masses on digital tomosynthesis mammograms: preliminary experience. Radiology. 2005;237:1075.
32. Andersson I, Ikeda DM, Zackrisson S, et al. Breast tomosynthesis and digital mammography: a comparison of breast cancer visibility and BIRADS classification in a population of cancers with subtle mammographic findings. Eur Radiol. 2008;18:2817.
33. Stavros AT, Thickman D, Rapp CL, et al. Solid breast nodules: use of sonography to distinguish between benign and malignant lesions. Radiology. 1995;196(1):123–34.
34. Parker SH, Jobe WE, Dennis MA, Stavros AT, Johnson KK, Yakes WF, Truell JE, Price JG, Kortz AB, Clark DG. US-guided automated large-core breast biopsy. Radiology. 1993;187:507–11.
35. Evans A, Whelehan P, et al. Quantitative shear wave ultrasound elastography: initial experience in solid breast masses. Breast Cancer Res. 2010;12(6):R104.
36. Itoh A, Ueno E, Tohno E, et al. Breast disease: clinical application of US elastography for diagnosis. Radiology. 2006;239(2):341–50.
37. Athanasiou A, Tardivon A, Tanter M, Sigal-Zafrani B, Bercoff J, Deffieux T, Gennisson JL, Fink M, Neuenschwander S. Breast lesions: quantitative elastography with supersonic shear imaging – preliminary results. Radiology. 2010;256(1):297–303.
38. Burnside ES, Hall TJ, Sommer AM, et al. Differentiating benign from malignant solid breast masses with US strain imaging. Radiology. 2007;245(2):401–10.
39. Berg WA, Cosgrove DO, Dore CJ, et al. Shear-wave elastography improves the specificity of breast US: the BE1 multinational study of 939 masses. Radiology. 2012;262:435–49.
40. Kolb TM, Lichy J, Newhouse JH. Occult cancer in women with dense breasts: detection with screening US—diagnostic yield and tumor characteristics. Radiology. 1998;207:191–9.
41. Berg WA, Blume JD, Cormack JB, et al. Combined screening with ultrasound and mammography vs mammography alone in women at elevated risk of breast cancer. JAMA. 2008;299(18):2151–63.
42. Berg WA, Zhang Z, Lehrer D, et al. ACRIN 6666 investigators. Detection of breast cancer with addition of annual screening ultrasound, or a single screening MRI to mammography in women w elevated breast cancer risk. JAMA. 2012;307:1394–404.
43. Scheel JR, Lee JM, Sprague BL, Lee CI, Lehman CD. Screening ultrasound as an adjunct to mammography in women with mammographically dense breasts. Am J Obstet Gynecol. 2015;212(1):9–17.
44. Hooley RJ, Greenberg KL, Stackhouse RM, Geisel JL, Butler RS, Philpotts LE. Screening US in patients with mammographically dense breasts: initial experience with connecticut public act 09-41. Radiology. 2012;265:59–69.
45. Freer P. Mammographic breast density: impact on breast cancer risk and implications for screening. Radiographics. 2015;35(2):302–15.
46. Furman-Haran E, Grobgeld D, Kelcz F, Degani H. Critical role of spatial resolution in dynamic contrast-enhanced breast MRI. See comment in PubMed commons below. J Magn Reson Imaging. 2001;13(6):862–7.

47. Kriege M, Brekelmans C, Boetes C, et al. Magnetic resonance imaging screening study group. Efficacy of MRI and mammography for breast cancer screening in women with a familial or genetic predisposition. N Engl J Med. 2004;351:427–37.
48. Kuhl C, Weigel S, Schrading S, et al. Prospective multicenter cohort study to refine management recommendations for women at elevated familial risk of breast cancer: the EVA trial. J Clin Oncol. 2010;28:1450–7.
49. ACR practice parameter for the performance of contrast-enhanced magnetic resonance imaging (MRI) of the breast. http://www.acr.org/~/media/2a0eb28eb59041e2825179afb72ef624.pdf (accessed 8.16.16).
50. Melnikow J, Fenton JJ, Whitlock EP, et al. Supplemental screening for breast cancer in women with dense breasts: a systematic review for the U.S. preventive services task force. Ann Intern Med. 2016;164:268.
51. Chiarelli AM, Prummel MV, Muradali D, et al. Effectiveness of screening with annual magnetic resonance imaging and mammography: results of the initial screen from the Ontario high risk breast screening program. J Clin Oncol. 2014;32:2224–30.
52. Warner E, Plewes DB, Hill KA, et al. Surveillance of BRCA1 and BRCA2 mutation carriers with magnetic resonance imaging, ultrasound, mammography, and clinical breast examination. JAMA. 2004;292:1317–25.
53. Kriege M, Brekelmans CT, Boetes C, et al. Differences between first and subsequent rounds of the MRISC breast cancer screening program for women with a familial or genetic predisposition. Cancer. 2006;106:2318–26.
54. Leach MO, Boggis CR, Dixon AK, et al. Screening with magnetic resonance imaging and mammography of a UK population at high familial risk of breast cancer: a prospective multicentre cohort study (MARIBS). Lancet. 2005;365:1769–78.
55. Kuhl CK, Schrading S, Leutner CC, et al. Mammography, breast ultrasound, and magnetic resonance imaging for surveillance of women at high familial risk for breast cancer. J Clin Oncol. 2005;23:8469–76.
56. Lehman CD, Blume JD, Weatherall P, et al. Screening women at high risk for breast cancer with mammography and magnetic resonance imaging. Cancer. 2005;103:1898–905.
57. Sardanelli F, Podo F, Santoro F, et al. Multicenter surveillance of women at high genetic breast cancer risk using mammography, ultrasonography, and contrast-enhanced magnetic resonance imaging (the high breast cancer risk Italian 1 study): final results. Investig Radiol. 2011;46:94–105.
58. Kriege M, Brekelmans CT, Obdeijn IM, Boetes C, Zonderland HM, Muller SH, et al. Factors affecting sensitivity and specificity of screening mammography and MRI in women with an inherited risk for breast cancer. Breast Cancer Res Treat. 2006;100:109–19.
59. Kuhl CK, Schrading S, Strobel K, Schild HH, Hilgers RD, Bieling HB. Abbreviated breast magnetic resonance imaging (MRI): first postcontrast subtracted images and maximum-intensity projection-a novel approach to breast cancer screening with MRI. J Clin Oncol. 2014;32:2304–10.
60. Gutierrez RL, DeMartini WB, Silbergeld JJ, et al. High cancer yield and positive predictive value: outcomes at a center routinely using preoperative breast MRI for staging. AJR. 2011;196:W93–9.
61. Tillman GF, Orel SG, Schnall MD, Schultz DJ, Tan JE, Solin LJ. Effect of breast magnetic resonance imaging on the clinical management of women with early-stage breast carcinoma. J Clin Oncol. 2002;20:3413–342.
62. Weinstein SP, Orel SG, Heller R, et al. MR imaging of the breast in patients with invasive lobular carcinoma. AJR Am J Roentgenol. 2001;176(2):399–406.
63. Mann RM, Hoogeveen YL, Blickman JG, Boetes C. MRI compared to conventional diagnostic work-up in the detection and evaluation of invasive lobular carcinoma of the breast: a review of existing literature. Breast Cancer Res Treat. 2008;107(1):1–14.
64. Dialani V, Chadashvili T, Slanetz PJ. Role of imaging in neoadjuvant therapy for breast cancer. Ann Surg Oncol. 2015;22(5):1416–24.

65. Paran Y, Bendel P, Margalit R, Degani H. Water diffusion in the different microenvironments of breast cancer. NMR Biomed. 2004;17:170–80.
66. Min Q, Shao K, Zhai L, Liu W, Zhu C, Yuan L, et al. Differential diagnosis of benign and malignant breast masses using diffusion-weighted magnetic resonance imaging. World J Surg Oncol. 2015;13:32.
67. Bansal R, Shah V, Aggarwal B. Indian J Radiol Imaging. 2015;25(4):397–403.
68. Pereira F, Martins G, Figueiredo E, Domingues M, et al. Assessment of breast lesions with diffusion-weighted MRI: comparing the use of different b values. Am J Roentgenol. 2009;193:1030–5.
69. Rubesova E, Grell AS, De Maertelaer V, Metens T, Chao SL, Lemort M. Quantitative diffusion imaging in breast cancer: a clinical prospective study. J Magn Reson Imaging. 2006;24:319–24.
70. Abe H, Mori N, Tsuchiya K, Schacht DV, Pineda FD, Jiang Y, Karczmar GS. Kinetic analysis of benign and malignant breast lesions with ultrafast dynamic contrast-enhanced MRI: comparison with standard kinetic assessment. AJR Am J Roentgenol. 2016;17:1–8.
71. Dromain C, Balleyguier C, Adler G, Garbay JR, Delaloge S. Contrast-enhanced digital mammography. Eur J Radiol. 2009;69(1):34–42.
72. Jong RA, Yaffe MJ, Skarpathiotakis M, Shumak RS, Danjoux NM, Gunesekara A, Plewes DB. Contrast-enhanced digital mammography: initial clinical experience. Radiology. 2003;228(3):842–50.
73. Weidner N, Semple JP, Welch WR, Folkman J. Tumor angiogenesis and metastasis correlation in invasive breast carcinoma. N Engl J Med. 1991;324:1–7.
74. Sogani J, Morris EA, Kaplan JB, D'Alessio D, Goldman D, Moskowitz CS, Jochelson MS. Comparison of background parenchymal enhancement at contrast-enhanced spectral mammography and breast MR imaging. Radiology. 2016;4:160284.
75. Jochelson MS, Dershaw DD, Sung JS, et al. Bilateral contrast-enhanced dual-energy digital mammography: feasibility and comparison with conventional digital mammography and MR imaging in women with known breast carcinoma. Radiology. 2013;266(3):743–51.
76. Dromain C, Thibault F, Muller S, et al. Dual-energy contrast-enhanced digital mammography: initial clinical results. Eur Radiol. 2011;21(3):565–74.
77. Francescone MA, Jochelson MS, Dershaw DD, et al. Low energy mammogram obtained in contrast-enhanced digital mammography (CEDM) is comparable to routine full-field digital mammography (FFDM). Eur J Radiol. 2014;83(8):1350–5.
78. Lewin JM, Isaacs PK, Vance V, Larke FJ. Dual-energy contrast-enhanced digital subtraction mammography: feasibility. Radiology. 2003;229(1):261–8.
79. Philips J. Personal communication 9/1/16.
80. Barr RG. Breast elastrography. New York: Thieme Medical Publishers Inc; 2014.

Nipple-Sparing Mastectomy

2

Suzanne B. Coopey and Barbara L. Smith

Abbreviations

NSM	Nipple-sparing mastectomy
NCCN	National Comprehensive Cancer Network
cm	Centimeter
BRCA	Breast cancer susceptibility gene
NAC	Nipple areola complex
DIEP	Deep inferior epigastric perforator

Introduction

Although the term "mastectomy" implies removal of all breast tissue, a variety of mastectomy techniques have been used, which vary based on indication and extent of skin and glandular tissue excised. There has been continuing reduction in the extent of surgery required for successful treatment of breast cancer over the last 50 years. This has included the transition from the radical mastectomy to the modified radical mastectomy then to the simple (or total) mastectomy [1]. Breast reconstruction techniques were developed over time, initially applied only as delayed reconstructions performed 1–2 years after mastectomy due to concerns

S.B. Coopey, MD (✉)
Division of Surgical Oncology, Massachusetts General Hospital,
55 Fruit Street, Yawkey 7B, Boston, MA 02114, USA
e-mail: scoopey@partners.org

B.L. Smith, MD, PhD
Division of Surgical Oncology, Massachusetts General Hospital,
55 Fruit Street, Yawkey 9A, Boston, MA 02114, USA
e-mail: blsmith1@partners.org

M. Howard-McNatt (ed.), *Changing Paradigms in the Management of Breast Cancer*, DOI 10.1007/978-3-319-60336-0_2

that reconstruction would delay detection of recurrent cancer or have other negative effects on oncologic outcomes. As the safety of delayed reconstruction was recognized, options for immediate reconstruction at the time of mastectomy were explored. It became clear the preservation of more breast skin could improve cosmetic outcomes.

The subcutaneous mastectomy technique was first described by Rice and Strickler in 1951 for risk reduction or treatment of benign disease. A subcutaneous mastectomy intentionally leaves glandular tissue beneath the nipple areola complex to preserve its blood supply [2]. The actual term "subcutaneous mastectomy" was coined by Freeman in 1962 and was endorsed strictly for benign disease or risk reduction [3]. Retention of this amount of subareolar and subcutaneous breast tissue is less effective for risk reduction, and there are numerous reports of breast cancer occurrences after subcutaneous mastectomy, especially in BRCA mutation carriers [4, 5]. This approach has largely been abandoned in favor of more modern nipple-sparing techniques.

In 1991, the skin-sparing mastectomy was formally introduced by Toth and Lappert [6]. With this technique, the nipple areola complex and all visible glandular tissue are removed, but the rest of the skin envelope and inframammary fold are preserved. This facilitates immediate breast reconstruction and improves cosmetic outcomes. Studies comparing skin-sparing mastectomy plus immediate or delayed reconstruction to mastectomy without reconstruction have shown equivalent local recurrence rates, confirming the safety of skin-sparing mastectomy for breast cancer treatment [7].

Although nipple reconstruction with skin grafts, local flaps, and tattooing improves cosmetic outcomes, only a limited approximation of the native nipple appearance is possible. This led to renewed interest in developing oncologically safe nipple-sparing mastectomy techniques. In contrast to the old subcutaneous mastectomy, today's nipple sparing, or total skin-sparing mastectomy, strives to leave no glandular tissue behind the nipple areola complex or under the skin flaps. Successful NSM requires careful patient selection, proper technique to maintain nipple perfusion and minimize complications, and meticulous removal of glandular tissue.

Oncologic Safety

Occult Nipple Involvement

Historical rates of occult nipple involvement identified in nipple-sacrificing mastectomies are as high as 50%, leading to concerns about the safety of saving the nipple [3]. However, many older studies predated the use of screening mammography and included nipples with worrisome clinical findings, such as nipple retraction. In addition, the definition of nipple involvement varied in different studies; in some studies, nipples were considered positive if they contained lobular carcinoma in situ, now considered benign atypia, or if cancer was found as far as 2 cm from the nipple [3, 8–11]. Brachtel and colleagues at our institution examined 316 mastectomies with clinically uninvolved nipples in a more modern series and found occult cancer in 21% of nipples [12].

Despite high rates of nipple involvement in nipple-sacrificing mastectomy specimens, rates of positive nipple margins in modern nipple-sparing mastectomy series are much lower. In more recent series of NSM performed for cancer treatment, rates of positive nipple margins range from 2.5 to10%, likely reflecting careful patient selection [13–19].

Patient Selection for Nipple-Sparing Mastectomy

Initially patients with tumors greater than 2 cm or with tumor-to-nipple distances less than 2 cm were excluded from NSM, because these features were found to increase the likelihood of occult nipple involvement [20]. With experience and observation of low rates of nipple involvement, eligibility for NSM has expanded to include the majority of patients undergoing mastectomy [21, 22]. Few absolute contraindications to nipple sparing remain; these include direct involvement of the nipple areola complex on preoperative clinical exam or imaging or the presence of pathologic nipple discharge (Fig. 2.1).

In some centers, even patients with locally advanced breast cancer are considered eligible for nipple sparing. In a recent study of 139 patients with stage 2B or stage 3 breast cancer treated with NSM, only 5% of patients developed an isolated

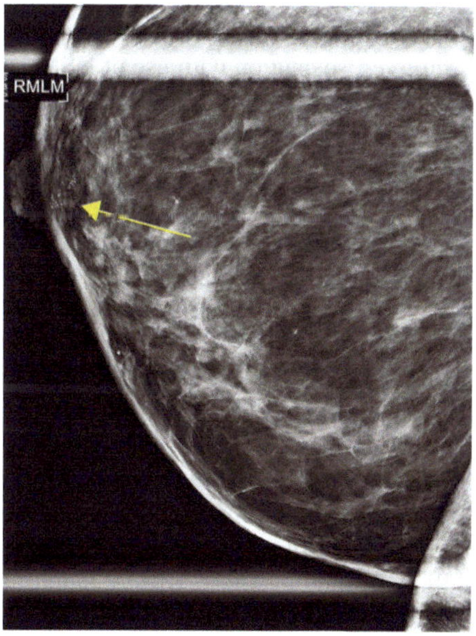

Fig. 2.1 Mammogram showing microcalcifications under nipple in a 45-year-old patient with ductal carcinoma in situ

local recurrence at a mean follow-up of 41 months and no recurrence involved the retained nipple areola complex [23]. The authors concluded that with appropriate multimodality therapy, nipple sparing does not increase risk of local recurrence, even in patients with locally advanced disease.

Patients who have had prior radiation or who need post-mastectomy radiation are also candidates for NSM. Although prior radiation and post-mastectomy radiation increase risk for complications with any reconstruction, most patients who undergo NSM with radiation do well [24]. Tang and colleagues at our institution compared 816 NSM with no radiation to 69 NSM in previously irradiated breasts [24]. Prior radiation increased the rate of skin necrosis from 4.5 to 11.6% and increased risk of total nipple necrosis from 0.9 to 4.3% [24]. Among 97 NSM that received post-mastectomy radiation, 10.3% had skin necrosis and 4.1% had total nipple necrosis. Rates of implant loss were 2.2% without radiation, 2.9% with prior radiation, and 8.2% with post-mastectomy radiation [24]. Risk factors for complications with radiation included smoking, age >55, breast volume >800 cm^3, and periareolar incision placement [24]. It was concluded that prior radiation or the need for post-mastectomy radiation are not absolute contraindications to NSM and that complications could be minimized with appropriate patient selection [24].

Cosmetic factors are also considered when assessing eligibility for NSM. Nipple sparing is contraindicated in patients for whom the retained nipple would be in an unacceptable position on the reconstructed breast. Marked breast ptosis or very large breast size may result in poor nipple position if the nipple is preserved. Salgarello and colleagues advise against NSM in patients with bra size larger than a D cup and for D cup breasts with grade 3 ptosis, that is, ptosis with the nipple well below the inframammary fold [25]. In addition, an excised breast weight of more than 750 g and a sternal notch-to-nipple distance of greater than 26 cm have been found to increase skin flap complications in patients undergoing skin-sparing mastectomies, so caution with use of NSM is also advised in these patients [26].

Nipple Mastectomy for Risk Reduction

NSM for risk reduction is endorsed by the most recent NCCN guidelines [27] (Fig. 2.2). Risk reduction surgery should be considered in women with a known BRCA 1 or BRCA 2 mutation, or another gene mutation with a significantly increased risk of breast cancer, or a compelling family history of breast cancer [27]. In a retrospective analysis of 639 women treated with bilateral prophylactic subcutaneous mastectomy from 1960 to 1993 for a family history of breast cancer, Hartmann and colleagues noted a 90% reduction in breast cancer at 14-year median follow up [4]. Twenty-six of these patients were later found to have BRCA 1 or BRCA2 mutations; 23 had been treated with subcutaneous mastectomy and three with simple mastectomy [28]. No cancers had developed at 13.4-year median follow-up among these BRCA mutation carriers. Using published data for the likelihood of breast cancer in BRCA1 and BRCA2 mutation carriers, they would have expected six to nine breast cancers to develop during the follow-up period

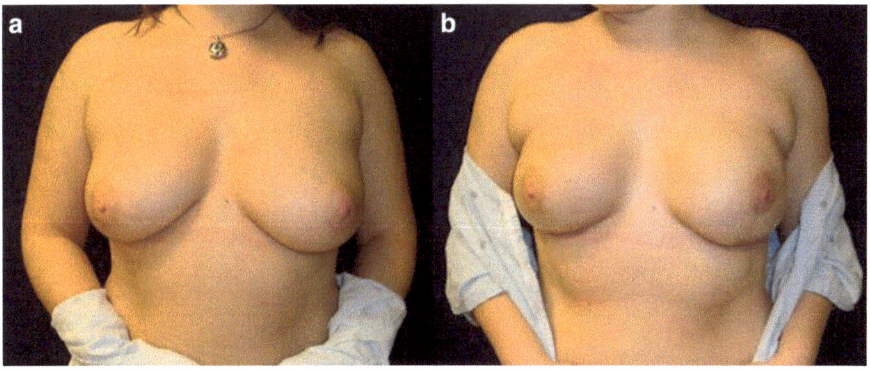

Fig. 2.2 Prophylactic NSM with single-stage direct to implant in BRCA mutation carrier with inferolateral incision, preop (**a**) and 1 month postop (**b**)

with no intervention. Their results suggest that the risk of breast cancer is reduced by 89.5–100.0% in BRCA1 and BRCA2 mutation carriers after prophylactic subcutaneous mastectomy [28]. With current NSM techniques that excise all subareolar tissue, even greater risk reduction may be possible.

Yao et al. reported on NSM in 397 breasts of 201 BRCA1 and BRCA2 carriers, 125 had a BRCA1 mutation, and 76 had a BRCA2 mutation; 150 (74.6%) patients underwent NSM solely for risk reduction and 51 (25.4%) underwent NSM for unilateral cancer and contralateral risk reduction [29]. Incidental cancers were found in four (2.7%) of the 150 risk reduction patients and two (3.9%) of the 51 cancer patients. The nipple areola complex was involved with cancer in three (5.8%) of the cancer patients. No prophylactic mastectomy had a positive nipple margin. With a mean follow-up of 32.6 months, no patient developed a recurrence at the NAC, although four patients (three cancer patients and one prophylactic) experienced cancers elsewhere – two locally and two in the axilla [29]. When Peled and colleagues reviewed outcomes of 26 BRCA mutation carriers who underwent NSM for risk reduction and 27 BRCA mutation carriers who underwent NSM for unilateral breast cancer and contralateral risk reduction, they found no evidence of new or recurrent cancers, respectively, at 51-month mean follow-up [30]. In a recent multi-institutional study of risk-reducing NSM in 348 patients with BRCA mutations, Jakub et al. reported no evidence of cancer at 56-month mean follow-up [31]. Although follow-up in NSM series is limited, to date NSM appears to be a safe approach for risk reduction and for cancer treatment in high-risk patients.

Oncologic Outcome of Therapeutic Nipple-Sparing Mastectomy

Despite increasing use of NSM in the last 5–10 years, concerns remain about oncologic safety given the lack of long-term follow-up. Sites potentially at risk for new or recurrent breast cancer after NSM include the retained nipple areola complex

Table 2.1 Oncologic outcomes of nipple-sparing mastectomies for cancer

Author	Institution	Year	# Breasts	Follow-up (months)	Locoregional recurrence (%)	NAC recurrence
Orzalesi	Italian Nat'l Database	2016	755	36	2.9	5
Krajewski	Mayo Clinic	2015	226	24	1.7	0
Coopey	Mass General	2013	156	22	2.6	0
Lohsiriwat	European Inst. of Oncology	2012	861	50	4.2	7
Peled	UCSF	2012	412	28	2	0
Boneti	University AR	2011	152	25	4.6	0
Filho	MSKCC	2011	157	10	0	0
Jenson	John Wayne	2011	127	60	0	0

and skin flaps, particularly at the periphery of the breast where visualization may be difficult with incisions used for NSM. Review of 297 NSM for cancer at Massachusetts General Hospital found a 3.0% risk of locoregional recurrence at 42-month median follow-up, with no recurrence involving the retained nipple areola complex [32]. These results are consistent with oncologic outcomes in other NSM series reported over the last 5 years, summarized in Table 2.1. Locoregional recurrence rates after NSM range from 0 to 4.6% at 10–60 months of follow-up [14, 15, 21, 22, 30, 33–36].

Only two modern studies report any tumor recurrences in the retained nipple after NSM. Lohsiriwat and colleagues from Italy performed 861 NSM for cancer and seven patients (0.8%) developed recurrences in the nipple areola complex with 50 months median follow-up [35]. The mean time to nipple recurrence was 32 months, and in all cases the nipple areola complex was removed. At a mean of 47 months after nipple removal, no patient developed any further local or distant recurrence. Lohsiriwat et al. describe leaving at least 5 mm of glandular tissue beneath the nipple areola complex to prevent necrosis and giving a single dose of radiation to the nipple areola complex and 1 cm beyond, a technique which is different than those used in North American studies [35]. Recently, Orzalesi et al. reviewed a national multi-institutional registry of NSM performed in Italy which included 1,006 patients [36]. Of 755 cases included in the locoregional recurrence analysis, 5 (0.7%) developed a recurrence of the nipple areola complex at a mean 36-month follow-up. In this series, no particular technique was described for dissection under the nipple areola complex [36].

In a review of 20 NSM series, De La Cruz and colleagues found disease-free survival in series with <3-year follow-up, 3–5-year follow-up, and >5-year follow-up was 93.1%, 92.3%, and 76.1%, respectively [37]. Many of the studies with >5 years of follow-up included patients treated in the mid-1980s and 1990s [38, 39]. More recent retrospective cohort studies comparing NSM plus immediate reconstruction to mastectomy without reconstruction have shown no significant difference in local or distant recurrence rates with NSM [40, 41]. When Adam et al. matched 67 NSM plus reconstruction patients to 203 mastectomy without reconstruction patients, they found no significant difference in estimated 5-year disease-free survival (94.1 and 82.5%, $p = 0.068$) or in overall survival (OS) (96.2 and 91.3%, $p = 0.166$) between them [40]. In fact, they noted a nonsignificant trend toward worse outcomes in the mastectomy without reconstruction group and concluded that NSM with reconstruction was a safe alternative. Similarly, when Park and colleagues compared 114 patients who underwent skin-sparing or nipple-sparing mastectomy plus immediate reconstruction to a matched control group of patients who underwent mastectomy with no reconstruction, they found no significant difference in 5-year locoregional recurrence-free survival between the two groups, 96.4% and 96.1%, respectively ($p = 0.552$) [41].

Surgical Technique

Incision Placement

The ideal incision for NSM would allow thorough resection of all of the breast tissue by the breast surgeon and ease of reconstruction for the plastic surgeon, through an aesthetically favorable scar [42]. In addition, preservation of nipple and areola blood supply is critical to successful nipple sparing. Following mastectomy, blood is supplied to the NAC from the periphery of the breast through the subdermal plexus in the skin flaps. Incisions used for NSM must preserve inflow to the nipple.

There are six basic types of incisions for NSM: inferolateral, inframammary, lateral radial, inferior radial, periareolar, and through extension of a prior scar. With the inferolateral incision, the incision begins on the lateral border of the breast at the same horizontal level as the nipple (3 o'clock position on the left breast and 9 o'clock position on the right breast). The incision is curved inferomedially along the outer border of the breast. The incision continues medially until it intersects with an imaginary vertical line through the nipple at the 6 o'clock position [42] (Fig. 2.3).

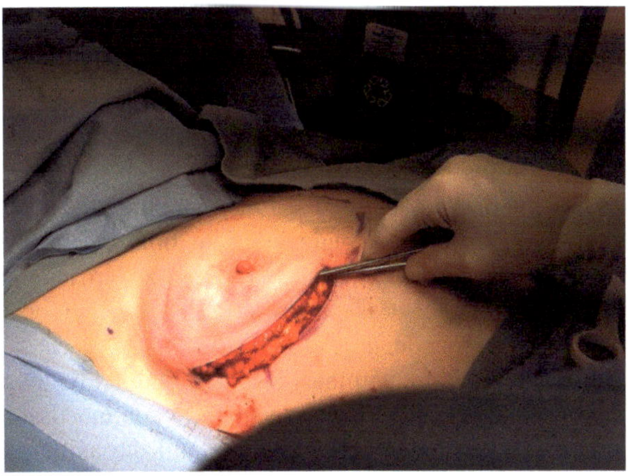

Fig. 2.3 Inferolateral incision placement

The incision length is typically 10–12 cm and must be long enough to accommodate the surgeon's hand. This incision preserves the internal mammary perforators that supply the medial skin flaps and provides easy access to the axilla. The inferolateral incision provides a favorable cosmetic result, but its inferior location can make dissection of the superomedial breast more challenging [43]. Access to the superior and medial aspects of the breast is facilitated by separating the breast from the pectoralis muscle.

The inframammary fold incision remains in the inferior portion of the breast along the inframammary fold, centered beneath the nipple, and spans 12–14 cm [44]. It is useful for DIEP flap reconstructions as it provides good medial exposure for the anastomosis of the deep inferior epigastric vessels to the internal mammary vessels. This incision also has the cosmetic advantage of being completely hidden by the breast in the upright position. It has the disadvantage of giving a more challenging exposure and usually requires a longer scar, which could interfere with blood supply to the nipple or inferior skin flap [42]. Another disadvantage of this incision is that a separate axillary incision is usually required for axillary staging [44].

The lateral radial and inferior radial incisions are more similar to incisions used for standard skin-sparing mastectomies and may be technically easier than the inferolateral and inframammary incisions. However, both leave visible scars prominent on the breast, and the lateral radial incision has been known to cause deviation of the nipple toward the scar [45]. On the other hand, an inferior radial incision is sometimes favored if a patient has larger breasts and would benefit from skin excision to raise the nipple to a more superior position on the reconstructed breast. A periareolar incision placed either along the superior or inferior half of the areola and usually with a lateral radial extension can also be utilized [43]. This approach may be technically easier for the surgeon as it is similar to the traditional skin-sparing mastectomy approach. Not surprisingly, however, placing an incision along the edge of the areola has been associated with a higher risk of nipple necrosis and nipple loss. Some authors believe that incisions in this location should be avoided, although others have found it an acceptable approach [33, 46].

Overview of Technique

Decisions about incision placement should be made in collaboration with the plastic surgeon and, to the extent possible, take patient preference into account. At our institution the majority of NSM are performed via an inferolateral approach; this allows the mastectomy and sentinel lymph node biopsy or axillary dissection to be performed through a single incision. Inferolateral and inferior incisions require modifications in technique compared to standard skin-sparing mastectomy incisions which are more centrally located on the breast. In our inferolateral approach, after the incision is made, a short flap is raised to the chest wall inferiorly and laterally, preserving the inframammary fold. If a sentinel lymph node biopsy with frozen section is planned, dissection can then be continued along the lateral border of the breast and serratus anterior muscle until the axillary fat pad is encountered. The sentinel lymph node can then be obtained, and frozen section performed while the mastectomy is completed.

Next, we have found it helpful to define the inferior edge of the pectoralis major muscle and to separate the breast from the underlying pectoralis muscle medially to the sternum and superiorly to the clavicle early in the procedure. This allows for easier retraction and manipulation of the breast tissue to aid in visualization of the Cooper's ligament dissection plane, particularly in the medial and superior skin flaps. The anterior dissection occurs at the junction of the hypodermis and the anterior mammary fascia, dividing Cooper's ligaments, identical to that of a skin-sparing mastectomy. Facelift or "bear claw" retractors may be used to elevate the skin edge and provide countertraction on the breast tissue to aid in the dissection. Once the dissection continues farther medially and superiorly, lighted retractors or a technique of eversion of the skin flap with the surgeon's hand while the assistant puts traction on the breast tissue is also helpful. During all retraction maneuvers, care is taken to avoid trauma to the skin flaps and nipple.

It is important to avoid making excessively thin flaps that compromise blood supply to the skin and nipple. If the dissection is maintained in the Cooper's ligament plane and not in the subcutaneous fat itself, perfusion to the skin flaps is usually preserved. Studies of skin-sparing mastectomies have shown that skin flaps of 4–5 mm in thickness lead to rates of skin necrosis up to 17% whereas skin flaps >10 mm have skin necrosis rates of less than 5% [47]. For superficial tumors, it is better to take a separate anterior margin from the skin flap directly over the tumor rather than make the entire skin flap too thin.

At the level of the nipple, we use a technique where areolar skin flaps are raised, leaving the nipple duct bundle intact. This can be done with blunt dissection using a curved clamp as there are no Cooper's ligaments under the areola and minimizes trauma to the areola skin. A curved clamp is then passed around the duct bundle just beneath the areola, as is done when isolating a vessel bundle for ligation. A second clamp is used to grasp the nipple duct bundle immediately below the nipple and areola dermis, and the external skin is examined to be sure that no skin is included in the clamp. The clamp is rotated 90° away from the skin toward the surgeon to pull additional ductal tissue down from the nipple papilla, and the bundle is then sharply divided, first on the superficial surface of the clamp and then on the deep side of the clamp (Fig. 2.4). The contents of the clamp constitute the nipple margin specimen for pathology assessment. This technique removes most of the ductal tissue within the nipple papilla and leaves an anterior margin that is the underside of the nipple and areola dermis, leaving no ductal tissue or breast tissue beneath the nipple areola complex (Fig. 2.4b).

Nipple Margin Assessment

Based on pathology evaluation of cancer-containing nipples, we know that invasive cancer and ductal carcinoma in situ generally spread by direct extension sequentially into the retroareolar tissues and subareolar ducts and then into the nipple

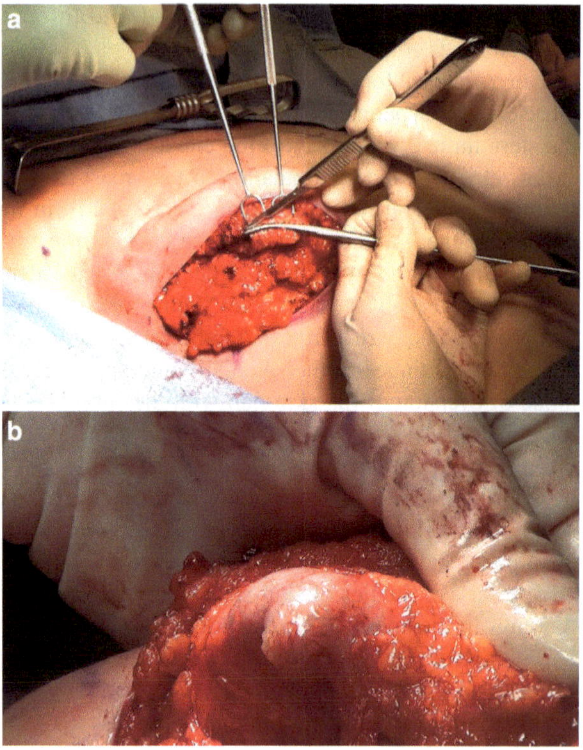

Fig. 2.4 (**a**) Technique for obtaining nipple margin specimen. (**b**) Nipple areola skin margin after duct bundle removal

papilla itself [12]. Therefore, safe nipple preservation requires adequate sampling and pathology analysis of excised tissue from within the nipple and immediately beneath the areola, to be sure that no tumor remains in the retained nipple.

Histological assessment of the nipple margin specimen may be performed on frozen section, which allows for immediate management of a positive margin, or on permanent section. Accurate nipple margin assessment on frozen section is difficult, and distinguishing benign atypia from intraductal carcinoma is challenging, potentially resulting in unnecessary nipple excision. Therefore, permanent section analysis of nipple margins appears to be the best strategy for maximizing nipple preservation [19, 48]. With permanent section assessment, the management of a positive nipple margin can be determined in the context of complete pathologic staging and with knowledge of the full treatment plan.

If the nipple margin contains invasive cancer or ductal carcinoma in situ, it is considered positive, and the nipple should be removed. Nipple removal is not required for atypia or lobular carcinoma in situ. Rates of positive nipple margins in therapeutic NSM range from 2.5 to 10% [13–19]. In our series of 37 nipples excised for positive nipple margins, the excised nipple contained cancer only 30% of the time [17]. Recently, our group has transitioned from complete nipple areola complex excision for positive nipple margins to excision of just the nipple papilla with retention of most of the areola skin. In general, we have found that if the areola can be saved, reconstruction of the nipple is easier and the cosmetic result is better. With 36-month follow-up using this technique, we have had no recurrences at the site of nipple removal or in any retained areola [17].

Complications

Nipple Necrosis

In a recent systematic review of NSM, Piper and colleagues identified 23 studies which reported nipple necrosis rates [49]. Of 2980 cases, 263 (8.8%) reported some degree of nipple necrosis, either partial or total. Complete nipple loss due to necrosis occurred in 2% of cases overall, with a range of 0–10% across series [49].

Mastectomy Skin Flap Necrosis

Mastectomy skin flaps can undergo a spectrum of ischemic changes postoperatively. Changes can range from mild color change, either erythema or cyanosis, suggesting decreased perfusion, to partial thickness necrosis with epidermolysis, and to full-thickness necrosis with eschar formation [50]. In a systemic review of 16 studies, the rate of partial or full-thickness skin flap necrosis was 9.5% [49]. Colwell and colleagues found that increasing body mass index, smoking, periareolar incisions, and preoperative radiation were significant predictors of NSM complications [46].

Implant Loss

In a systemic review of 16 studies, the rate of expander-implant loss was 3.9% [49]. Rates of skin ischemia and implant loss decrease with experience. In a recent review of nearly 500 NSM plus implant or tissue expander reconstructions at Massachusetts General Hospital, the rate of implant loss was only 1.9%, despite nearly 60% of reconstructions being single-stage direct to implant [46].

Patient Satisfaction

Cosmetic Outcome

Patient reported satisfaction measures after NSM for both risk reduction and cancer treatment are consistently favorable [51] (Fig. 2.5). Using BREAST-Q scores, Howard and colleagues found that patient satisfaction with breast appearance and overall psychosocial well-being were higher after NSM with reconstruction than at the preoperative, baseline assessment [51]. When Metcalfe looked at outcomes

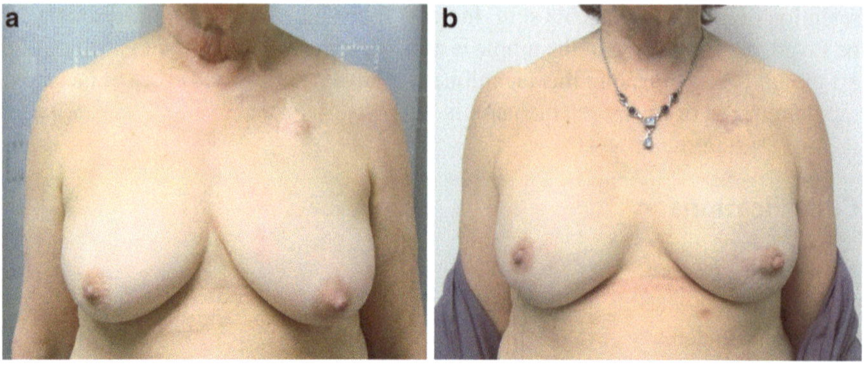

Fig. 2.5 64-year-old female s/p bilateral NSM for left breast cancer. (**a**) Preop; (**b**) 1 year postop

among NSM and skin-sparing mastectomy patients 4 years after surgery, they found that patients undergoing NSM had higher satisfaction with their reconstructed breasts and higher sexual well-being scores compared to skin-sparing mastectomy patients [52]. It is important to remember to inform patients preoperatively that their nipples and central breast skin will be numb after nipple-sparing mastectomy.

Conclusion

Eligibility for nipple-sparing mastectomy for risk reduction and for breast cancer treatment continues to increase. Meticulous surgical technique is essential to preserve blood supply to the nipple and skin flaps, while also ensuring adequate excision of the breast tissue. In appropriately selected patients, nipple-sparing mastectomy is oncologically safe and the risk of complications is acceptably low.

References

1. Sakorafas GH, Safioleas M. Breast cancer surgery: an historical narrative. Part III. From the sunset of the 19th to the dawn of the 21st century. Eur J Cancer Care. 2010;19:145–66.
2. Rice CO, Strickler JH. Adeno-mammectomy for benign breast lesions. Surg Gynecol Obstet. 1951;93(6):759–62.
3. Rusby JE, Smith BL, Gui GPH. Nipple sparing mastectomy. Br J Surg. 2010;97:305–16.
4. Hartmann LC, Schaid DJ, Woods JE, et al. Efficacy of bilateral prophylactic mastectomy in women with a family history of breast cancer. N Engl J Med. 1999;340:77–84.
5. Kasprzak L, Mesurolle B, Tremblay F, Galvez M, Halwani F, Foulkes WD. Invasive breast cancer following bilateral subcutaneous mastectomy in a BRCA2 mutation carrier: a case report and review of the literature. World J Surg Oncol. 2005;3:52.
6. Toth BA, Lappert P. Modified skin incisions for mastectomy: the need for plastic surgical input in preoperative planning. Plast Reconstr Surg. 1991;87(6):1048–53.

7. Yi M, Kronowitz SJ, Meric-Bernstam F, et al. Local, regional, and systemic recurrence rates in patients undergoing skin-sparing mastectomy compared with conventional mastectomy. Cancer. 2011;117:916–24.
8. Smith J, Payne WS, Carney JA. Involvement of the nipple and areola in carcinoma of the breast. Surg Gynecol Obstet. 1976;143:546–8.
9. Lagios MD, Gates EA, Westdahl PR, Richards V, Alpert BS. A guide to the frequency of nipple involvement in breast cancer. A study of 149 consecutive mastectomies using a serial subgross and correlated radiographic technique. Am J Surg. 1979;138:135–42.
10. Wertheim U, Ozzello L. Neoplastic involvement of nipple and skin flap in carcinoma of the breast. Am J Surg Pathol. 1980;4:543–9.
11. Andersen JA, Gram JB, Pallesen RM. Involvement of the nipple and areola in breast cancer. Value of clinical findings. Scand J Plast Reconstr Surg. 1981;15:39–42.
12. Brachtel EF, Rusby JE, Michaelson JS, Chen LL, Muzikansky A, Smith BL, et al. Occult nipple involvement in breast cancer: clinicopathologic findings in 316 consecutive mastectomy specimens. J Clin Oncol. 2009;27:4948–54.
13. Crowe JP, Patrick RJ, Yetman RJ, Djohan R. Nipple-sparing mastectomy update: one hundred forty-nine procedures and clinical outcomes. Arch Surg. 2008;143(11):1106–10.
14. Boneti C, Yuen J, Santiago C, et al. Oncologic safety of nipple skin-sparing or total skin-sparing mastectomies with immediate reconstruction. J Am Coll Surg. 2011;212:686–95.
15. Filho PA, Capko D, Barry JM, et al. Nipple-sparing mastectomy for breast cancer and risk-reducing surgery: the memorial Sloan-Kettering Cancer Center experience. Ann Surg Oncol. 2011;18:3117–22.
16. Petit JY, Veronisi U, Orecchia R, et al. Nipple sparing mastectomy with nipple areola intraoperative radiotherapy: one thousand and one cases of a five years experience at the European institute of oncology of Milan (EIO). Breast Cancer Res Treat. 2009;117:333–8.
17. Tang R, Coopey SB, Merrill AL, et al. Positive nipple margins in nipple-sparing mastectomies: rates, management, and oncologic safety. J Am Coll Surg. 2016;222:1149–55.
18. Camp MS, Coopey SB, Tang R, et al. Management of positive sub-areolar/nipple duct margins in nipple-sparing mastectomies. Breast J. 2014;20:402–7.
19. Amara D, Peled AW, Wang F, et al. Tumor involvement of the nipple in total skin-sparing mastectomy: strategies for management. Ann Surg Oncol. 2015;22:3803–8.
20. Rusby JE, Brachtel EF, Othus M, et al. Development and validation of a model predictive of occult nipple involvement in women undergoing mastectomy. Br J Surg. 2008;95:1356–61.
21. Coopey SB, Tang R, Lei L, et al. Increasing eligibility for nipple-sparing mastectomy. Ann Surg Oncol. 2013;20:3218–22.
22. Krajewski AC, Boughey JC, Degnim AC, et al. Expanded indications and improved outcomes for nipple-sparing mastectomy over time. Ann Surg Oncol. 2015;22:3317–23.
23. Peled AW, Wang F, Foster FD, et al. Expanding the indications for total skin-sparing mastectomy: is it safe for patients with locally advanced disease? Ann Surg Oncol. 2016;23:87–91.
24. Tang R, Coopey SB, Colwell AS, et al. Nipple-sparing mastectomy in irradiated breasts: selecting patients to minimize complications. Ann Surg Oncol. 2015;22:3331–7.
25. Salgarello M, Visconti G, Barone-Adesi L. Nipple-sparing mastectomy with immediate implant reconstruction: cosmetic outcomes and technical refinements. Plast Reconstr Surg. 2010;126:1460–71.
26. Davies K, Allan L, Roblin P, Ross D, Farhadi J. Factors affecting post-operative complications following skin sparing mastectomy with immediate breast reconstruction. Breast. 2011;20:21–5.
27. NCCN Clinical Practice Guidelines: Breast cancer risk reduction v1.2016 [Internet]. Available from: https://wwwnccnorg/professionals/physician_gls/pdf/breast_riskpdf. 2016.
28. Hartmann LC, Sellers TA, Schaid DJ, et al. Efficacy of bilateral prophylactic mastectomy in BRCA1 and BRCA2 gene mutation carriers. J Natl Cancer Inst. 2001;93:1633–7.
29. Yao K, Liederbach E, Tang R, et al. Nipple-sparing mastectomy in BRCA1/2 mutation carriers: an interim analysis and review of the literature. Ann Surg Oncol. 2015;22:370–6.

30. Peled AW, Irwin CS, Hwang ES, Ewing CA, Alvarado M, Esserman LJ. Total skin-sparing mastectomy in BRCA mutation carriers. Ann Surg Oncol. 2014;21:37–41.
31. Jakub J, Peled A, Gray R, et al. Multi-institutional study of the oncologic safety of prophylactic nipple-sparing mastectomy in a BRCA population [Abstract]. In: Proceedings from the 17th annual meeting of the American Society of Breast Surgeons. 2016 April 13–17, Dallas.
32. Coopey SB, Tang R, Rai U, et al. Oncologic safety of nipple sparing mastectomy in women with breast cancer [Abstract]. In: Proceedings from the 17th annual meeting of the American Society of Breast Surgeons. 2016 April 13–17, Dallas.
33. Peled AW, Foster RD, Stover AC, et al. Outcomes after Total skin-sparing mastectomy and immediate reconstruction in 657 breasts. Ann Surg Oncol. 2012;19:3402–9.
34. Jensen JA, Orringer JS, Giuliano AE. Nipple-sparing mastectomy in 99 patients with a mean follow-up of 5 years. Ann Surg Oncol. 2011;18:1665–70.
35. Lohsiriwat V, Martella S, Rietjens M. Paget's disease as a local recurrence after nipple-sparing mastectomy: clinical presentation, treatment, outcome, and risk factor analysis. Ann Surg Oncol. 2012;19:1850–5.
36. Orzalesi L, Casella D, Santi C, et al. Nipple sparing mastectomy: surgical and oncological outcomes from a national multicentric registry with 913 patients (1006 cases) over a six year period. Breast. 2016;25:75–81.
37. De La Cruz L, Moody AM, Tappy EE, Blankenship SA, Hecht EM. Overall survival, disease-free survival, local recurrence, and nipple–areolar recurrence in the setting of nipple-sparing mastectomy: a meta-analysis and systematic review. Ann Surg Oncol. 2015;22:3241–9.
38. Gerber B, Krause A, Dieterich M, Kundt G, Reimer T. The oncological safety of skin sparing mastectomy with conservation of the nipple-areola complex and autologous reconstruction: an extended follow-up study. Ann Surg. 2009;249:461–8.
39. Benediktsson KP, Perbeck L. Survival in breast cancer after nipple sparing subcutaneous mastectomy and immediate reconstruction with implants: a prospective trial with 13 years median follow-up in 216 patients. Eur J Surg Oncol. 2008;34:143–8.
40. Adam H, Bygdeson M, De Boniface J. The oncological safety of nipple-sparing mastectomy: a Swedish matched cohort study. Eur J Surg Oncol. 2014;40:1209–15.
41. Park SH, Han W, Yoo TK, et al. Oncologic safety of immediate breast reconstruction for invasive breast cancer patients: a matched case control study. J Breast Cancer. 2016;19:68–75.
42. Colwell AS, Gadd M, Smith BL, Austen WG. An inferolateral approach to nipple-sparing mastectomy. Ann Plast Surg. 2010;65:140–3.
43. Sacchini V, Pinotti JA, Barros ACSD, et al. Nipple-sparing mastectomy for breast cancer and risk reduction: oncologic or technical problem? J Am Coll Surg. 2006;203:704–14.
44. Harness JK, Vetter TS, Salibian AH. Areola and nipple–areola sparing mastectomy for breast cancer treatment and risk reduction: report of an initial experience in a community hospital setting. Ann Surg Oncol. 2011;18:917–22.
45. Djohan R, Gage E, Gatherwright J, et al. Patient satisfaction following nipple-sparing mastectomy and immediate breast reconstruction: an 8-year outcome study. Plast Reconstr Surg. 2010;125:818–29.
46. Colwell AS, Tessler O, Lin AM, et al. Breast reconstruction following nipple-sparing mastectomy: predictors of complications, reconstruction outcomes, and 5-year trends. Plast Reconstr Surg. 2014;133:496–506.
47. Robertson SA, Rusby JE, Cutress RI. Determinants of optimal mastectomy skin flap thickness. Br J Surg. 2014;101:899–911.
48. Rusby JE, Kirstein LJ, Brachtel EF, et al. Nipple-sparing mastectomy: lessons from ex vivo procedures. Breast J. 2008;14:464–70.
49. Piper M, Peled AW, Foster RD, Moore DH, Esserman LJ. Total skin-sparing mastectomy: a systematic review of oncologic outcomes and postoperative complications. Ann Plast Surg. 2013;70:435–7.
50. Lemaine V, Hoskin TL, Farley DR, et al. Introducing the SKIN score: a validated scoring system to assess severity of mastectomy skin flap necrosis. Ann Surg Oncol. 2015;22:2925–32.

51. Howard MA, Sisco M, Yao K, et al. Patient satisfaction with nipple-sparing mastectomy: a prospective study of patient reported outcomes using the BREAST-Q. J Surg Oncol. 2016;114:416–22.
52. Metcalfe KA, Cil TD, Semple JL, et al. Long-term psychosocial functioning in women with bilateral prophylactic mastectomy: does preservation of the nipple-areolar complex make a difference? Ann Surg Oncol. 2015;22:3324–30.

Contralateral Prophylactic Mastectomy: Current Perspectives

3

Katharine Yao

Introduction

In 1991 the National Institutes of Health published a consensus statement [1] that stated that breast conservation surgery (BCS) was "preferable" for early-stage breast cancer because it provided equivalent survival to mastectomy [2–8]. Shortly after this statement, the rate of breast conservation surgery increased [9]. However, over the past decade, we have witnessed a shift back toward mastectomies, particularly bilateral mastectomy for patients with unilateral breast cancer or contralateral prophylactic mastectomy (CPM). This trend has surfaced despite the absence of randomized trials for CPM and any official consensus statement endorsing CPM. Current NCCN guidelines [10] discourage CPM for patients with unilateral breast cancer, and a recent consensus statement for the American Society of Breast Surgeons states that CPM should be discouraged in average risk women [11, 12].

However, the decision context for breast surgery has become much more complex over the past decade and is heavily influenced by multiple external and internal factors. Improved access to breast reconstruction, increased use of breast MRI, and more referrals for genetic counseling and/or genetic testing have all become much more commonplace now then 10 years ago, and these factors have all been associated with increased CPM rates [13–16]. Lastly, patients have more exposure to breast cancer thru the media and patient advocacy groups and access to many more different sources of information. Patients are also taking more proactive roles in treatment decisions and seeking more opinions, not only from doctors but also friends, family, and other breast cancer survivors. Patients are mainly driving the

K. Yao, MD (✉)
Division of Surgical Oncology, Department of Surgery, NorthShore University HealthSystem, Evanston, IL, USA

Pritzker School of Medicine, University of Chicago, Chicago, IL, USA
e-mail: kyao@northshore.org

M. Howard-McNatt (ed.), *Changing Paradigms in the Management of Breast Cancer*, DOI 10.1007/978-3-319-60336-0_3

increased use of CPM, hoping to improve their outcomes and to avoid recurrences. Whether justified or not, the increased use of CPM has not abated, and surgeons will need to learn how to effectively counsel patients on decisions for CPM.

Trends in CPM

Some of the first studies to examine the increasing CPM rate came from the Surveillance Epidemiology End Results (SEER) database. A 2007 and 2009 study two reported that the rate of CPM had increased 148% and 150% among all patients for noninvasive and invasive cancer, respectively [17, 18]. When patients undergoing mastectomy were examined, there was a 188% and 162% increase, respectively. These two studies were the first in a string of studies examining the increasing CPM rate across the United States (Table 3.1) [15, 17–23]. In 2010, a report from the National Cancer Data Base (NCDB) showed an increase in CPM from 0.4% in 1998

Table 3.1 Studies examining trends in contralateral prophylactic mastectomy in the United States

Study	Year published	Study period	Percentage increase in CPM of all patients over the study period	Percentage increase in CPM of all mastectomy patients over the study period	Data source
Tuttle et al. [17], (invasive cancer)	2007	1998–2003	2.7%	6.8%	SEER
Tuttle et al. [18], (DCIS)	2009	1998–2005	3.1%	12.0%	SEER
Yao et al. [19]	2010	1998–2007	4.3%	NA	NCDB
Jones et al. [20]		1998–2007	NA	9.6%	Ohio state-NCCN network
King et al. [15]	2011	1997–2005	NA	17.5%	MSKCC single institution
Kummerow et al. [21]	2015	1998–2011	9.3%	24.3%	
Pesce et al. [23]	2014	2003–2010	5.6%	NA	NCDB
Kurian et al. [22]	2014	1998–2011	10.3%	NA	California cancer registry
Wong et al. [24]	2016	1998–2012	8.8%	NA	SEER

SEER Surveillance Epidemiology End Results, *NCDB* National Cancer Data Base, *MSKCC* Memorial Sloan Kettering Cancer Center, *NCCN* National Comprehensive Cancer Network, *NA* not available

to 4.7% in 2007 [19]. A 2011 study from Memorial Sloan Kettering reported that 6.7% of mastectomy patients underwent CPM in 1997 which increased to 24.2% in 2005 [15]. A recent SEER study showed that the CPM rate had more than tripled from 2002 to 2012 [24]. Interestingly, increasing CPM rates were documented across all stages, different areas of the country, all ages, insurance types, and facility types; however, certain common characteristics were seen. CPM rates are highest among Caucasians, patients with higher socioeconomic status, with private insurance and treated at high volume centers [17–19]. Race and socioeconomic status also play a role in CPM [25]; CPM is twice as common in Caucasians than other races [26] despite adjusting for socioeconomic factors. Patient age has consistently been shown to be the strongest factor associated with the increasing CPM rate. A NCDB study showed that CPM rates in 2011 were 9.7% among all age groups, but this percentage increased to 26% among those younger than 45 years old [23]. In a study of the California Cancer Registry [22], over 30% of women <40 years old underwent CPM in 2011. Another NCDB study published in 2015 showed that anywhere from 60% to 80% of women <=40 years old were undergoing CPM despite different tumor sizes [21]. However, this increasing trend for CPM has not been as evident in other countries. An article focused on Europe [27] did not show an increase in European CPM rates; however, one article reported that CPM rates in Britain have been increasing [28]. These findings underscore how cultural perceptions about CPM can have a profound effect on treatment preferences.

Contralateral Prophylactic Mastectomy and Survival

Although multiple single and multi-institutional studies published over the past 10–15 years in the United States have shown that CPM improved overall and disease-free survival, none are prospective randomized studies (Table 3.2), and therefore all studies are subject to selection bias [22, 29–36]. It is unlikely that a randomized trial of CPM versus UM or lumpectomy will be done in the near future. A Cochrane analysis published in 2009 concluded that CPM did not provide a survival benefit [37]. Four single [29, 32, 36, 38] and three multi-institution [30, 31, 35] retrospective studies demonstrated a disease-free survival benefit for CPM, while two single [32, 39] and three multi-institution [30, 34, 35] retrospective studies showed an overall survival benefit. A recent SEER study [35] showed that when CBC cases were removed from the analysis, it had little impact on CPM's survival benefit which shows that CBC has little to do with survival. In another SEER study of stages I–III patients, CPM was associated with breast cancer specific, all-cause and noncancer survival benefit, but its greatest effect was on noncancer survival [40]. Patients who undergo CPM may be more healthy and more compliant with their treatment regimens and have access to more advanced treatments then patients who do not undergo CPM.

On the other hand, CPM may truly benefit those who have a high CBC risk such as those patients who test positive for a genetic mutation. Retrospective studies have shown that BRCA mutation carriers derive a survival benefit from CPM [41], which

Table 3.2 Single and multi-institutional studies examining disease-free and overall survival in patients undergoing contralateral prophylactic mastectomy

Study	Year published	No pts CPM	Data source	DFS/DSS (adjusted)	OS (adjusted)	Follow-up
Peralta E et al. [29]	2000	64	Retrospective Single institution	DFS: 71% CPM vs. 53% control ($p = 0.06$)	64% CPM vs. 48% control ($p = 0.26$)	Mean: 6.8 years
Herrinton LJ et al. [30]	2005	1072	Cancer Research Network, Kaiser Permanente	Disease-specific survival: HR = 0.57 (95% CI, 0.45–0.72)	All-cause mortality: HR = 0.60 (95% CI, 0.50–0.72)	Median: 5.7 years
Bedrosian I et al. [31]	2010	8900	SEER	HR = 0.63 (95% CI, 0.57–0.69)	NA	Median 47 months
Brewster AM et al. [32]	2012	532	Retrospective Single institution	DFS: HR = 0.75 (95% CI, 0.59–0.97)	OS: HR-0.74 (95% CI 0.56–0.99)	Median: 4.5 years
Boughey J et al. [36]	2011	385	Retrospective Single institution	DFS: HR = 0.67 (95% CI, 0.54–0.84)	OS: HR = 0.77 (95% CI, 0.60–0.98)	Median: 17.3 years
Chung A et al. [33]	2012	177	Retrospective Single institution	No difference in DFS between unilateral mastectomy and unilateral mastectomy/CPM ($p = 0.081$)	No difference in OS between unilateral and unilateral mastectomy/CPM ($p = 0.42$)	Median: 61 months
Yao et al. [34]	2013	14,994	NCDB	NA	OS: HR = 0.88 (95% CI, 0.83–0.93)	Median: 5 years
Kruper et al. [35]	2014	26,526	SEER	DSS: HR = 0.83 (95% CI 0.77–0.90)	OS: HR = 0.77 (95% CI, 0.73–0.82)	NA
Kurian et al. [22]	2014	11,692	California Cancer Registry	NA	OS: HR = 1.02 (95% CI, 0.94–1.11)	Median: 89.1 months
Wong et al. [24]	2016	226,914	SEER	DSS: HR = 1.08 (95% CI 1.01–1.16–0.97)	OS: HR = 1.08 (95% CI 1.03–1.14)	Median 8.25 years

DFS disease-free survival, *DSS* disease-specific survival, *OS* overall survival, *NA* not available, *HR* hazard ratio, *SEER* Surveillance Epidemiology End Results, *NCDB* National Cancer Data Base

is understandable given the high CBC risk for BRCA carriers [42–44]. There have been no randomized prospective studies of BRCA carriers. CBC risk for other gene mutation carriers who have a breast cancer are not well studied although two studies have shown a higher CBC rate for CHEK2 1100delC mutation carriers [45, 46]. Insufficient data exist to routinely recommend CPM for gene carriers besides BRCA1 and BRCA2.

Contralateral Breast Cancer Risk

Many women choose CPM to reduce their risk of a contralateral cancer [72], but they often overestimate their CBC risk [47] at 30% at 10 years when most population based studies show a 5% or less risk at 10 years for average risk patients [48, 49]. Population-based studies and clinical trials (Table 3.3) [30, 48–56] that track CBC rates have shown that the CBC risk at 10 years is <=5%. CBC risk is lower for ER positive tumors, likely related to the protective effect of hormonal therapy on the contralateral breast. A SEER study from 2009 showed that CBC rates have been dropping 3%/year, likely secondary to the use of hormonal therapy [49]. An EBCTCG overview quotes a 0.4% and 0.5% annual risk of CBC for estrogen receptor (ER) positive and negative patients [57]. This translates into an approximate 4% risk at 10 years for ER positive tumors versus a 5% risk for an ER negative tumor. Younger patients are at higher risk for CBC, presumably because of their longer life span. A SEER study [61] reported that the 10-year CBC risk for a woman 25–29 years old with an ER negative tumor is 1.26 per 100/year compared to 0.45 per 100/year for an ER positive tumor. In contrast, the 10 year risk for a 50-year-old women with an ER negative tumor is 0.45 per 100/year compared to 0.26 per 100/year for an ER positive tumor. Family history also influences CBC rates. A Women's Environmental Cancer and Radiation Epidemiology [54] study showed that women with a first degree relative with breast cancer have a CBC risk at 10 years of 14.7% for those 30 years old, but this risk decreases to 6.7% for women in their 50s. These data demonstrate a differential risk for CBC according to patient age, ER status, and family history, but future studies are needed to determine other clinical factors that could influence CBC risk.

Characteristics of Contralateral Breast Cancers and Survival of Those Patients Who Develop a Contralateral Breast Cancer

Many studies have shown that CBCs tend to have more favorable tumor characteristics than the primary tumor [58–62]. Studies have also shown that patients who develop a CBC have worse survival especially if the CBC develops in a short interval from the primary cancer [60, 63–65]. Patients who had worse survival with a CBC were young patients, patients with large tumors, and node positive patients [60, 63, 64]. It is not clear if the reported worse survival is because these CBCs represent aggressive biology of the primary tumor, distant metastatic disease, or perhaps just older, inferior systemic treatments [60, 63, 64].

Table 3.3 Studies examining contralateral breast cancer rates

Study	Publication year	Data source	Follow-up	CBC risk
I. Soerjomataram et al. [50]	2005	Eindhoven Cancer Registry	4.9 years	SIR 3.5 (CI 3.2–3.8)
Gao et al. [48]	2003	SEER	5 years	3.0%
			10 years	6.1%
			15 years	9.1%
			20 years	12%
Herrinton L et al. [30]	2005	Cancer Research Network	5.7 years	2.7%
		Kaiser Permanente		
Cuzick et al. [51]	2010	ATAC trial	5 years	1–1.8%
			10 years	3.2% armidex arm
				4.9% tamoxifen arm
Nichols et al. [49]	2011	SEER	10 years	0.26 per 100/year (50 years old ER positive)
				0.45 per 100/year (50 years old ER negative)
Perez EA et al. [52]	2011	Herceptin trials	4 years	0.5–1.0% control arm
		NCCTG N9831 and NSABP B31		0.7–0.9% herceptin arm
Wapnir IL et al. [53]	2011	NSABP B17/B24	15 years	10% lumpectomy
				10.2–10.8% lumpectomy/XRT
				7.3% lumpectomy + Tamoxifen
Reiner et al. [54]	2012	WECARE	10 years	4.6–15.6% depending on family history
		Non-BRCA carriers with family hx		
Pilewskie M et al. [55]	2014	Single institution	8 years	3.5% MRI
		MKSCC		5.1% no MRI
McCormick B. et al. [56]	2015	RTOG 9804	7 yrs	4.8% tamoxifen + observation
		DCIS patients		3.9% tamoxifen + radiation

SIR standardized incidence ratio, *SEER* Surveillance Epidemiology End Results, *WECARE* Women's Environmental Cancer and Radiation Epidemiology Study, *MRI* magnetic resonance imaging, *ATAC* Arimidex, Tamoxifen, Alone, or in Combination Trial, *ER* estrogen receptor, *NCCTG* North Central Cancer Treatment Group, *NSABP* National Surgical Adjuvant Bowel and Breast Project, *RTOG* Radiation Therapy Oncology Group, *MSKCC* Memorial Sloan Kettering Cancer Center, *DCIS* ductal carcinoma in situ

Patient Perspectives on CPM

Patient Motivations for Choosing CPM

Although up to 10–20% of all women are undergoing CPM in the current era, half of all women consider CPM somewhere in the preoperative setting [66]. This preference was associated with higher levels of cancer worry, young age, and low knowledge about breast cancer [66]. The most common reasons to choose CPM revolve around a perceived survival benefit from CPM and fear of a second breast cancer in the contralateral breast. In a multi-institutional study of 123 young women, "desire to lower the chance of getting cancer in the other breast" was ranked as the most important reason women chose CPM with 98% of women stating it was extremely or very important in their decision to undergo CPM [67]. The third most common reason was to "improve survival" with 94% stating it was extremely or very important and desire to prevent cancer from spreading to other parts of the body was the fourth most common reason with 85% stating it was extremely or very important. Other studies have confirmed these findings [68–70]. Many patients have high levels of preoperative "cancer worry" and fear of recurrence [66, 67], and cancer worry has been associated with CPM interest and the performance of CPM [66]. Anxiety and worry are also likely a cause of cognitive dissonance; women choosing CPM to improve survival often correctly answer questions regarding the lack of CPM's association with recurrence and survival [67]. At the same time, there are many other reasons that women choose CPM. These include family history, avoiding screening mammograms and biopsies [67–69], cosmetic concerns, and for "peace of mind". Symmetry concerns were extremely or very important to 57% of participants in the young women study [67] and 59% of women in another study stated that reconstructive surgery availability influenced their decision [13]. Friends, family, and spouses also influence patients [68, 70], particularly if one of these individuals has been through breast cancer or another cancer.

Patient Satisfaction and Quality of Life with CPM

Most studies have shown that women are generally very satisfied with their decision to undergo CPM. Satisfaction rates with CPM range from 80 to 97%, and the same percentage would have chosen CPM again if given the choice [39, 67–69]. Even studies with longer follow-up show a high satisfaction rate with CPM [71]. However, retrospective studies have shown that QOL is similar between CPM and non-CPM patients. Less contentment with QOL was associated with poor health perception overall, not the decision to undergo CPM [72]. A recent study cross-sectional study of over 7000 women at approximately 5 years after surgery showed that although psychosocial well-being was statistically higher in the CPM group versus other surgery groups, the difference was too small to be clinically significant [73].

Nonetheless, women do report dissatisfaction with CPM related to reconstructive procedures or unexpected subsequent procedures and cosmetic outcomes.

Nearly a third reported that CPM had a negative effect on body appearance [71]. A report with longer follow-up showed that body appearance, feelings of femininity, and sexual relationships were negatively affected in 23–31% of patients [74]. A recent report also showed that nearly 40% of those who had reconstruction had at least one unplanned reoperation [39]. Reoperation was associated with lower satisfaction with CPM, lower likelihood of undergoing reconstruction again, and lower likelihood of choosing CPM. In a more recent study of young women, approximately 30% reported that surgical outcomes were worse than expected, especially regarding chest wall numbness and the need for multiple procedures [67]. A more recent study utilizing the Breast Q assessed patient's satisfaction with breast appearance and outcomes between CPM and UM patients with implant reconstruction [75]. They reported that CPM was an independent predictor of satisfaction with the breasts but not breast reconstruction outcome satisfaction. One prospective study conducted in Sweden showed that QOL, anxiety, depression, and sexuality were no different before and after CPM but that approximately 50% of women reported at least one body image problem postoperatively [76]. Despite high satisfaction with CPM, women do report negative effects as well.

Patient Knowledge About CPM

Patients often lack knowledge about their CBC risk and how CPM affects their outcomes. Studies have shown that patients' lack of knowledge regarding CPM has been associated with preoperative CPM interest [66]. Women often overestimate their CBC risk at approximately 30% at 10 years [47, 77]. Interestingly, the perceived CBC risk was not different between CPM, UM, and BCS patients [47]. Patients often have the misperception that CPM will eliminate risk of any type of breast cancer recurrence [67]. Seventy three percent of women in one study stated that there was no difference in survival between surgical options, but of the 27% that felt there was a difference, approximately 60% felt that BM patients would live longest [67]. Qualitative interviews with breast cancer patients revealed that women often felt that CPM would "insure a better survival" [70]. These knowledge deficits are significant because knowledge is a critical component of decision making and these deficits demonstrate that patients are not informed of how certain surgical procedures can impact their overall outcome.

Surgeon Perspectives About CPM

There is little data in the literature on physician's CPM knowledge and perceptions. One Australian study [78] reported that surgeon age and gender were not related to CPM rates, contrasting another study that showed higher CPM rates among female surgeons [79]. Most physicians report that patient motivations drive the decision to undergo CPM with surgeons discussing it with patients only 5–20% of the time

[78]. Surgeons stated that "fear and anxiety" was the most common reason women requested a CPM [78]. When asked when they would recommend a CPM, surgeons stated BRCA carrier status and strong family history were the most common reasons with patient initiative as the third most common. In another study based in the United States [80], over half of surgeons stated they were at some point uncomfortable performing CPM and roughly a third said they were comfortable performing CPM on an average risk patient. Another study from the same survey showed that approximately 40% of surgeons had "low knowledge" about CPM particularly about CBC risk in certain patient subgroups. Understanding physician's knowledge base and perceptions is crucial to understanding how physicians inform their patients and what influence they have on a patient's decision to undergo CPM. Indeed, Rosenberg's study showed that physicians were the most important source of information and have an enormous influence on patient decision making [67]. Future studies further examining the role and influence of the surgeon in the patient decision making process for CPM are needed.

Counseling Patients on Contralateral Prophylactic Mastectomy: Insuring Informed Consent

There are three critical factors that make up a high-quality decision: decisions should be informed and shared between physician and patient and reflective of patient's values and concerns. Applying these principles to the surgical decision making process is feasible. Previous trials of decision aids for breast cancer surgery decisions have shown that decision aids improve knowledge, decrease decisional regret, and improve decisional satisfaction [81–84], but few decision aids address decision making surrounding CPM. A recent consensus statement from the American Society of Breast Surgeons [11, 12] outlines the impact of CPM on patient reported outcomes and survival outcomes and outlines considerations for CPM and against CPM. CPM is generally recommended for those patients who are at higher risk for a CBC such as BRCA carriers, strong family history, or previous chest wall radiation but not for those at average risk for CBC (Table 3.4). Important to the discussion of CPM with patients are not only how CPM impacts survival and CBC risk but how CPM affects other patient outcomes such as sexuality and physical side effects. Understanding patient's values and preferences for radiation therapy, cosmesis, future screening, and how important it is to keep their breast will also facilitate shared decision making between the patient and physician. Other statements and guidelines [10, 85] have also stressed the importance of an informed discussion with patients about CPM. It is important to consider all the "pros" and "cons" when discussing the option of CPM with patients (Table 3.5) because the reasons to choose CPM may vary between different patients. The key component to each patient's decision is to insure patients are given the information, time, and resources to make a decision that is concordant with their wishes and values and safe for their health.

Table 3.4 Reasons to consider or not consider a CPM [11]

Reasons to consider a CPM	Reasons to not consider a CPM
BRCA carrier (there is insufficient evidence to support CPM for other pathogenic gene mutations such as CHEK2, PALB2, CDH1, etc.)	Average risk for a CBC
Suspicious family history suggestive of a hereditary component	Multiple comorbidities that would add to already increased operative risk
Previous chest wall radiation	Male breast cancer
	Negative testing for BRCA in a BRCA positive family (true negative)
	Advanced stage disease

CPM contralateral prophylactic mastectomy, *CBC* contralateral breast cancer

Table 3.5 Pros and cons of CPM

Pros of undergoing CPM	Cons of undergoing CPM
Decrease risk of a contralateral breast cancer	No improvement in survival
Improved symmetry with reconstruction for some patients whose primary tumor is not amenable to breast conservation	Decreased sensation along the chest wall
Avoid future screening mammograms and possible biopsies	Longer recovery time
"Peace of mind"	Increase in operative complications
	Loss of breasts
	Possible negative effects on sexuality, intimacy

CPM contralateral prophylactic mastectomy

References

1. NIH consensus conference. Treatment of early-stage breast cancer. JAMA. 1991;265(3):391–5.
2. Fisher B, Bauer M, Margolese R, et al. Five-year results of a randomized clinical trial comparing total mastectomy and segmental mastectomy with or without radiation in the treatment of breast cancer. N Engl J Med. 1985;312(11):665–73.
3. Blichert-Toft M, Rose C, Andersen JA, et al. Danish randomized trial comparing breast conservation therapy with mastectomy: six years of life-table analysis. Danish Breast Cancer Cooperative Group. J Natl Cancer Inst Monogr. 1992;11:19–25.
4. Veronesi U, Cascinelli N, Mariani L, et al. Twenty-year follow-up of a randomized study comparing breast-conserving surgery with radical mastectomy for early breast cancer. N Engl J Med. 2002;347(16):1227–32.
5. Sarrazin D, Le MG, Arriagada R, et al. Ten-year results of a randomized trial comparing a conservative treatment to mastectomy in early breast cancer. Radiother Oncol: J Eur Soc Ther Radiol Oncol. 1989;14(3):177–84.
6. van Dongen JA, Bartelink H, Fentiman IS, et al. Randomized clinical trial to assess the value of breast-conserving therapy in stage I and II breast cancer, EORTC 10801 trial. J Natl Cancer Inst Monogr. 1992;11:15–8.
7. Early Breast Cancer Trialists' Collaborative Group. Effects of radiotherapy and surgery in early breast cancer. An overview of the randomized trials. N Engl J Med. 1995;333(22):1444–55.

8. Morris AD, Morris RD, Wilson JF, et al. Breast-conserving therapy vs mastectomy in early-stage breast cancer: a meta-analysis of 10-year survival. Cancer J Sci Am. 1997;3(1):6–12.
9. Lazovich D, Solomon CC, Thomas DB, Moe RE, White E. Breast conservation therapy in the United States following the 1990 National Institutes of Health Consensus Development Conference on the treatment of patients with early stage invasive breast carcinoma. Cancer. 1999;86(4):628–37.
10. NCCN Guidelines. 2015; http://www.nccn.org/professionals/physician_gls/f_guidelines.asp#site. 2015.
11. Boughey JC, Attai DJ, Chen SL, et al. Contralateral prophylactic mastectomy consensus statement from the American Society of Breast Surgeons: additional considerations and a framework for shared decision making. Ann Surg Oncol. 2016;23(10):3106–11.
12. Boughey JC, Attai DJ, Chen SL, et al. Contralateral Prophylactic Mastectomy (CPM) consensus statement from the American Society of Breast Surgeons: data on CPM outcomes and risks. Ann Surg Oncol. 2016;23(10):3100–5.
13. Hawley ST, Jagsi R, Morrow M, Katz SJ. Correlates of contralateral prophylactic mastectomy in a population based sample. J Clin Oncol: Off J Am Soc Clin Oncol. 2011;29:6010.
14. Katipamula R, Degnim AC, Hoskin T, et al. Trends in mastectomy rates at the Mayo Clinic Rochester: effect of surgical year and preoperative magnetic resonance imaging. J Clin Oncol: Off J Am Soc Clin Oncol. 2009;27(25):4082–8.
15. King TA, Sakr R, Patil S, et al. Clinical management factors contribute to the decision for contralateral prophylactic mastectomy. J Clin Oncol: Off J Am Soc Clin Oncol. 2011;29(16):2158–64.
16. Wang F, Amara D, Peled AW, et al. Negative genetic testing does not deter contralateral prophylactic mastectomy in younger patients with greater family histories of breast cancer. Ann Surg Oncol. 2015;22(10):3338–45.
17. Tuttle TM, Habermann EB, Grund EH, Morris TJ, Virnig BA. Increasing use of contralateral prophylactic mastectomy for breast cancer patients: a trend toward more aggressive surgical treatment. J Clin Oncol: Off J Am Soc Clin Oncol. 2007;25(33):5203–9.
18. Tuttle TM, Jarosek S, Habermann EB, et al. Increasing rates of contralateral prophylactic mastectomy among patients with ductal carcinoma in situ. J Clin Oncol: Off J Am Soc Clin Oncol. 2009;27(9):1362–7.
19. Yao K, Stewart AK, Winchester DJ, Winchester DP. Trends in contralateral prophylactic mastectomy for unilateral cancer: a report from the National Cancer Data Base, 1998–2007. Ann Surg Oncol. 2010;17(10):2554–62.
20. Jones NB, Wilson J, Kotur L, Stephens J, Farrar WB, Agnese DM. Contralateral prophylactic mastectomy for unilateral breast cancer: an increasing trend at a single institution. Ann Surg Oncol. 2009;16(10):2691–6.
21. Kummerow KL, Du L, Penson DF, Shyr Y, Hooks MA. Nationwide trends in mastectomy for early-stage breast cancer. JAMA Surg. 2015;150(1):9–16.
22. Kurian AW, Lichtensztajn DY, Keegan TH, Nelson DO, Clarke CA, Gomez SL. Use of and mortality after bilateral mastectomy compared with other surgical treatments for breast cancer in California, 1998–2011. JAMA. 2014;312(9):902–14.
23. Pesce CE, Liederbach E, Czechura T, Winchester DJ, Yao K. Changing surgical trends in young patients with early stage breast cancer, 2003 to 2010: a report from the National Cancer Data Base. J Am Coll Surg. 2014;219(1):19–28.
24. Wong SM, Freedman RA, Sagara Y, Aydogan F, Barry WT, Golshan M. Growing use of contralateral prophylactic mastectomy despite no improvement in long-term survival for invasive breast cancer. Ann Surg. 2017;265(3):581–9.
25. Brown D, Shao S, Jatoi I, Shriver CD, Zhu K. Trends in use of contralateral prophylactic mastectomy by racial/ethnic group and ER/PR status among patients with breast cancer: a SEER population-based study. Cancer Epidemiol. 2016;42:24–31.
26. Grimmer L, Liederbach E, Velasco J, Pesce C, Wang CH, Yao K. Variation in contralateral prophylactic mastectomy rates according to racial groups in young women with breast cancer, 1998 to 2011: a report from the National Cancer Data Base. J Am Coll Surg. 2015;221(1):187–96.

27. Guth U, Myrick ME, Viehl CT, Weber WP, Lardi AM, Schmid SM. Increasing rates of contralateral prophylactic mastectomy – a trend made in USA? Eur J Surg Oncol: J Eur Soc Surg Oncol Br Assoc Surg Oncol. 2012;38(4):296–301.
28. Neuburger J, Macneill F, Jeevan R, van der Meulen JH, Cromwell DA. Trends in the use of bilateral mastectomy in England from 2002 to 2011: retrospective analysis of hospital episode statistics. BMJ Open. 2013;3(8):e003179.
29. Peralta EA, Ellenhorn JD, Wagman LD, Dagis A, Andersen JS, Chu DZ. Contralateral prophylactic mastectomy improves the outcome of selected patients undergoing mastectomy for breast cancer. Am J Surg. 2000;180(6):439–45.
30. Herrinton LJ, Barlow WE, Yu O, et al. Efficacy of prophylactic mastectomy in women with unilateral breast cancer: a cancer research network project. J Clin Oncol: Off J Am Soc Clin Oncol. 2005;23(19):4275–86.
31. Bedrosian I, Hu CY, Chang GJ. Population-based study of contralateral prophylactic mastectomy and survival outcomes of breast cancer patients. J Natl Cancer Inst. 2010;102(6):401–9.
32. Brewster AM, Bedrosian I, Parker PA, et al. Association between contralateral prophylactic mastectomy and breast cancer outcomes by hormone receptor status. Cancer. 2012;118(22):5637–43.
33. Chung A, Huynh K, Lawrence C, Sim MS, Giuliano A. Comparison of patient characteristics and outcomes of contralateral prophylactic mastectomy and unilateral total mastectomy in breast cancer patients. Ann Surg Oncol. 2012;19(8):2600–6.
34. Yao K, Winchester DJ, Czechura T, Huo D. Contralateral prophylactic mastectomy and survival: report from the National Cancer Data Base, 1998–2002. Breast Cancer Res Treat. 2013;142(3):465–76.
35. Kruper L, Kauffmann RM, Smith DD, Nelson RA. Survival analysis of contralateral prophylactic mastectomy: a question of selection bias. Ann Surg Oncol. 2014;21(11):3448–56.
36. Boughey JC, Hoskin TL, Degnim AC, et al. Contralateral prophylactic mastectomy is associated with a survival advantage in high-risk women with a personal history of breast cancer. Ann Surg Oncol. 2010;17(10):2702–9.
37. Lostumbo L, Carbine N, Wallace J, Ezzo J. Prophylactic mastectomy for the prevention of breast cancer. Cochrane Database Syst Rev. 2004;4:CD002748.
38. Lee JS, Grant CS, Donohue JH, Crotty TB, Harmsen WS, Ilstrup DM. Arguments against routine contralateral mastectomy or undirected biopsy for invasive lobular breast cancer. Surgery. 1995;118(4):640–7. discussion 647–648
39. Boughey JC, Hoskin TL, Hartmann LC, et al. Impact of reconstruction and reoperation on long-term patient-reported satisfaction after contralateral prophylactic mastectomy. Ann Surg Oncol. 2015;22(2):401–8.
40. Jatoi I, Parsons HM. Contralateral prophylactic mastectomy and its association with reduced mortality: evidence for selection bias. Breast Cancer Res Treat. 2014;148(2):389–96.
41. Heemskerk-Gerritsen BA, Rookus MA, Aalfs CM, et al. Improved overall survival after contralateral risk-reducing mastectomy in BRCA1/2 mutation carriers with a history of unilateral breast cancer: a prospective analysis. Int J Cancer J Int Cancer. 2015;136(3):668–77.
42. Mavaddat N, Peock S, Frost D, et al. Cancer risks for BRCA1 and BRCA2 mutation carriers: results from prospective analysis of EMBRACE. J Natl Cancer Inst. 2013;105(11):812–22.
43. van der Kolk DM, de Bock GH, Leegte BK, et al. Penetrance of breast cancer, ovarian cancer and contralateral breast cancer in BRCA1 and BRCA2 families: high cancer incidence at older age. Breast Cancer Res Treat. 2010;124(3):643–51.
44. Verhoog LC, Brekelmans CT, Seynaeve C, et al. Survival in hereditary breast cancer associated with germline mutations of BRCA2. J Clin Oncol: Off J Am Soc Clin Oncol. 1999;17(11):3396–402.
45. Weischer M, Nordestgaard BG, Pharoah P, et al. CHEK2*1100delC heterozygosity in women with breast cancer associated with early death, breast cancer-specific death, and increased risk of a second breast cancer. J Clin Oncol: Off J Am Soc Clin Oncol. 2012;30(35):4308–16.
46. Kriege M, Hollestelle A, Jager A, et al. Survival and contralateral breast cancer in CHEK2 1100delC breast cancer patients: impact of adjuvant chemotherapy. Br J Cancer. 2014;111(5):1004–13.

47. Abbott A, Rueth N, Pappas-Varco S, Kuntz K, Kerr E, Tuttle T. Perceptions of contralateral breast cancer: an overestimation of risk. Ann Surg Oncol. 2011;18(11):3129–36.
48. Gao X, Fisher SG, Emami B. Risk of second primary cancer in the contralateral breast in women treated for early-stage breast cancer: a population-based study. Int J Radiat Oncol Biol Phys. 2003;56(4):1038–45.
49. Nichols HB, Berrington de Gonzalez A, Lacey JV Jr, Rosenberg PS, Anderson WF. Declining incidence of contralateral breast cancer in the United States from 1975 to 2006. J Clin Oncol: Off J Am Soc Clin Oncol. 2011;29(12):1564–9.
50. Soerjomataram I, Louwman WJ, Lemmens VE, de Vries E, Klokman WJ, Coebergh JW. Risks of second primary breast and urogenital cancer following female breast cancer in the south of The Netherlands, 1972–2001. Eur J Cancer. 2005;41(15):2331–7.
51. Cuzick J, Sestak I, Baum M, et al. Effect of anastrozole and tamoxifen as adjuvant treatment for early-stage breast cancer: 10-year analysis of the ATAC trial. Lancet Oncol. 2010;11(12):1135–41.
52. Perez EA, Romond EH, Suman VJ, et al. Four-year follow-up of trastuzumab plus adjuvant chemotherapy for operable human epidermal growth factor receptor 2-positive breast cancer: joint analysis of data from NCCTG N9831 and NSABP B-31. J Clin Oncol: Off J Am Soc Clin Oncol. 2011;29(25):3366–73.
53. Wapnir IL, Dignam JJ, Fisher B, et al. Long-term outcomes of invasive ipsilateral breast tumor recurrences after lumpectomy in NSABP B-17 and B-24 randomized clinical trials for DCIS. J Natl Cancer Inst. 2011;103(6):478–88.
54. Reiner AS, John EM, Brooks JD, et al. Risk of asynchronous contralateral breast cancer in noncarriers of BRCA1 and BRCA2 mutations with a family history of breast cancer: a report from the Women's Environmental Cancer and Radiation Epidemiology Study. J Clin Oncol: Off J Am Soc Clin Oncol. 2013;31(4):433–9.
55. Pilewskie M, Olcese C, Eaton A, et al. Perioperative breast MRI is not associated with lower locoregional recurrence rates in DCIS patients treated with or without radiation. Ann Surg Oncol. 2014;21(5):1552–60.
56. McCormick B, Winter K, Hudis C, et al. RTOG 9804: a prospective randomized trial for good-risk ductal carcinoma in situ comparing radiotherapy with observation. J Clin Oncol: Off J Am Soc Clin Oncol. 2015;33(7):709–15.
57. Davies C, Godwin J, Gray R, et al. Relevance of breast cancer hormone receptors and other factors to the efficacy of adjuvant tamoxifen: patient-level meta-analysis of randomised trials. Lancet. 2011;378(9793):771–84.
58. Liederbach E, Piro R, Hughes K, Watkin R, Wang CH, Yao K. Clinicopathologic features and time interval analysis of contralateral breast cancers. Surgery. 2015;158(3):676–85.
59. Huo D, Melkonian S, Rathouz PJ, Khramtsov A, Olopade OI. Concordance in histological and biological parameters between first and second primary breast cancers. Cancer. 2011;117(5):907–15.
60. Vichapat V, Garmo H, Holmberg L, et al. Prognosis of metachronous contralateral breast cancer: importance of stage, age and interval time between the two diagnoses. Breast Cancer Res Treat. 2011;130(2):609–18.
61. Diaz R, Munarriz B, Santaballa A, Palomar L, Montalar J. Synchronous and metachronous bilateral breast cancer: a long-term single-institution experience. Med Oncol. 2012;29(1):16–24.
62. Quan G, Pommier SJ, Pommier RF. Incidence and outcomes of contralateral breast cancers. Am J Surg. 2008;195(5):645–50. discussion 650
63. Font-Gonzalez A, Liu L, Voogd AC, et al. Inferior survival for young patients with contralateral compared to unilateral breast cancer: a nationwide population-based study in the Netherlands. Breast Cancer Res Treat. 2013;139(3):811–9.
64. Vichapat V, Garmo H, Holmqvist M, et al. Tumor stage affects risk and prognosis of contralateral breast cancer: results from a large Swedish-population-based study. J Clin Oncol: Off J Am Soc Clin Oncol. 2012;30(28):3478–85.
65. Liederbach E, Sisco M, Wang C, et al. Wait times for breast surgical operations, 2003–2011: a report from the National Cancer Data Base. Ann Surg Oncol. 2015;22(3):899–907.

66. Parker PA, Peterson SK, Bedrosian I, et al. Prospective study of surgical decision-making processes for contralateral prophylactic mastectomy in women with breast cancer. Ann Surg. 2016;263(1):178–83.
67. Rosenberg SM, Tracy MS, Meyer ME, et al. Perceptions, knowledge, and satisfaction with contralateral prophylactic mastectomy among young women with breast cancer: a cross-sectional survey. Ann Intern Med. 2013;159(6):373–81.
68. Soran A, Ibrahim A, Kanbour M, et al. Decision making and factors influencing long-term satisfaction with prophylactic mastectomy in women with breast cancer. Am J Clin Oncol. 2015;38(2):179–83.
69. Han E, Johnson N, Glissmeyer M, et al. Increasing incidence of bilateral mastectomies: the patient perspective. Am J Surg. 2011;201(5):615–8.
70. Covelli AM, Baxter NN, Fitch MI, McCready DR, Wright FC. 'Taking control of cancer': understanding women's choice for mastectomy. Ann Surg Oncol. 2015;22(2):383–91.
71. Frost MH, Schaid DJ, Sellers TA, et al. Long-term satisfaction and psychological and social function following bilateral prophylactic mastectomy. JAMA. 2000;284(3):319–24.
72. Geiger AM, West CN, Nekhlyudov L, et al. Contentment with quality of life among breast cancer survivors with and without contralateral prophylactic mastectomy. J Clin Oncol: Off J Am Soc Clin Oncol. 2006;24(9):1350–6.
73. Hwang ES, Locklear TD, Rushing CN, et al. Patient-reported outcomes after choice for contralateral prophylactic mastectomy. J Clin Oncol: Off J Am Soc Clin Oncol. 2016;34(13):1518–27.
74. Frost MH, Hoskin TL, Hartmann LC, Degnim AC, Johnson JL, Boughey JC. Contralateral prophylactic mastectomy: long-term consistency of satisfaction and adverse effects and the significance of informed decision-making, quality of life, and personality traits. Ann Surg Oncol. 2011;18(11):3110–6.
75. Koslow S, Pharmer LA, Scott AM, et al. Long-term patient-reported satisfaction after contralateral prophylactic mastectomy and implant reconstruction. Ann Surg Oncol. 2013;20(11): 3422–9.
76. Unukovych D, Sandelin K, Liljegren A, et al. Contralateral prophylactic mastectomy in breast cancer patients with a family history: a prospective 2-years follow-up study of health related quality of life, sexuality and body image. Eur J Cancer. 2012;48(17):3150–6.
77. Portschy PR, Kuntz KM, Tuttle TM. Survival outcomes after contralateral prophylactic mastectomy: a decision analysis. J Natl Cancer Inst. 2014;106(8).
78. Musiello T, Bornhammar E, Saunders C. Breast surgeons' perceptions and attitudes towards contralateral prophylactic mastectomy. ANZ J Surg. 2013;83(7–8):527–32.
79. Arrington AK, Jarosek SL, Virnig BA, Habermann EB, Tuttle TM. Patient and surgeon characteristics associated with increased use of contralateral prophylactic mastectomy in patients with breast cancer. Ann Surg Oncol. 2009;16(10):2697–704.
80. Bellavance E, Peppercorn J, Kronsberg S, et al. Surgeons' perspectives of contralateral prophylactic mastectomy. Ann Surg Oncol. 2016;23(9):2779–87.
81. Goel V, Sawka CA, Thiel EC, Gort EH, O'Connor AM. Randomized trial of a patient decision aid for choice of surgical treatment for breast cancer. Med Decis Making Int J Soc Med Decis Making. 2001;21(1):1–6.
82. Street RL Jr, Voigt B, Geyer C Jr, Manning T, Swanson GP. Increasing patient involvement in choosing treatment for early breast cancer. Cancer. 1995;76(11):2275–85.
83. Whelan T, Levine M, Willan A, et al. Effect of a decision aid on knowledge and treatment decision making for breast cancer surgery: a randomized trial. JAMA. 2004;292(4):435–41.
84. Lam WW, Chan M, Or A, Kwong A, Suen D, Fielding R. Reducing treatment decision conflict difficulties in breast cancer surgery: a randomized controlled trial. J Clin Oncol: Off J Am Soc Clin Oncol. 2013;31(23):2879–85.
85. Giuliano AE, Boolbol S, Degnim A, Kuerer H, Leitch AM, Morrow M. Society of Surgical Oncology: position statement on prophylactic mastectomy. Approved by the Society of Surgical Oncology Executive Council, March 2007. Ann Surg Oncol. 2007;14(9):2425–7.

Management of the Axilla in Breast Cancer

4

Toan T. Nguyen and Judy C. Boughey

Introduction

In patients with breast cancer, axillary lymph node status is the most significant prognostic factor and predictor of long-term outcomes [1, 2]. Presence of nodal metastasis is associated with increased risk of locoregional recurrence and decreased overall survival. Patients who have nodal spread require more aggressive local and systemic therapy. Axillary lymph node dissection (ALND) was the standard of care for all patients presenting with breast cancer for much of the twentieth century for the purposes of staging and treatment. This procedure removes all the lymph nodes from level I and level II in the axilla and is associated with significant risk of functional disability of the ipsilateral arm, chronic pain, and lymphedema. It was not until the 1990s that a much less morbid procedure, sentinel lymph node (SLN) surgery was developed [3, 4]. SLN surgery has been proven to be safe and feasible for clinically node-negative patients while accurately determining nodal status (node positive versus node negative). Management of the axilla has since evolved at an accelerated pace in recent years. Numerous multi-institutional studies have provided strong evidence that less aggressive surgical treatment of the axilla in most patients provide similar prognostic data while maintaining similar locoregional control.

Anatomy and Physiology

Lymphatic drainage of the breast originates from the breast lobules and flows into a subareolar plexus, that was first described by Sappey in 1874 who injected mercury into the dermis of a cadaver to identify the lymphatic pathways [5]. The axillary lymph nodes receive over 80% of the lymphatic drainage from all quadrants of the

T.T. Nguyen, MD • J.C. Boughey, MD (✉)
Department of Surgery, Mayo Clinic, 200 First Street SW, Rochester, MN 55905, USA
e-mail: Boughey.judy@mayo.edu

M. Howard-McNatt (ed.), *Changing Paradigms in the Management of Breast Cancer*, DOI 10.1007/978-3-319-60336-0_4

breast. The internal mammary, infraclavicular, and supraclavicular lymph nodes receive the remainder of the drainage.

The axillary nodes are divided into three levels described in relationship to the pectoralis minor muscle. Level I nodes are inferior and lateral, level II nodes are posterior, and level III nodes are medial to pectoralis minor. A complete axillary dissection involves removing level I and level II lymph nodes and any gross disease in level III.

SLN surgery for breast cancer was introduced in the early 1990s as an alternative to an axillary dissection for clinically node-negative patients for staging purposes. This concept utilizes the theory that the lymphatic drainage of the breast and any tumors that develop will first drain into one or a few lymph node(s) before spreading to the rest of the axilla. Thus, by locating and removing these lymph node(s), called the sentinel lymph node(s), the status of the axilla can be determined. In experienced surgeons, this procedure carries an overall SLN detection rate of 99% and has a false-negative rate (FNR) between 5 and 10% [6].

The technique for SLN surgery involves injecting a tracer or two tracers into the breast to identify the SLNs. Most commonly used tracers are radioactive mapping agents and a blue dye (lymphazurin or methylene blue or patent blue dye). Numerous studies have shown that using dual agents increases SLN detection rates and minimizes SLN false-negative rates. The location of tracer injection was an area of debate in the past. Many surgeons initially injected the tracers around the tumor, with nonpalpable lesions being more difficult. However, several studies have shown that injecting in the subareolar space is easier, can be applied to multifocal tumors as well as nonpalpable tumors, and carries similar identification and accuracy rates to peritumoral injections [7, 8].

Clinically Node-Negative Patients

All patients initially diagnosed with breast cancer should undergo a complete history and physical. The physical should include an examination of the breast and axilla as well as the regional sites for lymphatic drainage, including the neck, supraclavicular, and infraclavicular regions. Unfortunately, physical examination alone is poor at assessing the axillary nodes as small metastatic lymph nodes may not be palpable and palpable lymph nodes may be reactive and not metastatic. Axillary ultrasound provides an extension of physical examination and provides a more reliable way to assess the axillary lymph nodes [9]. For this reason, an axillary ultrasound should be obtained and if any suspicious nodes are seen sonographically, a fine needle aspiration (FNA) biopsy or core needle biopsy should be performed. If the ultrasound-guided percutaneous biopsy does not show any metastatic involvement, patients are considered clinically node negative (cN0).

In the clinically node-negative patient with invasive breast cancer where surgery is the initial treatment, SLN surgery should routinely be performed to stage the axilla. Multiple randomized trials have proven that this is a safe and reliable technique, with equivalent overall and disease-free survival rates to ALND, but associated with much less morbidity.

The National Surgical Adjuvant Breast and Bowel Project (NSABP) B-32 randomized 5611 patients across 80 institutions to SLN surgery plus ALND versus SLN surgery and completion ALND only in cases where any of the SLN(s) were positive [10]. The SLN identification rate was 97% overall with a false-negative rate of 9.7% in the SLN plus ALND group. B-32 did not show any differences in overall survival, disease-free survival, or recurrence rates between the two groups. This study validated the use of SLN surgery in clinically node-negative patients and led to SLN surgery replacing ALND as the standard procedure in staging the axilla in these patients.

When SLN surgery replaced ALND in clinically node-negative patients, sentinel nodes containing metastasis found at the time of surgery required an ALND. However, clinicians observed that in the majority of patients where a SLN was positive and an ALND was subsequently performed, there was no further disease in the additional axillary nodes resected in addition to the disease identified in the SLN. Clearing negative lymph nodes is not thought to provide oncologic benefit. This begged the question of whether patients with minimal axillary metastatic burden require ALND.

The American College of Surgeons Oncology Group (ACOSOG) Z0011 trial by Dr. Armando Giuliano and colleagues challenged the dogma that patients with a positive SLN require an ALND [11, 12]. This trial randomized 891 patients who had a clinically negative axilla and were undergoing breast-conserving surgery for T1 or T2 tumors, planning adjuvant whole-breast radiation and were found to have only one or two positive sentinel lymph nodes into two groups: ALND versus no ALND. The majority of the patients received systemic adjuvant therapy. At a median follow-up time of 6.3 years, there were no significant differences in overall survival (91.8% versus 92.5%), disease-free survival (82.2% versus 83.9%), or axillary recurrence rates (0.9% versus 0.5%). More recently presented data provided longer follow-up results with a median of 9.25 years, showed that these results held true with longer follow-up. Nodal recurrence rates remained low and not significantly different between the two groups, 1.5% in the SLN group and 0.5% in the ALND group ($p = 0.28$) [13]. The authors concluded that in patients with early stage breast cancer with one or two positive sentinel lymph nodes undergoing breast-conserving surgery, SLN surgery alone is not inferior to ALND. The trial was criticized as the pre-specified accrual was not met, the majority of the patients had favorable tumor characteristics, and a significant number of patients were lost to follow-up in each group. In addition, the radiation fields were not documented and the degree of tangential radiation field coverage of the axilla or definitive radiation to the axilla is not known for the entire trial cohort. Radiation fields from a subgroup of 228 patients have been reviewed and showed that 19% of patients also had regional nodal irradiation, and this was more common in patients at higher risk for additional nodal involvement but, however, was not different between the two study arms [14]. Despite the criticism, the immediate impact Z0011 had on the national stage was irrefutable as surgeons have now adopted these findings into clinical practice and avoid ALND for patients meeting the Z0011 criteria.

The International Breast Cancer Study Group (IBCSG) 23-01 randomized T1 or T2 breast cancer patients that were clinically node negative who underwent BCT or mastectomy and had micrometastases (defined as <2 mm) in the SLN to ALND versus no ALND [15]. There were 464 patients in the ALND arm and 467 patients in the no ALND arm. The authors found no statistical differences between the two groups in terms of 5-year overall survival (97.6% ALND versus 97.5% no ALND) and 5-year locoregional recurrence rates (2.4% ALND versus 2.8% no ALND). These findings corroborate the Z0011 findings, although 23-01 was limited to micrometastatic nodal disease. The proportion of mastectomy patients was too low to provide meaningful extrapolation to patients undergoing mastectomy.

Together, these recent trials have provided strong, randomized, multi-institutional data that SLN surgery alone in patients undergoing breast-conserving surgery found to have minimal disease burden in the axilla (micrometastases, one or two positive lymph nodes) is not inferior to a complete axillary dissection. Since ALND is associated with a greater morbidity and long-term complications compared to SLN, surgeons should omit ALND in patients with low-burden axillary disease undergoing breast-conserving therapy with adjuvant whole-breast radiation. However, an ALND should still be performed in patients who have three or more positive sentinel lymph nodes, or have fixed matted nodes, and in patients who are undergoing a mastectomy with any positive axillary lymph nodes.

The European trial EORTC 10981-22023 AMAROS (After Mapping of the Axilla, Radiotherapy or Surgery) was a multi-institutional trial randomizing patients with a positive SLN to ALND versus axillary radiotherapy [16]. There were 744 patients in the ALND group and 681 patients in the axillary radiotherapy group. In this trial, unlike in Z0011, mastectomy patients were allowed to participate. The authors found no statistical differences between the two groups in terms of 5-year overall survival (93.3% in the ALND group versus 92.5% in the radiation group) as well as 5-year disease-free survival (86.9% in the ALND group versus 82.7% in the radiation group), suggesting that radiation can be equivalent to ALND in early node-positive patients. However, many of these patients met Z0011 criteria and could potentially avoid both ALND and axillary radiation.

Clinically Node-Positive Patients

Axillary ultrasound at the time of diagnosis on all patients with invasive breast cancer helps provide preoperative staging information. Patients with suspicious-appearing lymph nodes on imaging, and FNA biopsy or core biopsy of an axillary lymph node proves metastatic disease are considered to be clinically node positive and this is designated with an (f) suffix [e.g., cN1(f)]. Placement of a clip in the node should be considered for cases where the biopsy shows metastatic involvement.

Historically, many patients who were operable candidates proceeded directly to surgery, while patients who were inoperable received neoadjuvant chemotherapy. In the modern era, there has been significantly greater use of neoadjuvant chemotherapy even in the setting of operable disease. While there is no evidence for a survival benefit with the use of neoadjuvant chemotherapy, this practice often allows for a reduction in the primary tumor burden in the breast and the extent of disease in the axilla as well as allowing assessment of tumor response. Patients who are not candidates for breast-conserving surgery often become candidates after neoadjuvant chemotherapy and patients are less likely to require ALND after neoadjuvant chemotherapy than if they undergo primary surgery.

The accuracy and false-negative rates of SLN surgery performed after neoadjuvant chemotherapy are similar to when SLN is performed upfront in clinically node-negative patients. The advantages of performing SLN surgery after neoadjuvant chemotherapy are as follows: (1) it allows the breast and axillary surgery to be performed at one operation rather than two separate operations, (2) less patients overall are node positive so fewer axillary dissections are needed, and most importantly (3) it allows assessment of response to therapy. If the SLNs are removed prior to chemotherapy, assessment of axillary response to chemotherapy cannot be performed.

For patients with clinically node-positive disease, historically ALND has been recommended after neoadjuvant chemotherapy. However, improvements in chemotherapy and targeted therapy have resulted in rates of nodal response to neoadjuvant chemotherapy as high as 40–75% [17–19]. Therefore, much recent interest has focused on the accuracy and feasibility of staging axillary response with SLN surgery following treatment, and reserving ALND for patients with residual nodal involvement rather than committing all patients to an ALND. Early studies demonstrated a higher than acceptable FNR of SLN surgery in this setting. In the last decade, several large, multi-institutional trials have been completed focusing specifically on assessing the accuracy of SLN surgery in node-positive patients treated with neoadjuvant chemotherapy.

The ACOSOG Z1071 trial enrolled 756 patients who had biopsy-proven, node-positive disease in the axilla and were treated with neoadjuvant chemotherapy [20]. After neoadjuvant chemotherapy, each patient had their primary breast surgery and underwent SLN surgery and completion axillary dissection (regardless of the SLN result). The primary endpoint for the trial was to determine the false-negative rate of SLN surgery with resection of at least two SLNs. The predetermined threshold for the study was a FNR of less than 10%. The overall FNR in the study was 12.6%. Subset analysis showed that the FNR was significantly lower at 10.8% when dual tracers were used for SLN identification. Additionally, the FNR was lower when more sentinel nodes were removed, with a FNR of 9.1% with three or more SLNs. In addition, in patients where the lymph node that was originally biopsied and proven to be positive and had a clip placed, the FNR was 6.8% in cases where the clipped node was removed as part of the SLN surgery.

The SENTINA trial was undertaken at 103 institutions in Germany and Austria to study the optimal timing of SLN surgery in patients being treated with neoadjuvant therapy [21]. The trial had four study arms one of which (arm C) had 592 clinically node-positive patients treated with neoadjuvant chemotherapy that converted to a clinically and ultrasound node-negative axilla and underwent SLN surgery and ALND. The FNR of SLN in patients in arm C was 14.2%. The authors also showed a lower FNR with the use of dual-agent tracers versus one agent (8.6% versus 16.0%) as well as a lower FNR when more sentinel nodes were removed (24.3% with one node, 18.5% with two nodes, and 4.9% with three or more nodes).

The Canadian trial SN FNAC study analyzed 153 biopsy-proven, node-positive patients who received neoadjuvant chemotherapy and then subsequently had SLN surgery and ALND to determine the FNR [22]. They included patients with isolated tumor cells (ITCs) identified on immunohistochemistry in the SLN as node positive. With this definition, the FNR was 8.4%. If the cases with ITCs were counted as negative nodes, the FNR was 13.4%. They also showed that removing more SLNs was associated with a lower FNR (18.2% with one SLN versus 4.9% with two or more SLNs).

Interest has grown regarding the ability to identify and resect the biopsy-proven, positive node as part of the surgical staging procedure after chemotherapy. The Z1071 subgroup data showed a lower FNR when the biopsy-proven node was clipped and the clipped node was resected at SLN surgery. A group in the Netherlands reported on a technique called the MARI procedure (Marking Axillary Lymph Node with Radioactive Seeds) in 100 patients [23]. At diagnosis, a radioactive seed was placed in the positive node and after completion of chemotherapy, the seed localized node was resected. They reported a FNR of 7% with MARI, in the absence of SLN surgery. The MD Anderson group has reported on targeted axillary dissection (TAD): they place a clip in the biopsy-proven lymph node at diagnosis and then subsequently after chemotherapy localize the clipped node with a radioactive seed [24]. They combine SLN surgery with removal of the radioactive seed localized node. The FNR using TAD in their study was 2%. Some institutions have already adopted this technique as standard protocol for node-positive patients who have a clinically negative axilla after neoadjuvant chemotherapy.

These prospective, multi-institutional trials have paved the way to allow patients with node-positive breast cancer who have a great response to neoadjuvant chemotherapy to potentially avoid ALND. SLN surgery in these patients allows assessment of the nodal status of the axilla after chemotherapy. Several techniques can help minimize the false-negative rate in this setting including: use of dual tracer, resection of two or more SLNs, evaluation of the SLNs for treatment effect or biopsy changes and consideration of clip placement in the node at diagnosis with resection of the clipped node at surgery.

Role of Radiation

The management of breast cancer requires a multidisciplinary approach. The benefits of radiation to the breast in all patients treated with breast-conserving surgery and to the chest wall in selected patients treated with mastectomy have been proven in terms of recurrence and overall survival. The benefit of radiation to the axilla and regional nodal basins is more complex. Adding radiation therapy to the axilla increases morbidity, specifically lymphedema. The complexity in management increases even further as the multidisciplinary team considers axillary dissection versus axillary radiation versus using both axillary dissection and radiation.

Post-mastectomy patients with four or more metastatic axillary lymph nodes (pN2 disease) have a significantly higher risk of locoregional recurrence. These patients benefit from chest wall radiation with regional nodal irradiation (RNI), which includes the axilla, as well as the supraclavicular, infraclavicular, and internal mammary nodes [25–27]. Post-mastectomy radiation therapy (PMRT) is currently the standard of care in this setting and provides a significant reduction in locoregional recurrence and increase in breast-cancer specific survival and overall survival [28–30]. For patients treated with a mastectomy who have one to three positive nodes, earlier studies showed a significant decrease in local and regional recurrence and better survival for patients who received PMRT [31, 32]. More recent studies utilizing modern chemotherapy regimen showed that for post-mastectomy patients with one to three positive nodes, locoregional recurrence was in the range of 4–5% without additional radiotherapy [33, 34]. Current NCCN Guidelines recommend strong consideration of PMRT in post-mastectomy patients with one to three positive nodes.

For patients undergoing breast-conserving therapy, whole-breast irradiation (WBI) is standard treatment. In pathologically node-negative patients, specific nodal radiotherapy is unnecessary. However, it is estimated that the tangential fields in whole-breast radiation can cover up to 80% of level I and level II axillary lymph nodes. In pN2 patients, regional nodal irradiation (RNI) is indicated in addition to WBI. Controversy exists in patients with one to three positive lymph nodes undergoing breast-conserving therapy as the benefit of adding RNI to WBI is less clear. The recent NCIC-CTG MA.20 trial was undertaken to evaluate the role of RNI in these patients [35]. In this trial, 1832 women with node-positive or high-risk, node-negative breast cancer treated with lumpectomy and adjuvant systemic therapy were randomized to two arms: WBI versus WBI plus RNI. Eighty-five percent of the patients in this study had one to three positive nodes and 96% of patients had an ALND. At a median follow-up time of 9.5 years, there was no difference in survival (81.8% in the WBI group versus 82.8% in the WBI plus RNI group). However, there was a significant difference in disease-free survival (77.0% in the WBI group versus 82.0% in the WBI plus RNI group) and isolated locoregional disease-free survival (92.2% in the WBI group versus 95.2% in the WBI plus RNI group). The authors concluded that the addition of RNI to WBI in this select population did not alter overall survival but did reduce breast-cancer recurrences.

However, the MA.20 results and ACOSOG Z0011 results conflict, as the Z0011 study demonstrated that patients with one or two positive SLN(s) treated with lumpectomy and whole-breast radiation without regional nodal radiation do not require axillary dissection. Therefore, since there has been no clear overall survival advantage for the addition of RNI, the role of RNI for patients with one to three positive nodes treated with breast-conserving surgery remains a controversial topic. Current NCCN Guidelines recommend strongly considering RNI for these patients.

The benefit of radiation in node-positive patients that convert to pathologically node-negative with neoadjuvant chemotherapy becomes the next question to study. Two trials are currently accruing patients to address management of the axilla in node-positive patients treated with neoadjuvant chemotherapy. The NASBP B-51 trial is currently enrolling patients who have node-positive disease, treated with neoadjuvant chemotherapy, and have no evidence of residual nodal disease at the time of surgery (by SLN surgery or ALND) [36]. Patients in the trial are randomized to axillary radiation versus no axillary radiation. The Alliance trial A11202 is currently enrolling patients who present with node-positive disease, treated with neoadjuvant chemotherapy, and have residual node-positive disease by SLN surgery [37]. They are randomized to undergo ALND versus axillary radiation. End points in both trials are survival and recurrence. The results of these trials should elucidate a clearer picture for the optimal management of the axilla for node-positive patients undergoing neoadjuvant chemotherapy.

Ductal Carcinoma in Situ

Ductal carcinoma in situ (DCIS) is by definition noninvasive disease. There is theoretically no potential for metastatic spread. In patients with DCIS treated with breast conservation, routine nodal staging is not indicated. However, previous studies have documented an upstage rate from DCIS on core needle biopsy to invasive cancer at surgical resection of 15%. Cases where there is comedo necrosis, a large palpable mass, or DCIS involving more than 4 cm have a greater chance of finding invasive disease. In patients undergoing breast-conserving surgery that have a high risk for invasive disease, it is reasonable to consider SLN surgery at time of lumpectomy to avoid the need for a second operation. Additionally, in patients undergoing a mastectomy for DCIS, disruption of the lymphatic drainage of the breast occurs with the removal of the breast and the accuracy of SLN surgery after a mastectomy is unknown. Therefore, in patients undergoing a mastectomy for DCIS, SLN surgery is recommended [38].

Special Considerations

Inflammatory breast cancer (IBC) is an aggressive form of breast cancer, classically characterized by diffuse erythema and skin edema known as *peau d'orange*. Treatment consists of neoadjuvant chemotherapy, followed by a modified radical mastectomy, and post-mastectomy radiation. There are no prospective or large cohort studies to evaluate the accuracy or safety of performing SLN surgery in these patients. Since the rates of involved lymph nodes are high and the false-negative rate of SLN was high in the limited available studies, axillary dissection is recommended [39].

Breast cancer occurring in pregnant patients, or pregnancy associated breast cancer, is always a challenging clinical scenario. Some authors have advocated that ALND be the standard approach in all patients as previous studies showed that axillary lymph nodes are frequently positive and the safety or efficacy of radiolabeled tracers are uncertain. Blue dye should never be used in pregnant patients as it is a category C substance with significant teratogenic effects. However, the absorbed radiation dose with standard technetium 99m to the fetus are mostly below 20 μGy for 10–20 MBq (typical doses for a SLN injection) as assessed by experimental models, and falls well below the safety threshold for the developmental defects [40]. Therefore, clinically node-negative pregnant patients can undergo axillary staging with SLN surgery using morning of surgery, low-dose injection of radiolabeled tracer.

Patients with recurrent breast cancer who have had prior axillary nodal staging may have aberrant non-axillary drainage patterns due to the disruption of the original drainage pathways. Preoperative lymphoscintigraphy is helpful in these patients. Although repeat SLN surgery has been reported as feasible and accurate, this topic has not been well-studied [41–43]. In a meta-analysis reviewing 692 patients with recurrent breast cancer (301 after previous SLN surgery and 361 after previous ALND and 30 with no previous axillary surgery), a sentinel lymph node was identified in 452 of the 692 patients (65.3%). SLN identification rate was significantly higher in patients who had undergone previous SLN surgery compared to a previous ALND (81.0 versus 52.2%, $p < 0.0001$) [44]. In patients with successful lymphatic mapping, aberrant drainage pathways were visualized in 175 of 405 patients (43.2%), and this was more frequent after previous ALND than after previous SLN surgery (69.2 versus 17.4%, $p < 0.0001$). Thus for patients with recurrent breast cancer, SLN surgery can be attempted and lymphoscintigraphy to map the drainage should be performed. In cases where SLN fails to map, ALND should be considered for axillary staging.

Future Directions

The management of the axilla in breast cancer patients has advanced over the last decade allowing a less invasive surgical approach for many patients. The Z0011 study findings have been widely implemented into practice resulting in less ALNDs for women with clinically node-negative disease who are found to be sentinel node positive at time of breast-conserving surgery. More recent studies have led to the introduction of SLN surgery after neoadjuvant chemotherapy for node-positive disease.

The question arises whether in the future axillary surgery will be required for axillary staging. The SOUND trial in Italy is enrolling patients in an ongoing prospective randomized study comparing SLN surgery versus no axillary surgical staging in patients with small early stage breast cancer with a negative preoperative axillary ultrasound [45]. This study is questioning the benefit of SLN surgery in patients with early breast cancer. In addition, the group at MD Anderson is enrolling patients in a trial comparing FNA histology from a percutaneous biopsy to standard surgical evaluation of the lymph node after neoadjuvant chemotherapy in node-positive patients. The results of these and other similar trials might change the paradigm of surgical evaluation of the axilla in the near future.

Conclusion

We have moved from a historical approach of performing an axillary dissection for all patients diagnosed with breast cancer to a contemporary approach of sentinel lymph node surgery for most patients with clinically node-negative breast cancer and to omitting axillary dissection in selected node-positive patients. We could possibly be avoiding any axillary surgery at all in the future. The trend is moving toward less aggressive surgery in the axilla and individualizing the surgical approach to the axilla based on breast surgical procedure, extent of nodal disease, tumor biology, and response to therapy. Multidisciplinary team input is important and the impact of systemic and radiation plans should be considered together with the surgical approach to the axilla.

References

1. Carter CL, Allen C, Henson DE. Relation of tumor size, lymph node status, and survival in 24,740 breast cancer cases. Cancer. 1989 Jan 1;63(1):181–7.
2. Beenken SW, Urist MM, Zhang Y, Desmond R, Krontiras H., Medina H, et al. Axillary lymph node status, but not tumor size, predicts locoregional recurrence and overall survival after mastectomy for breast cancer. Ann Surg. 2003 May;237(5):732–8; discussion 738–9.
3. Giuliano AE, Kirgan DM, Guenther JM, Morton DL. Lymphatic mapping and sentinel lymphadenectomy for breast cancer. Ann Surg. 1994 Sep;220(3):391–8; discussion 398–401.
4. Giuliano AE, Jones RC, Brennan M, Statman R. Sentinel lymphadenectomy in breast cancer. J Clin Oncol. 1997 Jun;15(6):2345–50.
5. Sappey MPC. Anatomie, Physiologie, Pathologie des vaisseaux Lymphatiques consideres chez L'homme at les Vertebres. Paris: A. Delahaye and E. Lecrosnier; 1874.
6. Krag DN, Anderson SJ, Julian TB, Brown AM, Harlow SP, Ashikaga R, et al. Technical outcomes of sentinel-lymph-node resection and conventional axillary-lymphnode dissection in patients with clinically node-negative breast cancer: results from the NSABP B-32 randomised phase III trial. Lancet Oncol. 2007 Oct;8(10):881–8.
7. Klimberg VS, Rubio IT, Henry R, Cowan C, Colvert M, Korourian S. Subareolar versus peritumoral injection for location of the sentinel node. Ann Surg. 1999 Jun;229(6):860-4; discussion 864-5.
8. Kern KA. Sentinel lymph node mapping in breast cancer using subareolar injection of blue dye. J Am Coll Surg. 1999 Dec;189(6):539–45.
9. Al-Hilli Z, Hieken TJ, Boughey JC. Axillary ultrasound in the management of the newly diagnosed breast cancer patient. Breast J. 2015 Nov-Dec;21(6):634–41.
10. Krag DN, Anderson SJ, Julian TB, Brown AM, Harlow SP, Costantino JP, et al. Sentinel-lymph node resection compared with conventional axillary-lymph-node dissection in clinically node-negative patients with breast cancer: overall survival findings from the NSABP B-32 randomised phase 3 trial. Lancet Oncol. 2010 Oct;11(10):927–33.
11. Giuliano AE, McCall L, Beitsch P, Whitworth PW, Blumencranz P, Leitch AM, et al. Locoregional recurrence after sentinel lymph node dissection with or without axillary dissection in patients with sentinel lymph node metastases: the American College of Surgeons Oncology Group Z0011 randomized trial. Ann Surg. 2010 Sep;252(3):426–32; discussion 432–3.
12. Giuliano AE, Hunt KK, Ballman KV, Beitsch PD, Whitworth PW, Blumencranz PW, et al. Axillary dissection vs no axillary dissection in women with invasive breast cancer and sentinel node metastasis: a randomized clinical trial. JAMA. 2011 Feb 9;305(6):569–75.
13. Giuliano AE, Ballman K, McCall L, Beitsch P, Whitworth PW, Blumencranz P, et al. Locoregional recurrence after sentinel lymph node dissection with or without axillary dissection in patients with sentinel lymph node metastases: long-term follow-up from the American College of Surgeons Oncology Group (Alliance) ACOSOG Z0011 randomized trial. Ann Surg. 2016 Sep;264(3):413–20.
14. Jagsi R, Chadha M, Moni J, Ballman K, Laurie F, Buchholz TA, et al. Radiation field design in the ACOSOG Z0011 (Alliance) trial. J Clin Oncol. 2014 Nov 10;32(32):3600–6.
15. Galimberti V, Cole BF, Zurrida S, Viale G, Luini A, Veronesi P, et al. Axillary dissection versus no axillary dissection in patients with sentinel-node micrometastases (IBCSG 23-01): a phase 3 randomised controlled trial. Lancet Oncol. 2013 Apr;14(4):297–305.

16. Donker M, van Tienhoven G, Straver ME, Meijnen P, van de Velde CJ, Mansel RE, et al. Radiotherapy or surgery of the axilla after a positive sentinel node in breast cancer (EORTC 10981-22023 AMAROS): a randomised, multicentre, open-label, phase 3 non-inferiority trial. Lancet Oncol. 2014 Nov;15(12):1303–10.
17. Dominici L, Negron Gonzalez V, Buzdar A, Lucci A, Mittendorf EA, Le-Petross HT, et al. Cytologically proven axillary lymph node metastases are eradicated in patients receiving preoperative chemotherapy with concurrent trastuzumab for HER2-positive breast cancer. Cancer. 2010 Jun 15;116(12):2884–9.
18. Fisher B, Brown A, Mamounas E, Wieand S, Robidoux A, Margolese RG, et al. Effect of preoperative chemotherapy on local-regional disease in women with operable breast cancer: findings from National Surgical Adjuvant Breast and Bowel Project B-18. J Clin Oncol. 1997 Jul;15(7):2483-93.
19. Kuerer H, Sahin A, Hunt K, Newman LA, Breslin TM, Ames FC, et al. Incidence and impact of documented eradication of breast cancer axillary lymph node metastases before surgery in patients treated with neoadjuvant chemotherapy. Ann Surg. 1999 Jul;230(1):72–8.
20. Boughey JC, Suman VJ, Mittendorf EA, Ahrendt GM, Wilke LG, Taback B, et al. Sentinel lymph node surgery after neoadjuvant chemotherapy in patients with node-positive breast cancer: the ACOSOG Z1071 (Alliance) clinical trial. JAMA. 2013 Oct 9;310(14):1455–61.
21. Kuehn T, Bauerfeind I, Fehm T, Fleige B, Hausschild M, Helms G, et al. Sentinel-lymph-node biopsy in patients with breast cancer before and after neoadjuvant chemotherapy (SENTINA): a prospective, multicentre cohort study. Lancet Oncol. 2013 Jun;14(7):609–18.
22. Boileau JF, Poirier B, Basik M, Holloway CM, Gaboury L, Sideris L, et al. Sentinel node biopsy after neoadjuvant chemotherapy in biopsy-proven node-positive breast cancer: the SN FNAC study. J Clin Oncol. 2015 Jan;33(3):258–64.
23. Donker M, Straver ME, Wesseling J, Loo CE, Schot M, Drukker CA, et al. Marking axillary lymph nodes with radioactive iodine seeds for axillary staging after neoadjuvant systemic treatment in breast cancer patients: the MARI procedure. Ann Surg. 2015 Feb;261(2):378–82.
24. Caudle AS, Yang WT, Krishnamurthy S, Mittendorf EA, Black DM, Gilcrease MZ, et al. Improved axillary evaluation following neoadjuvant therapy for patients with node-positive breast cancer using selective evaluation of clipped nodes: implementation of targeted axillary dissection. J Clin Oncol. 2016 Apr 1;34(10):1072–8.
25. Clarke M, Collins R, Darby S, Davies C, Elphinstone P, Evans V, et al. Effects of radiotherapy and of differences in the extent of surgery for early breast cancer on local recurrence and 15-year survival: an overview of the randomised trials. Lancet. 2005 Dec 17;366(9503):2087–106.
26. Danish Breast Cancer Cooperative Group, Nielsen HM, Overgaard M, Grau C, Jensen AR, Overgaard J. Study of failure pattern among high-risk breast cancer patients with or without postmastectomy radiotherapy in addition to adjuvant systemic therapy: long-term results from the Danish Breast Cancer Cooperative Group DBCG 82 b and c randomized studies. J Clin Oncol. 2006 May 20;24(15):2268–75.
27. Ragaz J, Olivotto IA, Spinelli JJ, Phillips N, Jackson SM, Wilson KS, et al. Locoregional radiation therapy in patients with high-risk breast cancer receiving adjuvant chemotherapy: 20-year results of the British Columbia randomized trial. J Natl Cancer Inst. 2005 Jan 19;97(2):116–26.
28. Truong PT, Olivotto IA, Whelan TJ, Levine M, Steering Committee on Clinical Practice Guidelines for the Care and Treatment of Breast Cancer. Clinical practice guidelines for the care and treatment of breast cancer: 16. Locoregional post-mastectomy radiotherapy. CMAJ. 2004 Apr 13;170(18):1263–73.
29. Eifel P, Axelson JA, Costa J, Crowley J, Curran WJ Jr, Deshler A, et al. National Institutes of Health consensus development conference statement: adjuvant therapy for breast cancer, November 1–3, 2000. J Natl Cancer Inst. 2001 Jul 4;93(13):979–89.
30. Recht A, Edge SB, Solin LJ, Robinson DS, Estabrook A, Fine RE, et al. Postmastectomy radiotherapy: clinical practice guidelines of the American Society of Clinical Oncology. J Clin Oncol. 2001 March 1;19(5):1539–69.

31. Overgaard M, Nielsen HM, Overgaard J. Is the benefit of postmastectomy irradiation limited to patients with four or more positive nodes, as recommended in international consensus reports? A subgroup analysis of the DBCG 82 b&c randomized trials. Radiother Oncol. 2007 Mar;82(3):247–53.
32. Ragaz J, Jackson SM, Le N, Plenderleith IH, Spinelli JJ, Basco VE, et al. Adjuvant radiotherapy and chemotherapy in node-positive premenopausal women with breast cancer. N Engl J Med. 1997 Oct 2;337(14):956–62.
33. Moo TA, McMillan R, Lee M, Stempel M, Patil S, Ho A, et al. Selection criteria for postmastectomy radiotherapy in t1–t2 tumors with 1 to 3 positive lymph nodes. Ann Surg Oncol. 2013 Oct;20(10):3169–74.
34. McBride A, Allen P, Woodward W, Kim M, Kuerer HM, Drinka EK, et al. Locoregional recurrence risk for patients with T1,2 breast cancer with 1–3 positive lymph nodes treated with mastectomy and systemic treatment. Int J Radiat Oncol Biol Phys. 2014 Jun 1;89(2):392–8.
35. Whelan TJ, Olivotto IA, Parulekar WR, Ackerman I, Chua BH, Nabid A, et al. Regional nodal irradiation in early-stage breast cancer. N Engl J Med. 2015 Jul 23;373(4):307–16.
36. A randomized phase III clinical trial evaluation post-mastectomy chest wall and regional nodal XRT and post-lumpectomy regional nodal XRT in patients with positive axillary nodes before neoadjuvant chemotherapy who convert to pathologically negative axillary nodes after neoadjuvant chemotherapy. NSABP-51/RTOG 1304 Trial, NCT01872975 n.d.
37. Comparison of axillary lymph node dissection with axillary radiation for patients with node-positive breast cancer treated with chemotherapy. Alliance A11202 Trial, NCT01872975 n.d.
38. National Comprehensive Cancer Network (NCCN) guidelines version 2.2016. Ductal carcinoma in situ (DCIS). Available at: https://www.nccn.org/professionals/physician_gls/pdf/breast.pdf. Accessed 11 Sept 2016. n.d.
39. Kaufmann M, Morrow M, von Minckwitz G, Harris JR, Biedenkopf Expert Panel Members. Locoregional treatment of primary breast cancer: consensus recommendations from an International Expert Panel. Cancer. 2010 Mar 1;116(5):1184–91.
40. Pandit-Taskar N, Dauer LT, Montgomery L, St. Germain J, Zanzonico PB, Divgi CR. Organ and fetal absorbed dose estimates from 99mTc-sulfur colloid lymphoscintigraphy and sentinel node localization in breast cancer patients. J Nucl Med. 2006 Jul;47(7):1202–8.
41. Intra M, Trifirò G, Viale G, Rotmensz N, Gentilini OD, Soteldo J. Second biopsy of axillary sentinel lymph node for reappearing breast cancer after previous sentinel lymph node biopsy. Ann Surg Oncol. 2005 Nov;12(11):895–9.
42. Taback B, Nguyen P, Hansen N, Edwards GK, Conway K, Giuliano AE. Sentinel lymph node biopsy for local recurrence of breast cancer after breast-conserving therapy. Ann Surg Oncol. 2006 Aug;13(8):1099–104.
43. Newman EA, Cimmino VM, Sabel MS, Diehl KM, Frey KA, Change AE, et al. Lymphatic mapping and sentinel lymph node biopsy for patients with local recurrence after breast-conservation therapy. Ann Surg Oncol. 2006 Jan;13(1):52–7.
44. Maaskant-Braat AJ, Voogd AC, Roumen RM, Nieuwenhuijzen GA. Repeat sentinel node biopsy in patients with locally recurrent breast cancer: a systematic review and meta-analysis of the literature. Breast Cancer Res Treat. 2013 Feb;138(1):13–20.
45. A randomized trial comparing sentinel lymph node biopsy vs. no axillary surgical staging in patients with small breast cancer and a negative preoperative axillary assessment (IEO S637/311), NCT02167490. n.d.

Margins and Breast Cancer

5

Anees B. Chagpar

Introduction

A fundamental tenet of breast surgical oncology is the need to achieve clear margins as positive margins are associated with a higher local recurrence rate. The definition of what constitutes a clear margin has morphed over time, but recent consensus statements have shed some light on this controversy. Currently, there is a frenzy of activity to elucidate techniques and develop technologies that may aid surgeons in their quest to achieve negative margins at the initial procedure, so as to reduce re-excision rates. At the same time, however, the liberal use of systemic and radiation therapy may lead some to question how vociferously surgeons go after clear margins.

Definition of a Positive Margin

Invasive Cancer

For quite some time there has been debate over what constitutes an unacceptable margin for patients with invasive carcinoma. While the NSABP B-06 trial had defined a positive margin as "tumor at ink", [1] there has historically been significant variability in what surgeons consider a negative margin [2]. A recent meta-analysis demonstrated that while positive margin status, defined as tumor at the resection margin, was associated with a roughly twofold higher rate of local recurrence rate; margin distance, however, was not a significant factor [3]. Hence, a Society of Surgical Oncology (SSO)-American Society for Radiation Oncology

A.B. Chagpar, MD, MSc, MA, MPH, MBA (✉)
Department of Surgery, Yale University School of Medicine, 20 York Street, North Pavilion, First Floor, New Haven, CT 06510, USA
e-mail: anees.chagpar@yale.edu

M. Howard-McNatt (ed.), *Changing Paradigms in the Management of Breast Cancer*, DOI 10.1007/978-3-319-60336-0_5

(ASTRO) consensus panel reached the conclusion that a positive tumor should be defined as tumor at ink, with larger margin widths not conferring a significant improvement in local recurrence rates.

Ductal Carcinoma in Situ (DCIS)

Patients who present with pure DCIS, especially with an extensive intraductal component, are more at risk of having positive margins [4–6]. Given that DCIS can be discontinuous, some have advocated larger margins for these patients. Margin width is a factor that is part of the Van Nuys Prognostic Index, and patients who have margins >1 cm have been found to have a lower local recurrence rate at 10 years than those with margins 1–9 mm and those with margins <1 mm (72.1% vs. 85.0% vs. 94.5%, $p < 0.01$) [7]. The 2016 National Comprehensive Cancer Network (NCCN) guidelines echoed these data stating that "margins greater than 10 mm are widely accepted as negative (but may be excessive and may lead to a less optimal cosmetic outcome). Margins less than 1 mm are considered inadequate. With pathologic margins between 1 and 10 mm, wider margins are generally associated with lower local recurrence rates." [8] Most recently, an SSO-ASTRO-American Society of Clinical Oncology (ASCO) consensus evaluated data, including a meta-analysis, and reached the conclusion that achieving margins of 2 mm in patients with DCIS who will be undergoing whole breast radiation therapy reduces ipsilateral breast tumor recurrences more than narrower margins, but that wider margins did not significantly improve outcomes [9]. However, for patients with <2 mm margins (but with no tumor at ink), the consensus panel urged the use of clinical judgment in determining the need for re-excision.

Techniques to Improve Margin Clearance

While there has been considerable controversy regarding what constitutes a negative margin, it is clear that attainment of a negative margin at the initial definitive surgical procedure is optimal, as neither patients nor surgeons rejoice in having to return to the operating room for a re-excision to obtain clear margins. Despite their best efforts, most surgeons report a 20–40% rate of positive margins at the time of the initial surgery, [10, 11] although this rate may have reduced slightly due to a change in definition of what constitutes a negative margin [12]. There have been a number of techniques, both preoperatively and intraoperatively, that have been investigated to improve surgeons' ability to achieve clear margins at the initial surgical procedure.

Preoperative Imaging

Surgeons often obtain preoperative imaging to aid their surgical planning, and some have suggested that use of sensitive imaging techniques, such as Magnetic Resonance Imaging (MRI) may reduce the likelihood of having a positive margin at

Table 5.1 Preoperative MRI and positive margin rates

	Intervention		Positive margin rate		Re-excision rate	
Study	Arm	*n*	%	*p*-value	%	*p*-value
Comice	MRI	816	13%[a]	n/s	16%	0.77
	No MRI	807	15%[a]		19%	
Monet	MRI	74	n/s	n/s	45%[b]	0.069
	No MRI	75	n/s		28%[b]	
	SOC	116	34%		21%	

SOC standard of care, *n/s* not specified
[a]Positive margins stated are for invasive disease only
[b]Re-excision rate stated are for re-excision (breast conserving surgery) and conversion to mastectomy after initial surgery

the conclusion of the initial surgical procedure. To date, there have been two randomized controlled trials which have evaluated this hypothesis, neither of which found an improvement in positive margin rates with the use of MRI (Table 5.1). The COMICE trial [13] found no difference between the two arms, the MONET trial [14] paradoxically demonstrated an increase in positive margins associated with the use of preoperative MRI. An ongoing American College of Surgeons Oncology Group (ACOSOG)/American College of Radiology Imaging Network trial seeks to further evaluate the impact of MRI on surgical outcomes.

Some have argued that perhaps MRI is better for helping surgeons achieve negative margins in patients with DCIS, as these patients may be more likely to have positive margins. A meta-analysis which evaluated the use of MRI in patients with DCIS, however, concluded that MRI did not significantly affect margin status nor re-excision rates in these patients [15].

Localization Techniques for Non-palpable Tumors

With the widespread adoption of screening mammography, many of the malignancies we identify are not palpable. Indeed, even for those that present with palpable tumors, the use of neoadjuvant chemotherapy often renders these non-palpable. Hence, there has been increasing focus on whether different techniques for localization for these tumors may affect our ability to achieve negative margins at the initial surgical procedure. A recent Cochrane analysis found that there is no significant difference between wire localization, radio-occult lesion localization (ROLL) or radioactive seed localization (RSL) in terms of margin positivity and re-excision rates [16]. Several studies comparing these techniques and their impact on positive margin and re-excision rates are shown in Table 5.2.

The use of intraoperative ultrasound has also been evaluated as a means of localizing non-palpable tumors. A recent meta-analysis found that use of intraoperative ultrasound was significantly associated with a lower positive margin rate (OR from eight prospective studies: 1.63; 95% CI: 1.10–2.42, $p = 0.010$). This effect seems to be more pronounced in non-palpable tumors (OR: 1.47; 95% CI: 0.98–2.22,

Table 5.2 Type of localization for non-palpable lesions

Study	Intervention		Positive margin rate		Re-excision rate	
	Arm	*n*	%	*p*-value	%	*p*-value
Postma et al. [29]	ROLL	162	14%	0.644	12%	0.587
	WGL	152	12%		10%	
Duarte et al. [30]	ROLL	64	59%	n/s	25%	n/s
	WGL	65	60%		19%	
Gray et al. [31]	RSL	51	–	–	26%	0.02
	WGL	46	–		57%	
Rarick et al. [32]	RSL	44	23%	0.69	–	–
	WGL	62	24%		–	
Bloomquist et al. [33]	RSL	72	19.4%	0.53	–	–
	WGL	59	15.3%		–	
Sharek et al. [34]	RSL	114	–	–	21.1%	0.360
	WGL	118	–		26.3%	
Murphy et al. [35]	RSL	431	7.7%	0.38	23.0%	0.83
	WGL	256	5.5%		22.3%	
Hughes et al. [36]	RSL	383	27%	<0.001	8%	<0.001
	WGL	99	46%		25%	
Van der Noorda et al. [37]	RSL	128	19.5%	0.942	9.4%	0.801
	ROLL	275	18.5%		10.2%	
Donker et al. [38]	RSL	83	13%	n/s	8%	0.778
	ROLL	71	13%		7%	

ROLL radio-occult lesion localization, *RSL* radioactive seed localization, *WGL* wire-guided localization, *n/s* not specified

$p = 0.030$) than in palpable ones (OR: 2.36; 95% CI: 1.26–4.43, $p = 0.361$) [17]. Data from several other studies comparing ultrasound to either palpation or wire-guided localization are shown in Table 5.3.

Intraoperative Specimen Imaging

Several authors have suggested that intraoperative specimen radiography may help surgeons to identify close margins, such that additional tissue can be taken in the particular area that appears to be close. However, the absolute benefit is modest. For example, in their study of 174 patients who underwent breast conserving surgery with intraoperative specimen radiography, Hisada et al. found that 24 underwent intraoperative excision of a perceived close margin [18]. Of these, 5 (20.8%) were found to have histologically positive margins even after the intraoperative margin excision. Of the 150 patients who did not undergo intraoperative margin excision, 20 (20.0%) similarly had histologically positive margins at the conclusion of the operative procedure. McCormick et al. found that specimen radiography spared 6 of 93 patients an additional surgery to clear margins [19]. In the SHAVE trial, which

Table 5.3 Intraoperative ultrasound

	Intervention		Positive margin rate		Re-excision rate	
Study	Arm	*n*	%	*p*-value	%	*p*-value
Rahusen et al. [39]	US	26	11%	0.007	–	–
	WGL	23	45%		–	
Eggemann et al. [40]	US	90	12.2%	1.000	10.0%	0.798
	WGL	68	13.2%		11.8%	
James et al. [41]	US	96	10.4%	>0.05	20.8%	0.184
	WGL	59	11.9%		30.5%	
Moore et al. [42]	US	27	3.5%	<0.05	–	–
	SOC	24	29%		–	
COBALT [43]	US	65	3%	0.0093	2%	n/s
	Palpation	69	17%		11%	
Karanlik et al. [44]	US	84	17%	0.03	–	–
	Palpation	80	6%		–	
Fisher et al. [45]	US	73	–	–	23%	> 0.05
	Palpation	124	–		25%	
Davis et al. [46]	US	22	9%	0.01	9%	0.04
	Palpation	44	41%		34%	

US intraoperative ultrasound, *WGL* wire guided lumpectomy, *SOC* standard of care (i.e., no ultrasound, but otherwise localization technique not specified), *n/s*, not stated

allowed surgeons to take selective margins prior to randomization on the basis of intraoperative specimen radiography, patients who had selective margins taken were no less likely to have positive margins prior to randomization than those who did not (38% vs. 34%, $p = 0.53$) [6].

Some have argued that these results may be related to the concept that specimen radiography is two-dimensional. In a study in which orthogonal views were obtained of specimen radiographs, we found that initial margin positivity was reduced from 37.8 to 30.0% with the addition of standard specimen radiography and intraoperative re-excision; this was only reduced by another 1.1% by adding orthogonal views [20]. Still, some have lauded novel technology (like micro-CT scanners) to reduce margin positivity by improving intraoperative specimen radiography [21].

Novel Technology

In order to improve selective margin excision at the initial surgery, there has been considerable interest in novel technology to detect cancer at the margin. A radiofrequency probe, MarginProbe (Dune Medical), has been studied for a potential role in reducing margin positivity (Table 5.4). A number of other novel technologies are under current investigation.

Table 5.4 Novel technology

Study	Intervention		Positive margin rate		Re-excision rate	
	Arm	*n*	%	*p*-value	%	*p*-value
Schnabel et al. [58]	Device	298	30.9%	0.008	19.8%	0.097
	SOC	298	41.6%		25.8%	
Sebastian et al. [59]	Device	165	–	–	9.7%	<0.0001
	SOC	186	–		25.8%	
Thill et al. [60]	Device	42			17%	0.018
	SOC	67			39%	
Allweis et al. [61]	Device	143			12.6%	0.098
	SOC	150			18.6%	

Table 5.5 Routine cavity shave margins

Study	Type	Intervention		Re-excision rate	
		Arm	*n*	%	*p*-value
Kobbermann et al. [47]	Retrospective	CSM	69	21.7%	0.011
		SPM	69	42.0%	
Marudanayagam et al. [48]	Retrospective	CSM	394	5.58%	<0.01
		SPM	392	12.5%	
Unzeitig et al. [49]	Retrospective	CSM	67	23.9%	0.0003
		SPM	455	46.8%	
Janes et al. [50]	Retrospective	CSM	106	7.2%	0.001
		SPM	111	17.0%	
Huston et al. [51]	Retrospective	CSM	45	17.7%	n/s
		SCSM	77	32.5%	
		SPM	49	38.7%	
Chagpar et al. [6]	Prospective RCT	CSM	119	10.1%	0.02
		SPM	116	20.7%	

CSM cavity shave margins, *SPM* selective partial mastectomy, *SCSM* selective cavity shave margins, *n/s* not specified

Routine Cavity Shave Margins

Given that routine specimen radiography and resection of selective margins does not seem to significantly impact margin positivity, there has been significant interest in resection of routine cavity shave margins at the time of the initial surgery. There have been a number of retrospective studies, and now some randomized controlled trials, that have demonstrated that this technique can reduce positive margin and re-excision rates by 50% (Table 5.5). In addition, this technique has not been shown to adversely affect cosmetic outcomes, takes 10 min extra in the operating room, and may save healthcare dollars [22]. The American Society of Breast Surgeons endorsed routine cavity shave margins as one of the tools in the "toolbox" to reduce re-excision, but cautioned against "tiny shaves" that do not adequately excise the lumpectomy cavity [23]. A video of cavity shave margins that demonstrates complete cavity shave margins can be found here [24].

Table 5.6 Intraoperative pathologic examination of margins

Study	N	Technique	Without intervention	With intervention	*p*-value
Osako et al. [52]	1029	FS	30.3%[a]	5.9%[a]	n/s
Cendan et al. [53]	97	FS	25.8%[a]	18.6%[a]	n/s
Jorns et al. [54]	369	FS	14.9%[b]	50.5%[b]	n/s
Weber et al. [55]	111	FS	27.5%[a]	14.3%[a]	0.124
Esbona et al. [56]	–	FS	27%[b]	6%[b]	<0.0001
		IC	26%[b]	4%[b]	0.18
D'Halluin et al. [57]	400	IC	24.3%[b]	12.5%[b]	n/s

FS frozen section, *IC* imprint cytology
[a]Positive margin rate
[b]Re-excision rate for positive margins

Intraoperative Pathologic Evaluation of Margins

Several authors have proposed the concept of intraoperative pathologic evaluation of margins, either with frozen section or touch imprint cytology to reduce final positive margin rates (Table 5.6). Thill et al., in their review, noted the shortcomings of frozen section and touch imprint cytology. They note that frozen section is time consuming, prone to sampling error, and may further expend valuable tissue (particularly for small tumors) risking not having sufficient tissue for further histopathologic and biomarker evaluation [25]. Touch imprint cytology relies on superficial cells, thereby providing no information regarding margin width, relies on an experienced cytopathologist and does not allow for the distinction of DCIS versus invasive disease [25].

Conclusion

Re-excisions for positive margins has been described as an "epidemic" [26], and certainly no surgeon wants to return to the operating room. Still, that positive margins are associated with a higher risk of local recurrence, a number of techniques have been studied to reduce the positive margin and re-excision rate. The changing of the definition of a positive margin for invasive cancer to be "tumor at ink" may reduce the need for re-excision. While some have argued that focally positive margins may be acceptable in the current era of nearly ubiquitous systemic and radiation therapy [27], guidelines remain clear that obtaining negative margins is mandatory regardless of use of adjuvant therapy [28]. To date, no technique is perfect in the quest to eliminate the need for re-excisions and hence, the pursuit of surgical techniques to improve margin positivity rates continues.

References

1. Fisher B, Anderson S, Bryant J, Margolese RG, Deutsch M, Fisher ER, et al. Twenty-year follow-up of a randomized trial comparing total mastectomy, lumpectomy, and lumpectomy plus irradiation for the treatment of invasive breast cancer. N Engl J Med. 2002;347(16):1233–41.
2. Azu M, Abrahamse P, Katz SJ, Jagsi R, Morrow M. What is an adequate margin for breast-conserving surgery? Surgeon attitudes and correlates. Ann Surg Oncol. 2010;17(2):558–63.
3. Houssami N, Macaskill P, Marinovich ML, Morrow M. The association of surgical margins and local recurrence in women with early-stage invasive breast cancer treated with breast-conserving therapy: a meta-analysis. Ann Surg Oncol. 2014;21(3):717–30.
4. Toth D, Varga Z, Sebo E, Torok M, Kovacs I. Predictive factors for positive margin and the surgical learning curve in non-palpable breast cancer after wire-guided localization – prospective study of 214 consecutive patients. Pathol Oncol Res: POR. 2016;22(1):209–15.
5. Barentsz MW, Postma EL, van Dalen T, van den Bosch MA, Miao H, Gobardhan PD, et al. Prediction of positive resection margins in patients with non-palpable breast cancer. Eur J Surg Oncol: J Eur Soc Surg Oncol Br Assoc Surg Oncol. 2015;41(1):106–12.
6. Chagpar AB, Killelea BK, Tsangaris TN, Butler M, Stavris K, Li F, et al. A randomized, controlled trial of cavity shave margins in breast cancer. N Engl J Med. 2015;373(6):503–10.
7. Di Saverio S, Catena F, Santini D, Ansaloni L, Fogacci T, Mignani S, et al. 259 patients with DCIS of the breast applying USC/van Nuys prognostic index: a retrospective review with long term follow up. Breast Cancer Res Treat. 2008;109(3):405–16.
8. NCCN. NCCN clinical practice guidelines in oncology (NCCN guidelines). Breast Cancer. 2016;1.2016.
9. Morrow M, Van Zee KJ, Solin LJ, Houssami N, Chavez-MacGregor M, Harris JR, et al. Society of surgical oncology-American society for radiation oncology-American society of clinical oncology consensus guideline on margins for breast-conserving surgery with whole-breast irradiation in ductal carcinoma in situ. Ann Surg Oncol. 2016;6:287–95.
10. Wilke LG, Czechura T, Wang C, Lapin B, Liederbach E, Winchester DP, et al. Repeat surgery after breast conservation for the treatment of stage 0 to II breast carcinoma: a report from the National Cancer Data Base, 2004–2010. JAMA Surg. 2014;149(12):1296–305.
11. McCahill LE, Single RM, Aiello Bowles EJ, Feigelson HS, James TA, Barney T, et al. Variability in reexcision following breast conservation surgery. JAMA. 2012;307(5):467–75.
12. Schulman AM, Mirrielees JA, Leverson G, Landercasper J, Greenberg C, Wilke LG. Reexcision surgery for breast cancer: an analysis of the American Society of Breast Surgeons (ASBrS) MasterySM database following the SSO-ASTRO "No Ink on Tumor" guidelines. Ann Surg Oncol. 2016.
13. Turnbull L, Brown S, Harvey I, Olivier C, Drew P, Napp V, et al. Comparative effectiveness of MRI in breast cancer (COMICE) trial: a randomised controlled trial. Lancet. 2010;375(9714):563–71.
14. Peters NH, van Esser S, van den Bosch MA, Storm RK, Plaisier PW, van Dalen T, et al. Preoperative MRI and surgical management in patients with nonpalpable breast cancer: the MONET – randomised controlled trial. Eur J cancer (Oxford, England: 1990). 2011;47(6):879–86.
15. Fancellu A, Turner RM, Dixon JM, Pinna A, Cottu P, Houssami N. Meta-analysis of the effect of preoperative breast MRI on the surgical management of ductal carcinoma in situ. Br J Surg. 2015;102(8):883–93.
16. Chan BK, Wiseberg-Firtell JA, Jois RH, Jensen K, Audisio RA. Localization techniques for guided surgical excision of non-palpable breast lesions. Cochrane Database Syst Rev. 2015;12:CD009206.
17. Pan H, Wu N, Ding H, Ding Q, Dai J, Ling L, et al. Intraoperative ultrasound guidance is associated with clear lumpectomy margins for breast cancer: a systematic review and meta-analysis. PLoS One. 2013;8(9):e74028.

18. Hisada T, Sawaki M, Ishiguro J, Adachi Y, Kotani H, Yoshimura A, et al. Impact of intraoperative specimen mammography on margins in breast-conserving surgery. Mol Clin Oncol. 2016;5(3):269–72.
19. McCormick JT, Keleher AJ, Tikhomirov VB, Budway RJ, Caushaj PF. Analysis of the use of specimen mammography in breast conservation therapy. Am J Surg. 2004;188(4):433–6.
20. Chagpar AB, Butler M, Killelea BK, Horowitz NR, Stavris K, Lannin DR. Does three-dimensional intraoperative specimen imaging reduce the need for re-excision in breast cancer patients? A prospective cohort study. Am J Surg. 2015;210(5):886–90.
21. Tang R, Buckley JM, Fernandez L, Coopey S, Aftreth O, Michaelson J, et al. Micro-computed tomography (micro-CT): a novel approach for intraoperative breast cancer specimen imaging. Breast Cancer Res Treat. 2013;139(2):311–6.
22. Chagpar AB, Horowitz NR, Killelea BK, Tsangaris T, Longley P, Grizzle S, et al. Economic impact of routine cavity margins versus standard partial mastectomy in breast cancer patients: results of a randomized controlled trial. Ann Surg. 2016.
23. Landercasper J, Attai D, Atisha D, Beitsch P, Bosserman L, Boughey J, et al. Toolbox to reduce lumpectomy reoperations and improve cosmetic outcome in breast cancer patients: the American society of breast surgeons consensus conference. Ann Surg Oncol. 2015;22(10):3174–83.
24. Chagpar AB. Trial i. Cavity shave margins in breast cancer. N Engl J Med. 2015;373(22):2187–8.
25. Thill M, Baumann K, Barinoff J. Intraoperative assessment of margins in breast conservative surgery – still in use? J Surg Oncol. 2014;110(1):15–20.
26. Cody HS, 3rd, Van Zee KJ. Reexcision – the other breast cancer epidemic. N Engl J Med 2015;373(6):568–9.
27. McIntosh A, Freedman G, Eisenberg D, Anderson P. Recurrence rates and analysis of close or positive margins in patients treated without re-excision before radiation for breast cancer. Am J Clin Oncol. 2007;30(2):146–51.
28. Moran MS, Schnitt SJ, Giuliano AE, Harris JR, Khan SA, Horton J, et al. Society of surgical oncology-American society for radiation oncology consensus guideline on margins for breast-conserving surgery with whole-breast irradiation in stages I and II invasive breast cancer. Ann Surg Oncol. 2014;21(3):704–16.
29. Postma EL, Verkooijen HM, van Esser S, Hobbelink MG, van der Schelling GP, Koelemij R, et al. Efficacy of 'radioguided occult lesion localisation' (ROLL) versus 'wire-guided localisation' (WGL) in breast conserving surgery for non-palpable breast cancer: a randomised controlled multicentre trial. Breast Cancer Res Treat. 2012;136(2):469–78.
30. Duarte C, Bastidas F, de los Reyes A, Martinez MC, Hurtado G, Gomez MC, et al. Randomized controlled clinical trial comparing radioguided occult lesion localization with wire-guided lesion localization to evaluate their efficacy and accuracy in the localization of nonpalpable breast lesions. Surgery. 2016;159(4):1140–5.
31. Gray RJ, Salud C, Nguyen K, Dauway E, Friedland J, Berman C, et al. Randomized prospective evaluation of a novel technique for biopsy or lumpectomy of nonpalpable breast lesions: radioactive seed versus wire localization. Ann Surg Oncol. 2001;8(9):711–5.
32. Rarick J, Kimler BF, Tawfik O. Comparison of margin status and lesional size between radioactive seed localized vs conventional wire localized breast lumpectomy specimens. Ann Diagn Pathol. 2016;21:47–52.
33. Bloomquist EV, Ajkay N, Patil S, Collett AE, Frazier TG, Barrio AV. A randomized prospective comparison of patient-assessed satisfaction and clinical outcomes with radioactive seed localization versus wire localization. Breast J. 2016;22(2):151–7.
34. Sharek D, Zuley ML, Zhang JY, Soran A, Ahrendt GM, Ganott MA. Radioactive seed localization versus wire localization for lumpectomies: a comparison of outcomes. AJR Am J Roentgenol. 2015;204(4):872–7.
35. Murphy JO, Moo TA, King TA, Van Zee KJ, Villegas KA, Stempel M, et al. Radioactive seed localization compared to wire localization in breast-conserving surgery: initial 6-month experience. Ann Surg Oncol. 2013;20(13):4121–7.

36. Hughes JH, Mason MC, Gray RJ, McLaughlin SA, Degnim AC, Fulmer JT, et al. A multi-site validation trial of radioactive seed localization as an alternative to wire localization. Breast J. 2008;14(2):153–7.
37. van der Noordaa ME, Pengel KE, Groen E, van Werkhoven E, Rutgers EJ, Loo CE, et al. The use of radioactive iodine-125 seed localization in patients with non-palpable breast cancer: a comparison with the radioguided occult lesion localization with 99m technetium. Eur J Sur Oncol: J Eur Soc Surg Oncol Br Assoc Surg Oncol. 2015;41(4):553–8.
38. Donker M, Drukker CA, Valdes Olmos RA, Rutgers EJ, Loo CE, Sonke GS, et al. Guiding breast-conserving surgery in patients after neoadjuvant systemic therapy for breast cancer: a comparison of radioactive seed localization with the ROLL technique. Ann Surg Oncol. 2013;20(8):2569–75.
39. Rahusen FD, Bremers AJ, Fabry HF, van Amerongen AH, Boom RP, Meijer S. Ultrasound-guided lumpectomy of nonpalpable breast cancer versus wire-guided resection: a randomized clinical trial. Ann Surg Oncol. 2002;9(10):994–8.
40. Eggemann H, Costa SD, Ignatov A. Ultrasound-guided versus wire-guided breast-conserving surgery for nonpalpable breast cancer. Clin Breast Cancer. 2016;16(1):e1–6.
41. James TA, Harlow S, Sheehey-Jones J, Hart M, Gaspari C, Stanley M, et al. Intraoperative ultrasound versus mammographic needle localization for ductal carcinoma in situ. Ann Surg Oncol. 2009;16(5):1164–9.
42. Moore MM, Whitney LA, Cerilli L, Imbrie JZ, Bunch M, Simpson VB, et al. Intraoperative ultrasound is associated with clear lumpectomy margins for palpable infiltrating ductal breast cancer. Ann Surg. 2001;233(6):761–8.
43. Krekel NM, Haloua MH, Lopes Cardozo AM, de Wit RH, Bosch AM, de Widt-Levert LM, et al. Intraoperative ultrasound guidance for palpable breast cancer excision (COBALT trial): a multicentre, randomised controlled trial. Lancet Oncol. 2013;14(1):48–54.
44. Karanlik H, Ozgur I, Sahin D, Fayda M, Onder S, Yavuz E. Intraoperative ultrasound reduces the need for re-excision in breast-conserving surgery. World J Surg Oncol. 2015;13:321.
45. Fisher CS, Mushawah FA, Cyr AE, Gao F, Margenthaler JA. Ultrasound-guided lumpectomy for palpable breast cancers. Ann Surg Oncol. 2011;18(11):3198–203.
46. Davis KM, Hsu CH, Bouton ME, Wilhelmson KL, Komenaka IK. Intraoperative ultrasound can decrease the re-excision lumpectomy rate in patients with palpable breast cancers. Am Surg. 2011;77(6):720–5.
47. Kobbermann A, Unzeitig A, Xie XJ, Yan J, Euhus D, Peng Y, et al. Impact of routine cavity shave margins on breast cancer re-excision rates. Ann Surg Oncol. 2011;18(5):1349–55.
48. Marudanayagam R, Singhal R, Tanchel B, O'Connor B, Balasubramanian B, Paterson I. Effect of cavity shaving on reoperation rate following breast-conserving surgery. Breast J. 2008;14(6):570–3.
49. Unzeitig A, Kobbermann A, Xie XJ, Yan J, Euhus D, Peng Y, et al. Influence of surgical technique on mastectomy and reexcision rates in breast-conserving therapy for cancer. Int J Sur Oncol. 2012;2012:725121.
50. Janes SE, Stankhe M, Singh S, Isgar B. Systematic cavity shaves reduces close margins and re-excision rates in breast conserving surgery. Breast. 2006;15(3):326–30.
51. Huston TL, Pigalarga R, Osborne MP, Tousimis E. The influence of additional surgical margins on the total specimen volume excised and the reoperative rate after breast-conserving surgery. Am J Surg. 2006;192(4):509–12.
52. Osako T, Nishimura R, Nishiyama Y, Okumura Y, Tashima R, Nakano M, et al. Efficacy of intraoperative entire-circumferential frozen section analysis of lumpectomy margins during breast-conserving surgery for breast cancer. Int J Clin Oncol. 2015;20(6):1093–101.
53. Cendan JC, Coco D, Copeland EM, 3rd. Accuracy of intraoperative frozen-section analysis of breast cancer lumpectomy-bed margins. J Am Coll Surg 2005;201(2):194–8.
54. Jorns JM, Visscher D, Sabel M, Breslin T, Healy P, Daignaut S, et al. Intraoperative frozen section analysis of margins in breast conserving surgery significantly decreases reoperative rates: one-year experience at an ambulatory surgical center. Am J Clin Pathol. 2012;138(5):657–69.

55. Weber WP, Engelberger S, Viehl CT, Zanetti-Dallenbach R, Kuster S, Dirnhofer S, et al. Accuracy of frozen section analysis versus specimen radiography during breast-conserving surgery for nonpalpable lesions. World J Surg. 2008;32(12):2599–606.
56. Esbona K, Li Z, Wilke LG. Intraoperative imprint cytology and frozen section pathology for margin assessment in breast conservation surgery: a systematic review. Ann Surg Oncol. 2012;19(10):3236–45.
57. D'Halluin F, Tas P, Rouquette S, Bendavid C, Foucher F, Meshba H, et al. Intra-operative touch preparation cytology following lumpectomy for breast cancer: a series of 400 procedures. Breast. 2009;18(4):248–53.
58. Schnabel F, Boolbol SK, Gittleman M, Karni T, Tafra L, Feldman S, et al. A randomized prospective study of lumpectomy margin assessment with use of MarginProbe in patients with nonpalpable breast malignancies. Ann Surg Oncol. 2014;21(5):1589–95.
59. Sebastian M, Akbari S, Anglin B, Lin EH, Police AM. The impact of use of an intraoperative margin assessment device on re-excision rates. SpringerPlus. 2015;4:198.
60. Thill M, Dittmer C, Baumann K, Friedrichs K, Blohmer JU. MarginProbe(R) – final results of the German post-market study in breast conserving surgery of ductal carcinoma in situ. Breast. 2014;23(1):94–6.
61. Allweis TM, Kaufman Z, Lelcuk S, Pappo I, Karni T, Schneebaum S, et al. A prospective, randomized, controlled, multicenter study of a real-time, intraoperative probe for positive margin detection in breast-conserving surgery. Am J Surg. 2008;196(4):483–9.

Percutaneous Ablation in the Treatment of Breast Cancer

6

Vivian J. Bea, Dalliah Black, and Kelly Hunt

Introduction

Breast screening programs have increased the detection of early breast cancer, making most patients eligible for breast-conserving therapy (BCT) with segmental mastectomy and radiation. BCT has similar survival and locoregional recurrence outcomes compared to mastectomy [1–3] with fewer complications [4]. However, segmental mastectomy is usually still performed in the operating room, requires an incision, and is not free of complications such as hematoma, infection, pain, cosmetic deformity, and wound healing problems [5, 6]. Given these limitations, percutaneous ablation techniques that have been used to treat other cancer sites and benign breast fibroadenomas are being evaluated for the treatment of early breast cancer.

Potential advantages of percutaneous ablation over surgical excision include a more favorable cosmetic result, lower recovery time, lower complications, and improved quality of life [7, 8]. If its long-term safety is proved, percutaneous ablation without surgical excision may also decrease healthcare costs. Several techniques have been developed for ablation of breast cancers: radiofrequency ablation (RFA), cryoablation, laser, high-intensity focused ultrasound, and focused microwave therapy. Given the broader experience with RFA and cryoablation, this chapter will focus mainly on these two techniques.

The original version of this chapter was revised. The correction to this chapter is available at https://doi.org/10.1007/978-3-319-60336-0_16

V.J. Bea, MD • D. Black, MD (✉) • K. Hunt, MD, FACS, BSC
Department of Breast Surgical Oncology, University of Texas MD Anderson Cancer Center, 1400 Pressler St., Unit 1434, FTC 7.5000, Houston, TX 77030, USA
e-mail: vjbea@mdanderson.org; dmblack@mdanderson.org; khunt@mdanderson.org

M. Howard-McNatt (ed.), *Changing Paradigms in the Management of Breast Cancer*, DOI 10.1007/978-3-319-60336-0_6

Cryoablation

Technique

Cryoablation can be performed in an office setting without sedation [7–9]. Briefly, with the patient in supine position and sterile technique, the tumor is visualized and measured with ultrasound guidance (Fig. 6.1). Since cold from the cryoablation system acts as a natural anesthetic, only local anesthesia is required. Under ultrasound guidance, the probe is inserted into the center of the tumor (Fig. 6.2). Freezing requires investing in a treatment system such as Visica 2 Treatment System (Sanarus Medical; Pleasanton, California) and also the availability of liquid nitrogen to achieve subzero temperatures [10]. The probe has a proximal insulated portion allowing protection of the overlying skin and a distal active freezing zone which forms an ice ball ranging from 4 to 7 cm in size with a discrete hyperechoic rim. Attention must be paid to inserting the probe at least 0.5 cm longer than the distal active freezing zone. The goal of cryoablation is to achieve tissue necrosis of the targeted area through a cycle of freeze, passive thaw followed by another freeze cycle with the entire procedure being done under ultrasound guidance (Fig. 6.3). This process takes approximately 10 min for each cycle with a total procedure time of approximately 30–40 min. Freezing causes cell death through osmotic shifts, cell membrane damage, lysis, and damage to blood vessels. To prevent

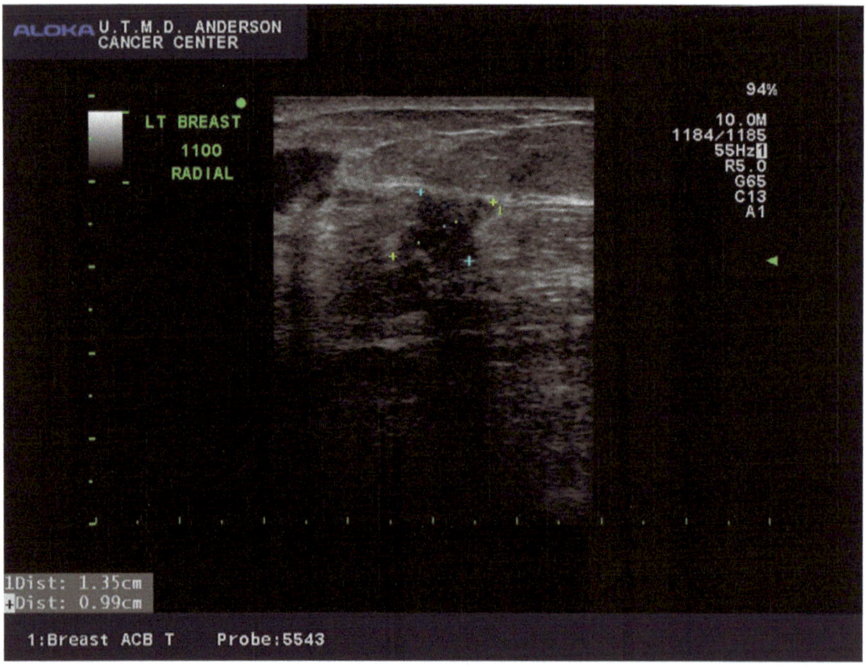

Fig. 6.1 Breast ultrasound prior to placement of cryoablation probe (Courtesy of Dr. Rosa Hwang)

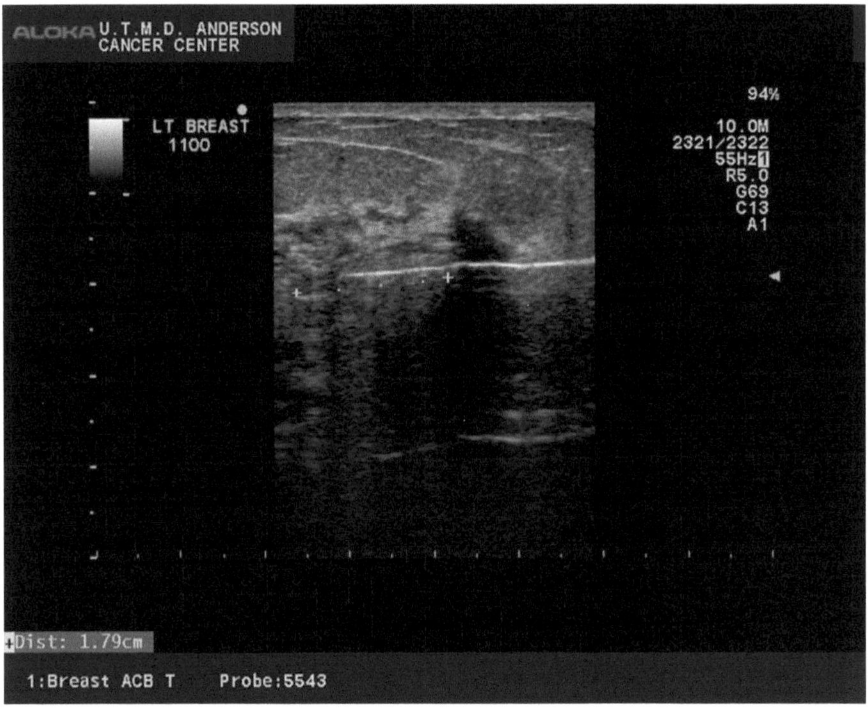

Fig. 6.2 Cryoablation probe inserted with ultrasound guidance through the center of the tumor with the tip extending past the tumor (Courtesy of Dr. Rosa Hwang)

skin damage, saline is injected between the ice ball and skin during freezing and particularly if the ice ball rim is <0.5 cm from the skin. Adequate skill in performing ultrasound-guided procedures is necessary for accurate probe placement.

Cryoablation and the Fibroadenoma Experience

Successful experience of cryoablating fibroadenomas provided a foundation for evaluating cryoablation to treat breast cancers. Cryoablation is Food and Drug Administration (FDA) approved for the treatment of fibroadenomas. In a study with 2.6-year follow-up, Kaufman et al. reported on 37 patients with ultrasound showing a 99% volume reduction in treated fibroadenomas with most (84%) remaining nonpalpable. Long-term results demonstrated excellent patient and physician satisfaction [11].

The larger multi-institutional FibroAdenoma Cryoablation Treatment (FACT) registry of 444 patients reported that the treatment area was palpable at 12 months in 60% of cases with high patient satisfaction (88%). Residual palpable areas were more common in lesions greater than 2 cm [10]. The fibroadenoma experience demonstrated cryoablation's safety and provided feasibility for applying this technique for breast cancer treatment.

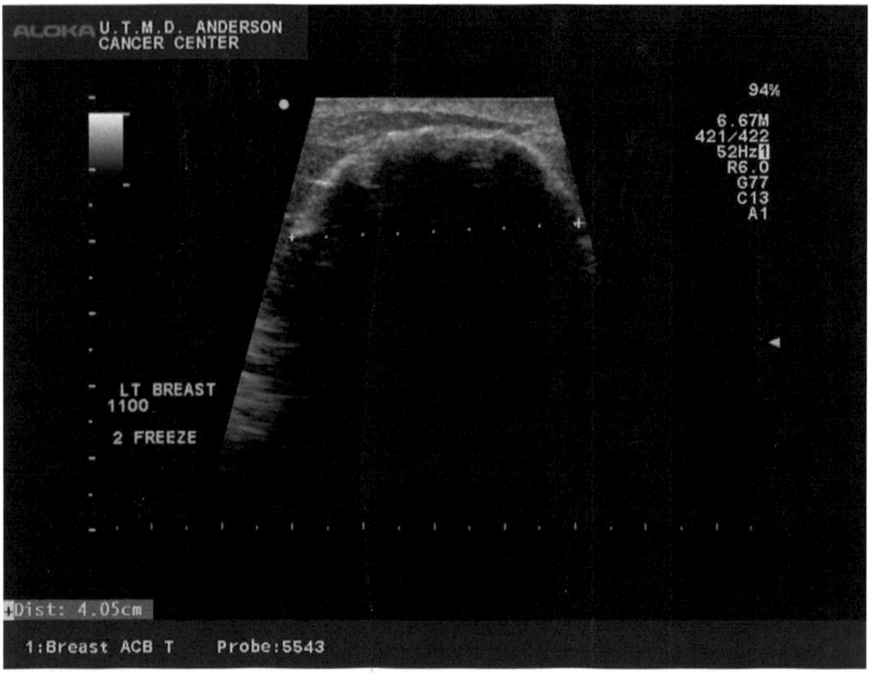

Fig. 6.3 Ultrasound image of ice ball formed after second freeze cycle with tumor cryoablation (Courtesy of Dr. Rosa Hwang)

Cryoablation for the Treatment of Invasive Breast Cancer

The concept of cryoablation was developed in the 1800s for palliative treatment of locally advanced uterine and breast cancers using iced saline solution [7, 12]. In recent decades, it has been utilized to treat select primary and metastatic cancers in the liver [13, 14]. For breast cancer, several parameters have been identified for successful cryoablation: unifocal ductal cancer measuring less than 1.5 cm, tumor location away from the skin, discrete tumor margins on imaging, and a visible posterior wall on ultrasound for evaluating the distal active freezing zone.

Small single-institution studies of ultrasound-guided cryoablation followed by surgical excision report variable success rates. With including a larger mean tumor size of 21 mm, Pfleiderer [15] reported limited success in treating 16 invasive cancers with cryoablation followed by surgical excision 5 days later. Five tumors measuring less than 16 mm did not have a remaining invasive component, but two specimens had residual ductal carcinoma in situ (DCIS). Eleven cancers measuring at least 23 mm had incomplete ablation demonstrated on surgical pathology.

A recent study incorporating pretreatment and posttreatment breast MRI demonstrated improved ablation outcomes, likely due to improved patient selection (Figs. 6.4 and 6.5). In 20 patients with invasive ductal cancer (IDC) measuring ≤15 mm, Poplack

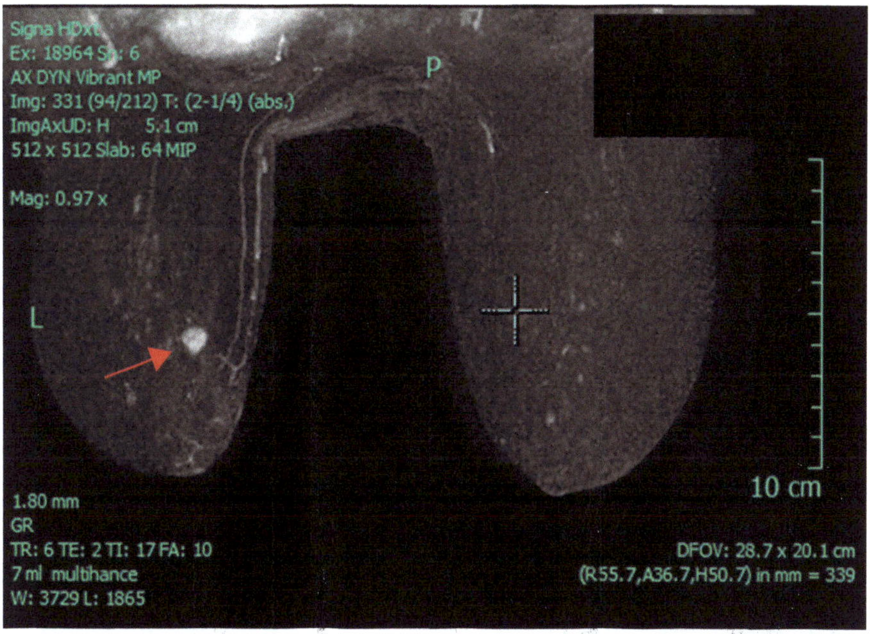

Fig. 6.4 Pre-cryoablation breast MRI demonstrating a unifocal tumor in the left breast (*arrow*) (Courtesy of Dr. Rosa Hwang)

et al. [16] reported 85% complete ablation. Posttreatment MRI had a 0% sensitivity and 88% specificity with a negative predictive value (NPV) of 83%.

A retrospective study preferred cryoablation when comparing it with radiofrequency ablation (RFA) for the treatment of IDC ≤2 cm in elderly patients [17]. Forty patients underwent cryoablation compared to 40 patients undergoing radiofrequency ablation with a mean age of 75 years. Post-ablation MRI was performed followed by surgical excision approximately 5 weeks later with 18-month mean follow-up. There was complete ablation in 75 patients (94%) on surgical excision, and this was accurately determined on MRI. Two patients undergoing cryoablation (95% success) and three patients undergoing RFA (93% success) had residual disease on surgical excision which was visualized on 4-week post-ablation MRI. The failures were thought to be due to incorrect positioning of the devices and inadequate necrosis area. There were no long-term cosmetic differences between the two groups, but there were two cases of skin necrosis in the RFA group. The authors preferred cryoablation given the analgesic affect from its cooling.

Studies of cryoablation without surgical excision of breast cancer are limited. However, this may become a treatment option for elderly patients with a short life expectancy. In a study of 23 patients with a median age of 85 years having invasive cancers ranging from 5 to 28 mm, there were five recurrences during the 14.6 month-median follow-up [18]. At 24-month follow-up, "complete tumor control" as evaluated on MRI was 9%. There were four hematomas and one skin burn.

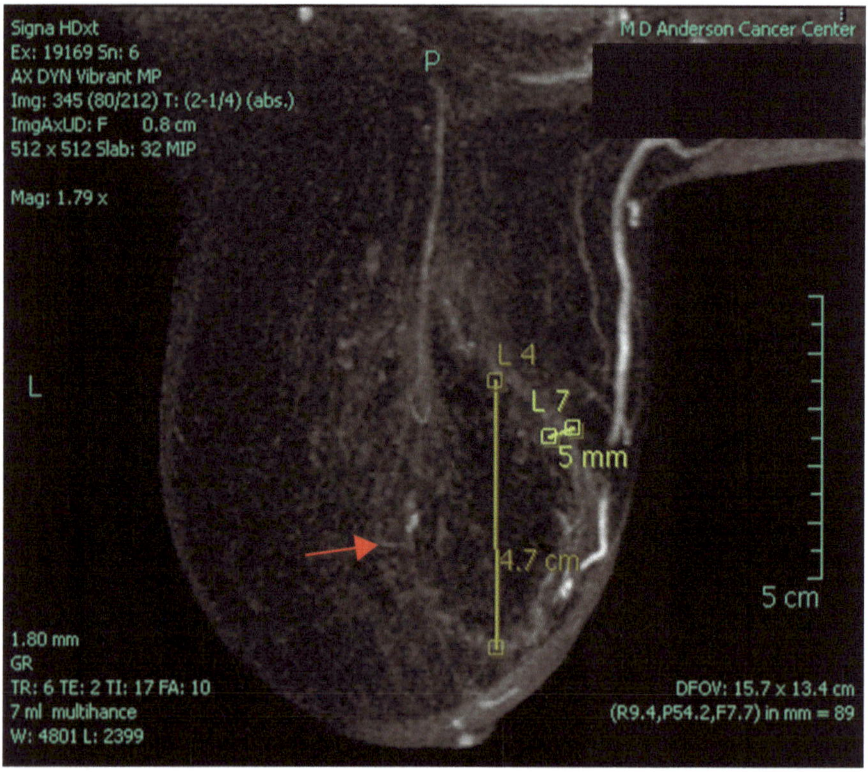

Fig. 6.5 Post-cryoablation breast MRI. *Red arrow* marks cryoablation halo cavity; no residual enhancing mass is seen

Multi-institutional Cooperative Cryoablation Trial: ACOSOG Z1072

The American College of Surgeons Oncology Group (ACOSOG) Z1072, a multi-institutional phase II trial, recently reported the effectiveness of cryoablation for treating invasive breast cancer [19]. The trial included patients with unifocal IDC ≤2 cm with a limited intraductal component (25%) and preoperative tumor enhancement on MRI. After undergoing cryoablation, patients underwent repeat breast MRI and surgical excision. Physicians were required to have a minimum of 20 ultrasound-guided procedures and 5 ultrasound-guided cryoablation procedures. Cryoablation successfully treated 66 of 87 (76%) of cancers with 16% other specimens having residual invasive cancer and 17% having residual DCIS. If multifocal disease was not defined as an ablation failure, 92% of tumors were successfully ablated. Postsurgical MRI had a negative predictive value of 81% with a 100% NPV for cancers <1.0 cm.

Cryoablation is a promising treatment for small unifocal invasive ductal cancers; however, improvements in imaging modalities for accurate identification of multifocal disease are needed to identify appropriate patients. Complications are low and include temporary site tenderness, hematoma, and skin necrosis [9, 19, 20]. A unique property of cryoablation compared to other ablation techniques is its production of antitumor immune responses. In animal models [21], it provides antigen presentation caused by pro-inflammatory cytokines. In theory, it is possible that the immune response induced by cryoablation may protect against local recurrences and possibly distant metastasis [7, 19]. Cryoablation has not been adequately evaluated as a treatment for invasive lobular carcinoma or extensive in situ disease [7, 22].

Radiofrequency Ablation

Radiofrequency ablation (RFA) is one of the most common percutaneous techniques in clinical practice for treating hepatocellular carcinoma, renal tumors, and metastasis usually to the liver [23–26]. The feasibility of using RFA for breast cancer was first reported by Jeffrey et al. in 1999 [27] in five patients with locally advanced invasive breast cancer. Surgical resection followed RFA. Analysis by immunohistochemistry demonstrated complete cell death in 80% of the breast tumors.

RFA must be performed in the operating room and under general anesthesia. The technique uses thermal energy through high-frequency alternating currents emitted from the non-insulated tip of a needle electrode. This transmits into the adjacent breast tissue, causing ionic vibrations as the ions attempt to follow the rapidly changing direction of the alternating current. Ionic agitation results in frictional heating to temperatures exceeding 100°C. This in turn causes cell death and coagulation necrosis of the tumor. Higher temperatures cause more destruction to tumor cells and the less exposure needed. Central placement of the electrode into the cancer is also important with this technique [28–30].

In a two-center pilot study of 26 patients with T1 and T2 invasive ductal, lobular, and tubular breast cancers, there was 96% complete tumor ablation [28]. One patient (4%) had a full-thickness skin burn. Our institution's feasibility study of more homogenous tumor pathology in 21 invasive cancers ≤2 cm (19 ductal histologies), there was complete ablation in all cases with no complications [29]. Limitations include the inability for real-time monitoring of the ablation edge to confirm complete ablation of the lesion with an adequate margin without damaging the skin.

To improve RFA temperature distribution and possible skin damage, Manenti et al. [31] utilized a cool-tip system in 34 patients with IDC ≤2 cm. Patients were evaluated with mammogram, breast ultrasound, and 3.0-T MRI before and after cool-tip RFA. Complete ablation occurred in 97% of tumors on histologic analysis, and post-ablation MRI showed no suspicious enhancement in 31 cases. Cosmesis was excellent in 28 patients, and there was a mild superficial skin burn in one patient with a tumor <1 cm to the skin edge. However, the cool-tip system also does not provide real-time monitoring.

RFA may also have a role in treating breast cancer patients who are elderly or not optimal surgical candidates [32, 33]. A recent study reported incorporating preoperative endocrine therapy in elderly patients followed by RFA. In 21 patients older than 70 years who had taken neoadjuvant endocrine therapy 6 months for cancers ≤3 cm, 1-year follow-up after RFA had one local failure [34]. None of the patients received irradiation. At 5-year follow-up of ten patients, three patients had local failures (two of the three patients had cancers with lobular histology) for an overall local recurrence rate of 19%. Four patients (19%) had skin burns, and there were four deaths during the study duration (two from cancer-related causes and two from non-cancer-related causes). Combining this study with others using preoperative endocrine therapy before RFA to evaluate outcomes of 104 patients but shorter follow-up (15–29 months), there was one local recurrence [30]. Future studies evaluating neoadjuvant endocrine therapy followed by RFA compared to endocrine therapy only in this select patient population is needed.

Additionally, a feasibility study by Klimberg et al. [35] evaluated RFA in treating the margins after vacuum-assisted excisional biopsy of breast cancer. Vacuum-assisted excisional biopsy with an 8-gauge probe has been reported to oftentimes completely remove the cancer. Leveraging the ability of large-gauge biopsies to remove the majority of a lesion, RFA (15 patients) or laser ablation (3 patients) was utilized to treat the cavity for possible residual disease at the margins. MRI was incorporated pre-procedure and after vacuum-assisted excisional biopsy. If residual or multicentric disease was noted on MRI, then patients underwent standard of care and were not included in the study. Otherwise, patients underwent excision as part of the study. Laser ablation was discontinued given unpredictability to create a consistent ablation area. Of the 15 patients undergoing RFA, all had successful complete ablation except one patient who had a 1-mm focus of atypia/DCIS distant to the immediate ablation field. Seven patients had no residual cancer on segmental mastectomy after vacuum-assisted excisional biopsy, and the other eight patients had nonviable tumor remaining at the tumor site.

Limitations of RFA

Due to the high variability of breast tissue density, the use of RFA has proven to be challenging. Oftentimes, the tissue surrounding breast masses is not homogenous and can cause differences in conductivity. Tissue impedance is affected leading to variation in treatment times to achieve total tumor ablation. This variation can lead to uncertainty in assessing the extent of tumor ablation [30].

The distance between the tumor, the skin, and chest wall should be at least 1 cm as RFA can cause skin or pectoralis muscle burns. In cases with borderline skin and chest wall distances, caution can be taken by subcutaneously injecting sterile water to avoid energy transmission to adjacent structures, applying lateral compression of the breast during the ablation procedure or ice cooling [29, 36]. Patients who undergo RFA must be counseled that a postprocedure palpable mass may remain even if they did not present with a palpable mass [31, 34]. A review of RFA studies reports a histologically confirmed successful ablation in 76–100% of studies with 1% pneumothorax, 5% skin burns, and 5% pectoralis muscle burns [30].

Percutaneous Microwave Coagulation

Percutaneous microwave coagulation (PMC) for the treatment of uterine fibroids and liver tumors [37, 38] led to the limited evaluation of percutaneous microwave coagulation (PMC) for the treatment of early breast cancers. PMC offers shorter ablation times, higher temperatures, and preferential heating of the cancer compared to normal breast tissue given that cancer has a higher water content. In a study of 41 patients with invasive ductal cancer clinically estimated to measure ≤3 cm, 95% of cases had complete coagulation on surgical pathology [39]. However, mean tumor volume was 5 cm^3 with a range of 0.09–14.14 cm^3. The mean coagulation time was 4.48 min. In three patients, a small epidermal burn or slight thermal injury to the pectoralis muscle occurred. Multi-institutional studies with long-term recurrence outcomes are not available.

High-Intensity Focused Ultrasound

There is less experience with high-intensity focused ultrasound (HIFU) utilizing ultrasound or MRI guidance for breast cancer ablation. HIFU has also been used in liver, prostate, kidney, and brain cancers [40]. An ultrasound beam transmits a pressure wave that produces temperature increases resulting in targeted coagulation necrosis and protein denaturation without harming adjacent tissue. In a meta-analysis of seven studies each having 6–28 patients, complete ablation was found in 46% of patients and near complete ablation (defined as less than 10% residual tumor) in 30% of patients. Treatment times were long, ranging from 78 to 171 min. Complications included pain (40%), skin burns (4%), and residual edema at the cancer site (17%). Further work to improve HIFU's ablation on histology and time are needed before becoming an option for routine clinical use.

Laser Ablation

Laser ablation is performed under local anesthetic by inserting the laser needle and a temperature sensing probe. The laser power is increased until the temperature probe reaches 60 °C. In a study of 54 patients (50 invasive and 4 in situ) [41], complete ablation was 70% with treatment time ranging 5–30 min with a median of 5900 J of laser energy used for median tumor size of 13 mm. These results included an initial learning and implementation period. After the learning period, the last 28 patients had 93–100% complete ablation. Continuous monitoring of the temperature was used to determine when adequate ablation was achieved as real-time imaging does not show tumor ablation changes. No significant complications were noted. Patients reported temporary sensitivity at the ablation site.

In a smaller study of 14 patients with T1 and T2 tumors [42], laser completely ablated 50% of tumors determined by NAD staining. Tumors less than 2 cm had higher complete ablation (88%). There was one skin burn and one small pneumothorax treated conservatively. Laser ablation's limitations and results from these and other small studies have limited further widespread evaluation of it as an option for percutaneous treatment of breast cancer.

The Role of Breast MRI in Percutaneous Ablation

In addition to mammogram and ultrasound, breast MRI has been utilized to determine patient eligibility by evaluating disease extent and the presence of multicentric disease and also to determine residual disease after ablation treatment [7, 19]. In a small study of 14 patients, Vilar et al. [43] compared tumor dimension on breast ultrasound with MRI before RFA and also correlated surgical pathology to a post-ablation MRI. Pre-RFA MRI measurements showed a statistically significant larger tumor volume compared to ultrasound in 80% of cases. After RFA, MRI accurately demonstrated no residual disease in all cases. In those cases with residual tumor remaining after RFA, MRI accurately measured the tumor dimensions compared to surgical pathology dimensions. In a similar study of 15 patients with invasive ductal cancer ≤15 mm [16], cryoablation was successful in 85% of the cases. MRI was performed with mammogram and ultrasound before ablation, and a repeat MRI was done 25–40 days after ablation, followed by surgical excision. MRI did not detect residual cancer at the ablation site in all three patients (sensitivity 0%) and had a specificity of 88%. The NPV was 83%.

In ACOSOG Z1072, tumor size ≤1 cm was associated with no residual MRI enhancement in 100% of cryoablation cases. However, for size >1 cm, 77% had complete ablation with no residual enhancement on MRI. MRI had a similar NPV of 81% for detecting residual disease after cryoablation [19]. Improvements in image detection of multifocal disease and extensive intraductal component are still needed.

Additional Considerations

Histopathologic confirmation with receptor subtyping should be obtained by core needle biopsy prior to ablation. Percutaneous ablation has not been adequately studied and should be used under study in patients who received neoadjuvant chemotherapy as viable tumor cells may still be present beyond the tumor compromising the ability to obtain local control. Percutaneous ablation techniques are also contraindicated in patients with extensive DCIS or lobular carcinoma. Physicians performing percutaneous ablation of breast cancers should have adequate experience in performing image-guided procedures [22, 30].

For patients undergoing percutaneous ablation for the primary tumor, axillary staging with sentinel node biopsy would still require a surgical procedure. Current research of nonoperatively assessing the axillary sentinel node with intradermal microbubble and contrast-enhanced ultrasound [44] may become an alternative for staging early breast cancers in patients undergoing percutaneous ablation of the primary cancer in an office setting. Less axillary surgery for the management of breast cancer is already becoming an acceptable approach. For example, ACOSOG Z0011 demonstrated that patients with invasive cancer ≤5 cm and one to two metastatic nodes on SLND do not benefit from axillary node dissection [45]. As the role of completion axillary dissection lessens for the management of early breast cancer, nonsurgical techniques to stage the axilla may complement percutaneous ablation in patients presenting with early breast cancer.

Defining appropriate long-term breast surveillance for patients undergoing percutaneous ablation is still needed but may likely include continued follow-up with detailed imaging as improvements in breast MRI and other newer modalities are made. Lastly, cost analysis to determine a potential economic benefit of percutaneous ablation may provide additional support for its use over surgical excision in the current setting of healthcare financial challenges.

Summary

Phase I and phase II studies evaluating different percutaneous ablation techniques, such as ACOSOG's multi-institutional 1071 trial, have overall reported a 70–100% success rate. Improvements in breast imaging are needed to better identify patients who may not be candidates for percutaneous ablation such as those having multicentric disease or extensive DCIS and for evaluating the effectiveness of an ablative treatment. Future studies evaluating the impact of cryoablation's immune-enhancing properties on local recurrence rates may also provide support for its preferential use. With further refinement in patient selection and imaging evaluation, percutaneous ablation may prove to be an effective treatment for patients with early breast cancer or those who are not surgical candidates.

References

1. Fisher B, Anderson S, Bryant J, et al. Twenty-year follow-up of a randomized trial comparing total mastectomy, lumpectomy, and lumpectomy plus irradiation for the treatment of invasive breast cancer. N Engl J Med. 2002;347(16):1233–41.
2. Veronesi U, Cascinelli N, Mariani L, et al. Twenty-year follow-up of a randomized study comparing breast-conserving surgery with radical mastectomy for early breast cancer. N Engl J Med. 2002;347(16):1227–32.
3. Early Breast Cancer Trialists. Effects of radiotherapy and surgery in early breast cancer. An overview of the randomized trials. N Engl J Med. 1995;333(22):1444–55.
4. El-Tamer MB, Ward BM, Schifftner T, Neumayer L, Khuri S, Henderson W. Morbidity and mortality following breast cancer surgery in women: national benchmarks for standards of care. Ann Surg. 2007;245(5):665–71. PubMed PMID: 17457156; PubMed Central PMCID: PMC1877061
5. Eck DL, Koonce SL, Goldberg RF, Bagaria S, Gibson T, Bowers SP, McLaughlin SA. Breast surgery outcomes as quality measures according to the NSQIP database. Ann Surg Oncol. 2012;19(10):3212–7. doi:https://doi.org/10.1245/s10434-012-2529-6. PubMed PMID: 22829006
6. Jagsi R, Li Y, Morrow M, Janz N, Alderman A, Graff J, Hamilton A, Katz S, Hawley S. Patient-reported quality of life and satisfaction with cosmetic outcomes after breast conservation and mastectomy with and without reconstruction: results of a survey of breast cancer survivors.

Ann Surg. 2015;261(6):1198–206. doi:https://doi.org/10.1097/SLA.0000000000000908. PubMed PMID: 25654742; PubMed Central PMCID: PMC4512928
7. Roubidoux MA, Yang W, Stafford RJ. Image-guided ablation in breast cancer treatment. Tech Vasc Interv Radiol. 2014;17(1):49–54. doi:https://doi.org/10.1053/j.tvir.2013.12.008. Review. PubMed PMID: 24636331
8. Sabel MS. Nonsurgical ablation of breast cancer: future options for small breast tumors. Surg Oncol Clin N Am. 2014;23(3):593–608. doi:https://doi.org/10.1016/j.soc.2014.03.009. Review. PubMed PMID: 24882353
9. Kaufman CS, Bachman B, Littrup PJ, White M, Carolin KA, Freman-Gibb L, Francescatti D, Stocks LH, Smith JS, Henry CA, Bailey L, Harness JK, Simmons R. Office-based ultrasound-guided cryoablation of breast fibroadenomas. Am J Surg. 2002;184(5):394–400. PubMed PMID: 12433600
10. Nurko J, Mabry CD, Whitworth P, Jarowenko D, Oetting L, Potruch T, Han L, Edwards MJ. Interim results from the FibroAdenoma Cryoablation Treatment Registry. Am J Surg. 2005;190(4):647–51. discussion 651-2. PubMed PMID:16164941
11. Kaufman CS, Littrup PJ, Freeman-Gibb LA, Smith JS, Francescatti D, Simmons R, Stocks LH, Bailey L, Harness JK, Bachman BA, Henry CA. Office-based cryoablation of breast fibroadenomas with long-term follow-up. Breast J. 2005;11(5):344–50. PubMed PMID: 16174156
12. Niu L, Zhou L, Xu K, Mu F. The role of cryosurgery in palliative care for cancer. Ann Palliat Med. 2013;2(1):26–34. doi:https://doi.org/10.3978/j.issn.2224-5820.2013.01.09. PubMed PMID: 25841740
13. Ravikumar TS, Buenaventura S, Salem RR, D'Andrea B. Intraoperative ultrasonography of liver: detection of occult liver tumors and treatment by cryosurgery. Cancer Detect Prev. 1994;18(2):131–8. PubMed PMID: 8025895
14. Kerkar S, Carlin AM, Sohn RL, Steffes C, Tyburski J, Littrup P, Weaver D. Long-term follow up and prognostic factors for cryotherapy of malignant liver tumors. Surgery. 2004;136(4):770–9. PubMed PMID: 15467661
15. Pfleiderer SO, Freesmeyer MG, Marx C, Kühne-Heid R, Schneider A, Kaiser WA. Cryotherapy of breast cancer under ultrasound guidance: initial results and limitations. Eur Radiol. 2002;12(12):3009–14. PubMed PMID: 12439583
16. Poplack SP, Levine GM, Henry L, Wells WA, Heinemann FS, Hanna CM, Deneen DR, Tosteson TD, Barth RJ Jr. A pilot study of ultrasound-guided cryoablation of invasive ductal carcinomas up to 15 mm with MRI follow-up and subsequent surgical resection. AJR Am J Roentgenol. 2015;204(5):1100–8. doi:https://doi.org/10.2214/AJR.13.12325. PubMed PMID: 25905948; PubMed Central PMCID: PMC4836389
17. Manenti G, Scarano AL, Pistolese CA, Perretta T, Bonanno E, Orlandi A, Simonetti G. Subclinical breast cancer: minimally invasive approaches. Our experience with percutaneous radiofrequency ablation vs. cryotherapy. Breast Care (Basel). 2013;8(5):356–60. doi:https://doi.org/10.1159/000355707. PubMed PMID: 24415989; PubMed Central PMCID: PMC3861851
18. Cazzato RL, de Lara CT, Buy X, Ferron S, Hurtevent G, Fournier M, Debled M, Palussière J. Single-centre experience with percutaneous cryoablation of breast cancer in 23 consecutive non-surgical patients. Cardiovasc Intervent Radiol. 2015;38(5):1237–43. doi:https://doi.org/10.1007/s00270-015-1181-5. PubMed PMID: 26183466
19. Simmons RM, Ballman KV, Cox C, Carp N, Sabol J, Hwang RF, Attai D, Sabel M, Nathanson D, Kenler A, Gold L, Kaufman C, Han L, Bleznak A, Stanley Smith J, Holmes D, Fornage B, Le-Petross C, Hoda S, McCall L, Hunt KK, ACOSOG investigators. A phase II trial exploring the success of cryoablation therapy in the treatment of invasive breast carcinoma: results from ACOSOG (alliance) Z1072. Ann Surg Oncol. 2016;23(8):2438–45. doi:https://doi.org/10.1245/s10434-016-5275-3. Epub 2016 May 24. PubMed PMID: 27221361
20. Edwards MJ, Broadwater R, Tafra L, Jarowenki D, Mabry C, Beitsch P, Whitworth P, Martin RC, Oetting L. Progressive adoption of cryoablative therapy for breast fibroadenoma in community practice. Am J Surg. 2004;188(3):221–4. PubMed PMID: 15450823

21. Sabel MS, Su G, Griffith KA, Chang AE. Rate of freeze alters the immunologic response after cryoablation of breast cancer. Ann Surg Oncol. 2010;17(4):1187–93. doi:https://doi.org/10.1245/s10434-009-0846-1. Epub 2009 Dec 22. PubMed PMID:20033323
22. Fornage BD, Hunt KK. Image-guided percutaneous ablation of small breast cancer: which technique is leading the pack? Technol Cancer Res Treat. 2015;14(2):209–11. doi:https://doi.org/10.7785/tcrt.2012.500395. PubMed PMID: 24325137; PubMed Central PMCID: PMC4423750
23. Raut CP, Izzo F, Marra P, Ellis LM, Vauthey JN, Cremona F, Vallone P, Mastro A, Fornage BD, Curley SA. Significant long-term survival after radiofrequency ablation of unresectable hepatocellular carcinoma in patients with cirrhosis. Ann Surg Oncol. 2005;12(8):616–28. PubMed PMID: 15965731
24. Long JA, Bernhard JC, Bigot P, Lanchon C, Paparel P, Rioux-Leclercq N, Albiges L, Bodin T, Nouhaud FX, Boissier R, Gimel P, Méjean A, Masson-Lecomte A, Grenier N, Cornelis F, Grassano Y, Comat V, Le Clerc QC, Rigaud J, Salomon L, Descotes JL, Sengel C, Roupret M, Verhoest G, Ouzaid I, Arnoux V, Bensalah K, French association of Urology Cancerology Comitee (CCAFU). Partial nephrectomy versus ablative therapy for the treatment of renal tumors in an imperative setting. World J Urol. 2016;35:649–56. PubMed PMID: 27498139
25. Babawale SN, Jensen TM, Frøkjær JB. Long-term survival following radiofrequency ablation of colorectal liver metastases: a retrospective study. World J Gastrointest Surg. 2015;7(3):33–8. doi:https://doi.org/10.4240/wjgs.v7.i3.33. PubMed PMID: 25848490; PubMed Central PMCID: PMC4381154
26. Bai H, Huangz X, Jing L, Zeng Q, Han L. The effect of radiofrequency ablation vs. liver resection on survival outcome of colorectal liver metastases (CRLM): a meta-analysis. Hepato-Gastroenterology. 2015;62(138):373–7. Review. PubMed PMID: 25916066
27. Jeffrey S, Birdwell R, Ikeda D, Daniel B, Nowels K, Dirbas F, Griffey S. Radiofrequency ablation of breast cancer. First report of an emerging technology. Arch Surg. 1999;134:1064–8.
28. Izzo F, Thomas R, Delrio P, Rinaldo M, Vallone P, DeChiara A, Botti G, D'Aiuto G, Cortino P, Curley SA. Radiofrequency ablation in patients with primary breast carcinoma: a pilot study in 26 patients. Cancer. 2001;92(8):2036–44. PubMed PMID: 11596017
29. Fornage BD, Sneige N, Ross MI, Mirza AN, Kuerer HM, Edeiken BS, Ames FC, Newman LA, Babiera GV, Singletary SE. Small (< or = 2-cm) breast cancer treated with US-guided radiofrequency ablation: feasibility study. Radiology. 2004;231(1):215–24. Epub 2004 Feb 27. PubMed PMID: 14990810
30. Grotenhuis BA, Vrijland WW, Klem TM. Radiofrequency ablation for early-stage breast cancer: treatment outcomes and practical considerations. Eur J Surg Oncol. 2013;39(12):1317–24. doi:https://doi.org/10.1016/j.ejso.2013.09.007. Epub 2013 Sep 14. Review. PubMed PMID: 24139998
31. Manenti G, Bolacchi F, Perretta T, Cossu E, Pistolese CA, Buonomo OC, Bonanno E, Orlandi A, Simonetti G. Small breast cancers: in vivo percutaneous US-guided radiofrequency ablation with dedicated cool-tip radiofrequency system. Radiology. 2009;251(2):339–46. doi:https://doi.org/10.1148/radiol.2512080905. Epub 2009 Mar 20. PubMed PMID: 19304918
32. Susini T, Nori J, Olivieri S, Livi L, Bianchi S, Mangialavori G, Branconi F, Scarselli G. Radiofrequency ablation for minimally invasive treatment of breast carcinoma. A pilot study in elderly inoperable patients. Gynecol Oncol. 2007;104(2):304–10. PubMed PMID: 17070572
33. Yamamoto N, Fujimoto H, Nakamura R, Arai M, Yoshii A, Kaji S, Itami M. Pilot study of radiofrequency ablation therapy without surgical excision for T1 breast cancer: evaluation with MRI and vacuum-assisted core needle biopsy and safety management. Breast Cancer. 2011;18(1):3–9. doi:https://doi.org/10.1007/s12282-010-0197-6. PubMed PMID: 20204556
34. Palussière J, Henriques C, Mauriac L, Asad-Syed M, Valentin F, Brouste V, Mathoulin-Pélissier S, Tunon de Lara C, Debled M. Radiofrequency ablation as a substitute for surgery in elderly patients with nonresected breast cancer: pilot study with long-term outcomes. Radiology. 2012;264(2):597–605. doi:https://doi.org/10.1148/radiol.12111303. Epub 2012 Jun 12. PubMed PMID: 22692040
35. Klimberg VS, Boneti C, Adkins LL, Smith M, Siegel E, Zharov V, Ferguson S, Henry-Tillman R, Badgwell B, Korourian S. Feasibility of percutaneous excision followed by ablation for local

control in breast cancer. Ann Surg Oncol. 2011;18(11):3079–87. doi:https://doi.org/10.1245/s10434-011-2002-y. Epub 2011 Sep 9. PubMed PMID:21904959; PubMed Central PMCID: PMC3280094
36. Burak WE Jr, Agnese DM, Povoski SP, Yanssens TL, Bloom KJ, Wakely PE, Spigos DG. Radiofrequency ablation of invasive breast carcinoma followed by delayed surgical excision. Cancer. 2003;98(7):1369–76. PubMed PMID: 14508822
37. Zhang J, Feng L, Zhang B, Ren J, Li Z, Hu D, Jiang X. Ultrasound-guided percutaneous microwave ablation for symptomatic uterine fibroid treatment – a clinical study. Int J Hyperth. 2011;27(5):510–6. doi:https://doi.org/10.3109/02656736.2011.562872. PubMed PMID: 21756048
38. Vogl TJ, Farshid P, Naguib NN, Zangos S, Bodelle B, Paul J, Mbalisike EC, Beeres M, Nour-Eldin NE. Ablation therapy of hepatocellular carcinoma: a comparative study between radiofrequency and microwave ablation. Abdom Imaging. 2015;40(6):1829–37. doi:https://doi.org/10.1007/s00261-015-0355-6. PubMed PMID: 25601438
39. Zhou W, Zha X, Liu X, Ding Q, Chen L, Ni Y, Zhang Y, Xu Y, Chen L, Zhao Y, Wang S. US-guided percutaneous microwave coagulation of small breast cancers: a clinical study. Radiology. 2012;263(2):364–73. doi:https://doi.org/10.1148/radiol.12111901. Epub 2012 Mar 21. PubMed PMID: 22438362
40. Peek MC, Ahmed M, Napoli A, ten Haken B, McWilliams S, Usiskin SI, Pinder SE, van Hemelrijck M, Douek M. Systematic review of high-intensity focused ultrasound ablation in the treatment of breast cancer. Br J Surg. 2015;102(8):873–82. doi:https://doi.org/10.1002/bjs.9793. discussion 882. Review. PubMed PMID: 26095255
41. Dowlatshahi K, Francescatti DS, Bloom KJ. Laser therapy for small breast cancers. Am J Surg. 2002;184(4):359–63. PubMed PMID: 12383903
42. van Esser S, Stapper G, van Diest PJ, van den Bosch MA, Klaessens JH, Mali WP, Borel Rinkes IH, van Hillegersberg R. Ultrasound-guided laser-induced thermal therapy for small palpable invasive breast carcinomas: a feasibility study. Ann Surg Oncol. 2009;16(8):2259–63. doi:https://doi.org/10.1245/s10434-009-0544-z. Epub 2009 Jun 9. PubMed PMID: 19506958; PubMed Central PMCID: PMC2711908.
43. Vilar VS, Goldman SM, Ricci MD, Pincerato K, Oliveira H, Abud TG, Ajzen S, Baracat EC, Szejnfeld J. Analysis by MRI of residual tumor after radiofrequency ablation for early stage breast cancer. AJR Am J Roentgenol. 2012;198(3):W285–91. doi:https://doi.org/10.2214/AJR.10.5581. PubMed PMID: 22358027
44. Cox K, Weeks J, Mills P, Chalmers R, Devalia H, Fish D, Sever A. Contrast-enhanced ultrasound biopsy of sentinel lymph nodes in patients with breast cancer: implications for axillary metastases and conservation. Ann Surg Oncol. 2016;23(1):58–64. doi:https://doi.org/10.1245/s10434-015-4606-0. PubMed PMID:25990967
45. Giuliano AE, Hunt KK, Ballman KV, Beitsch PD, Whitworth PW, Blumencranz PW, Leitch AM, Saha S, McCall LM, Morrow M. Axillary dissection vs no axillary dissection in women with invasive breast cancer and sentinel node metastasis: a randomized clinical trial. JAMA. 2011;305(6):569–75. doi:https://doi.org/10.1001/jama.2011.90. PubMed PMID: 21304082

New Technology and Techniques in Breast Reconstruction

7

Christine Velázquez and Ivo Alexander Pestana

Reconstruction Overview

The deformities commonly reconstructed include defects created by breast conservation surgery (BCS), or "lumpectomy," as well as the mastectomy defect resulting from the various forms of mastectomy. Regardless of the defect created, the goals of breast reconstruction remain consistent and include:

1. Creation of a breast mound that minimizes the perception of the breast deformity while using clothing
2. Use of techniques that do not hinder the diagnosis of new or recurrent breast disease
3. Employment of interventions that maintain patient quality of life similar to that prior to mastectomy

Techniques employed to achieve these goals include prosthetic-based procedures and tissue-based procedures.

C. Velázquez, MD (✉)
Department of General Surgery, Wake Forest University Baptist Medical Center, Medical Center Boulevard, Winston Salem, NC 27157, USA
e-mail: cvelazqu@wakehealth.edu

I.A. Pestana, MD, FACS
Department of Plastic and Reconstructive Surgery, Wake Forest University Baptist Medical Center, Medical Center Boulevard, Winston Salem, NC 27157, USA
e-mail: ipestana@wakehealth.edu

M. Howard-McNatt (ed.), *Changing Paradigms in the Management of Breast Cancer*, DOI 10.1007/978-3-319-60336-0_7

Implant-Based Breast Reconstruction

Dependent on the amount of remnant skin present at the completion of mastectomy, this technique most commonly involves at least two separate procedures. The first operation involves the placement of a tissue expander underneath the musculature of the anterior chest with or without the use of acellular dermal matrices (ADMs). This tissue expander is then accessed and inflated with saline or air every 1–2 weeks until the desired breast contour and volume is achieved. Once expansion is complete, the tissue expander is replaced with a permanent breast implant.

Benefits of this technique stem from the avoidance of scars on other parts of the body, quick recovery period, and shorter operations due to the technical ease of placing breast prosthetic devices. Disadvantages of the use of implants arise from the implant itself with common prosthetic problems including implant infection, malposition, rupture, and the development of capsular contracture.

Autologous Tissue Breast Reconstruction

Use of the patient's own tissue remains a common form of breast reconstruction. Donor sites employed are locations that frequently have excess soft tissue including the posterior thorax, abdomen, medial thighs, and upper or lower regions of the buttocks. Harvesting tissue from these sites allows for incisions to be well hidden in natural skin creases, which are obscured by standard undergarments and clothing.

The pedicled transverse rectus abdominis myocutaneous (pTRAM) flap and the latissimus dorsi myocutaneous (LDMC) flap remain the most commonly employed techniques for the creation of a breast with autogenous soft tissue. Benefits of autologous tissue breast reconstruction are the natural-appearing results that are associated with the utilization of vascularized soft tissue. Donor site morbidity such as muscle weakness and donor site contour irregularities are disadvantages associated with autologous reconstruction. In the case of the abdominal donor site, there remains a risk of ventral hernia or abdominal bulge in any intervention where the fascial system of the abdominal wall is interrupted. Due to the frequent paucity of excess soft tissue in the posterior thorax, the LDMC flap is commonly combined with the use of a breast prosthetic device to allow for the creation of a sufficient size breast mound.

Breast Reconstruction Decision-Making Process

Timing and technique are decisions made in planning breast reconstruction. Timing of breast reconstruction is considered "immediate" or "delayed." Immediate breast reconstruction is defined as the initiation of breast mound creation during the same operative episode as the mastectomy. This is commonly reserved for patients with benign breast disease or those with early-stage breast malignancies. Delayed breast

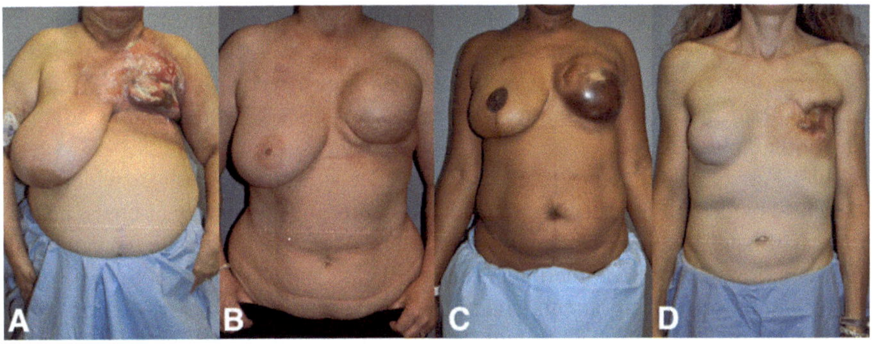

Fig. 7.1 Images demonstrating various forms of radiation injury affecting breast reconstruction. (**a**) Acute diffuse radiation injury characterized by erythema, edema, and desquamation of injured skin. (**b**) Fibrotic soft tissue coverage of underlying tissue expander preventing implant expansion. (**c**) Hyperpigmented and fibrotic skin with significant capsular contracture distorting the breast prosthesis. (**d**) Skin hyperpigmentation and contraction in association with poor wound healing and persistent wound after implant removal due to infection

reconstruction refers to breast mound creation once final pathology and adjuvant therapies are completed and typically occurs sometime after mastectomy.

The type and need for neoadjuvant and adjuvant therapies affect breast reconstruction decision-making. Previous chest irradiation and/or the need for post-mastectomy radiotherapy (PMRT) have a profound influence on both the timing and the technique used for reconstruction. Radiation of soft tissues results in fibrosis, decreased skin elasticity, skin hyperpigmentation, and telangiectasia development (Fig. 7.1). Radiated soft tissues are associated with derangements of the wound healing process resulting in a higher incidence of poor or delayed wound healing. Previous chest irradiation and loss of normal skin elasticity may prevent the ability to undergo tissue expansion to planned breast size and contour goals. Moreover, placement of a prosthetic device in the face of radiated chest soft tissues may result in poor wound healing and predispose the patient to implant exposure, infection, or prosthetic loss. Fibrotic soft tissues prevent the expansion of native skin to accommodate transferred autologous tissue and are commonly removed to allow for the creation of adequate breast mound size and contour.

Radiation following breast prosthetic placement is associated with a higher rate of complications, particularly capsular contracture [1]. Poor cosmetic result, expander extrusion, and eventual implant loss are all potential further complications. Patients receiving immediate implant reconstruction and subsequent radiation also have a high rate of reoperation for either correction of defects created by radiation or replacement of the reconstruction by an autologous flap [2]. Autogenous tissue utilized for breast reconstruction undergoes similar changes as native tissue when irradiated. Patients with radiated autologous breast reconstructions frequently require another flap to correct contour irregularities created by radiotherapy [3].

Due to the above, breast reconstruction should be delayed until after any planned radiation, if possible. In contrast, chemotherapy does not seem to increase the complication rate of implant-based or autologous breast reconstruction and may be safely performed on an immediate basis in patients who require adjuvant chemotherapy.

In the era of patient-centered care, a shared decision-making process which takes patient satisfaction into account is critical to improving the quality of breast healthcare. Ultimately, patient satisfaction in breast reconstruction is tied to the symmetry between breasts at the completion of reconstruction and is paramount to the process of technique selection. Patients undergoing unilateral breast reconstruction report higher patient satisfaction when autologous tissue techniques are employed for the unilateral reconstruction; however, bilateral mastectomy patients have equal satisfaction regardless of the technique chosen. This is due to the fact that breast symmetry is excellent when the same technique is used on both breasts [4].

New Techniques

Patient Education

Breast reconstruction options vary greatly and can be quite complex, making this a challenging decision for patients considering reconstruction. Preoperative patient education is one of the strongest predictors of patient satisfaction with breast reconstruction outcomes, and patient dissatisfaction with breast reconstruction information contributes to decision regret [5, 6]. Despite this understanding, approximately 20% of breast cancer survivors report they were never told about reconstruction [7]. Moreover, ethnic minority women appear to be the least informed about reconstruction [8]. Historically, breast reconstruction information was only available verbally and was provided by the oncologic surgeon or the reconstructive surgeon. Today, more information sources are available to mastectomy patients and include verbal, written, and digital/online options. Unfortunately, some of the most commonly used resources regarding breast reconstruction are written at a level that is too difficult for the average patient to understand [9]. In order to utilize patient education as a means to improve overall satisfaction, it is crucial not only to verify the quality and accuracy of resources provided but also to ensure that information is interpreted properly. Other factors affecting discussions regarding breast reconstructions include patient fear and anxiety regarding their diagnosis and oncologic management, cultural or language barriers, and the surgeon-patient relationship itself [5].

Currently, efforts are ongoing to maximize patient education and information quality by creating easy access, easy-to-use pre-consultation digital information regarding breast reconstruction that is then discussed and clarified during the meeting with the reconstructive surgeon. In order to reinforce information gained during the pre-consultation period and surgical consultation, opportunities for patients to speak to those who have completed the reconstruction process are becoming more common.

Patient Selection and Risk Management

Weight Loss and Its Role in Breast Reconstruction

Obesity, defined as a body mass index (BMI) above 30, is a worldwide epidemic. Selecting obese patients appropriate for breast reconstruction poses a challenge for the reconstructive surgeon due to the fact that this patient population is predisposed to other comorbidities (diabetes, hypertension, coronary artery disease, and lymphedema), as well as an increased risk of postoperative complications including seromas, skin and soft tissue infections, bronchopneumonia, and venous thromboembolism (VTE) [10]. In addition, operation-specific complications are more likely to occur in the obese patient. Understanding the risks associated with obese patients and each reconstruction option is critical to ensure a safe and appropriate method is chosen.

Implant-based breast reconstruction remains the most common type of breast reconstruction worldwide. When performed in the obese patient, there is a total complication rate ranging from 18 to 30%. The obese patient is twice as likely to suffer implant loss and seven times more likely to have reconstructive failure [11, 12]. Although flap survival rates are similar to autologous reconstruction in the nonobese patient, patients with a BMI >30 are significantly more likely to experience an abdominal donor site complication, including ventral hernias [13]. Examination of the NSQIP registry confirms an increased risk for postoperative morbidity in this patient population regardless of reconstruction technique [14].

Attempts to mitigate operative risk in the obese patient have included weight loss prior to operative intervention; however no clear evidence exists that this actually reduces postoperative complications [15]. Ozturk et al. examined 182 abdominal free flap-based breast reconstructions and reported significantly higher flap and donor site complications in obese patients than those with lower BMIs. Interestingly, the authors did not find preoperative weight loss to significantly reduce these complication rates [16]. Despite these results, obese patients should still be encouraged to lose weight prior to surgery due to the well-known health and psychological benefits of this practice and higher rates of patient satisfaction with respect to surgical outcomes [17].

Venous Thromboembolism (VTE) Risk Assessment

Postoperative venous thromboembolism (VTE) is a serious yet preventable disorder with the potential to cause short-term mortality and long-term morbidity. Early identification of VTE is critical to its successful management; however clinical signs are notoriously unreliable, which may lead to a delay in diagnosis [18, 19]. The potential for debilitating consequences secondary to VTE has fueled efforts to identify patients who are at high risk of VTE development and the institution of prophylactic measures when appropriate. The Caprini Risk Assessment Model (RAM) and guidelines provided by the American College of Chest Physicians (ACCP) have predominantly been applied to non-plastic surgical procedures to aid in identification of those patients who may benefit from chemical VTE prophylaxis. Recently, the Venous Thromboembolism Prevention Study (VTEPS) was completed in order to specifically apply the Caprini RAM as a screening tool to identify patients who would benefit from DVT prophylaxis after plastic and reconstructive surgical procedures. The Caprini RAM has been validated by the American Society of Plastic Surgeons (ASPS) and has been shown to decrease the rate of VTE events without an increased risk of postoperative bleeding complications. Similar to its use in non-plastic surgical procedures, a numerical score is assigned to each patient after review of different patient and operation-specific risk factors and recommends using chemical prophylaxis for "high risk" patients who have a Caprini score ≥7 [20].

Free Tissue Transfer Assessment

Preoperative Evaluation

Perforating vessels arising from the larger named blood vessels supplying the various breast reconstruction soft tissue donor sites have variations within an individual patient and among patients. Knowledge of these anatomic variations preoperatively aids in appropriate perforator selection and improves operative efficiency. Multiple diagnostic techniques including Doppler ultrasonography, computed tomography angiography (CTA), magnetic resonance angiography (MRA), and fluorescent angiography (FA) have been utilized to facilitate preoperative perforator mapping to provide reconstructive surgeons with invaluable information regarding vessel origin, caliber, branching patterns, and magnitude of flow [21, 22].

Doppler/duplex ultrasonography was first used in the 1990s to assist with perforator-based free flaps and is a cheap, widely available imaging modality that does not expose patients to radioactive or nephrotoxic contrast agents [23]. Despite these benefits, its known disadvantages include long study times, operator dependence, and the inability to reliably identify perforator caliber. Computed tomography angiography has supplanted ultrasound as the preferred method of preoperative perforator identification with sensitivities and specificities approaching 100% [24] (Fig. 7.2). Despite the established benefits of preoperative imaging with CTA, it can only provide a static view of the abdominal vasculature in its preoperative state, and it cannot provide information about flow within the perforators. In addition, radiation exposure and the potential to develop a contrast allergy may complicate the performance of this imaging test.

Magnetic resonance angiography has received recent attention as an option for perforator mapping [25]. The safer side effect profile of gadolinium and recent use of higher field strength scanners have improved the accuracy of MRA for perforator characterization [21]. With regard to perforator mapping, MRA has demonstrated high specificity when compared to CTA [26]. Furthermore, the image quality of MRA is generally considered to be inferior to that of CTA; however its muscle-to-vessel contrast ratio is excellent and most accurately delineates perforator intramuscular course. The disadvantages of MRA include its high cost, low availability, susceptibility to motion artifact, and limited capacity to detect perforators with a

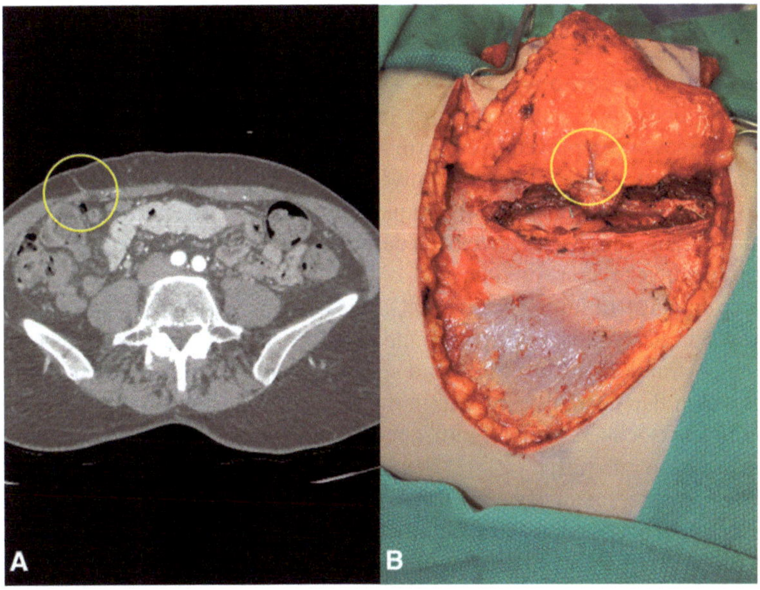

Fig. 7.2 (**a**) Computed tomography angiogram (CTA) image demonstrating right hemi-abdomen perforating vessels from the deep inferior epigastric pedicle. (**b**) Intraoperatively identified perforator correlating to preoperative perforator mapping with CTA

diameter <0.8 mm [25]. Although gadolinium is less likely to cause an anaphylactic reaction, it may produce nephrogenic systemic fibrosis limiting its use to a specific subset of patients including those with iodine allergies and impaired renal function. Additionally, MRA should be avoided in patients who are morbidly obese, those with pacemakers, and in patients who suffer from anxiety or claustrophobia.

Indocyanine green fluorescent angiography (ICGFA) is an accepted imaging technique newly applied to plastic and reconstructive surgery [27, 28]. This imaging technique allows direct visualization of macrovascular anastomoses, microvascular anastomoses, and tissue perfusion. The ICG fluorescent dye emits energy upon excitation by a light source (laser or LED light), which is then captured and recorded by a variety of image capture devices available creating real-time videos of blood flow and/or tissue perfusion. This unique feature allows images to be captured before, during, and after a flap is elevated, providing a live and continuous assessment of flap perfusion. Although the benefits of intraoperative fluorescent angiography are established, its role in the preoperative setting is being evaluated. A prospective study examining ICGFA perforator mapping of the abdominal wall in preparation for free tissue transfer breast reconstruction from the abdominal donor site demonstrated that skin blushes identified by ICGFA do not correlate with preoperative CTA or intraoperative perforator characteristics and therefore should not replace other forms of preoperative perforator mapping techniques [22].

Intraoperative Evaluation

Fluorescent Angiography (FA)

A growing body of literature supports intraoperative use of ICGFA. As discussed above, FA may be employed to confirm flow within vascular anastomoses. In addition, correlation between intraoperative FA and postoperative tissue perfusion-related complications has led to its frequent use in soft tissue perfusion assessment. Specific intraoperative uses have been described for both implant-based and autologous tissue breast reconstruction.

A common use of intraoperative ICGFA is determination of the viability of mastectomy skin flaps in the setting of immediate breast reconstruction. This technique has demonstrated high sensitivity and specificity in predicting postoperative mastectomy skin flap necrosis [29]. Similarly, Duggal et al. showed that intraoperative ICGFA was associated with a significant reduction in mastectomy skin flap necrosis and reoperation rate [30].

Perfusion assessment of breast reconstruction flap skin paddle and subcutaneous tissue is another common intraoperative use of ICGFA. Similar to its benefits in predicting skin loss for mastectomy flaps, ICGFA has been demonstrated to aid in intraoperative identification of poorly perfused portions of a flap, guiding soft tissue resection to minimize postoperative tissue loss [22].

Postoperative Evaluation

Implantable Doppler Monitoring

Loss of free tissue transplanted for breast reconstruction is a devastating complication. Intraoperative efforts to ensure flap survival are paramount and monitoring of these fragile procedures postoperatively is of equal importance. The goal of postoperative free flap monitoring is to maximize the potential for tissue salvage by focusing on early detection of microvascular complications before permanent flap injury occurs [31]. Although physical exam remains the gold standard for monitoring flap viability, early changes in a compromised flap can often be subtle. The use of adjunct technology can supplement clinical acumen and improve the accuracy and objectivity of flap monitoring.

The Cook-Swartz implantable Doppler system was first described by Swartz et al. in 1988 and pioneered real-time monitoring of blood flow through a vessel [32]. Continuous assessment of the microvascular anastomosis allows for early recognition of pedicle compromise. The Doppler consists of a 20 MHz ultrasonic Doppler crystal, a silicone cuff, and an external monitoring device. Intraoperatively, the probes may be placed on the vein, artery, or both. Direct pedicle monitoring is unique to this technique as other monitoring devices predominantly gauge flap viability through measurement of perfusion, oxygenation, or ischemia within the flap itself. Additionally, its invasive nature allows for the monitoring of buried flaps which are unexaminable from the body's surface. The success of this monitoring technique is measured by its ability to improve flap salvage/survival and decrease the rate of false-positive events, defined as a loss of signal without a true blood flow disruption [33]. Kind et al. evaluated a series of 147 free flaps monitored by implanted Doppler probe and reported a 100% rate of flap salvage with a 3.4% rate of false-positive events [34]. In addition, a meta-analysis of 547 patients demonstrated the Doppler probe to be a safe and effective monitoring technique after free flap reconstruction with a strong trend toward improved salvaged rates without increasing the rate of unnecessary reoperations [33]. The Flow Coupler is an advancement in the implantable Doppler probe concept as it represents a fusion between the venous coupler and a 20 MHz micro-Doppler probe and allows the surgeon to complete the microvascular anastomosis while simultaneously monitoring vascular patency [35, 36].

Several studies have demonstrated the implantable Doppler can be used as a trusted adjunct to clinical exam for close monitoring of blood flow after free flap reconstruction; however device implantation through placement of the cuff around the vein can be technically challenging and increase operative times [35]. Although published data regarding Flow Coupler is limited, its use can reliably identify a potential vascular crisis without requiring a separate procedure to apply the device.

Tissue Oximetry

Survival of microsurgical tissue transplants depends on tissue perfusion and oxygenation. Successful reperfusion of compromised flaps depends on early detection with quick reestablishment of blood flow. Flap salvage rates have an inverse relationship to the time interval marking the onset of ischemia and its clinical recognition. Tissue oximetry measurement using near-infrared spectroscopy is a noninvasive method of tissue monitoring and provides continuous, real-time numeric data in comparison to the qualitative information provided by the implantable Doppler [37]. The scattering and absorption of wavelengths of near-infrared light is measured by near-infrared spectroscopy and is related to the oxygen content of hemoglobin within the tissues being monitored. A surface probe is placed on the flap which allows measuring of the oxygen saturation within the cutaneous layer of the flap. The hemoglobin concentration of a flap is relatively constant; therefore changes in flap perfusion can be quickly detected prior to the development of obvious clinical signs [38]. Lin et al. support the routine use of tissue oximetry monitoring in postoperative patients, showing a significant decrease in the number of flaps requiring reoperation [39].

Mastectomy Modifications

Dramatic advancements have been made in the surgical management of breast malignancies since the introduction of the radical mastectomy by Halsted [40]. Radical mastectomy includes en bloc resection of the breast gland and skin, pectoralis muscles, and axillary lymph nodes in order to achieve local disease control. This approach successfully ensured patient survival but was associated with significant postoperative morbidity. Halsted's principles and radical mastectomy mark an important milestone in the history of breast cancer surgery and remained the standard surgical treatment for almost a century.

Over the last 50 years, the results of clinical trials as well as advancements in mammography and neoadjuvant therapies have helped revolutionize the surgical approach to breast cancer. Less aggressive versions of the radical mastectomy began to emerge starting with the modified radical mastectomy (MRM), also known as the non-skin-sparing mastectomy (NSSM) [41]. In contradistinction to the radical mastectomy, MRM removes all breast tissue and level I/II axillary lymph nodes while sparing the pectoralis musculature. By the early 1980s, it was established that BCS, consisting of wide local excision (lumpectomy) and subsequent radiation, has an equivalent survival rate when compared to mastectomy [42]. This observation, in addition to significantly decreased morbidity and improved cosmetic outcomes associated with BCS, secured its position as the treatment of choice for most low-grade invasive breast cancers for the past 20 years [43].

Despite the benefits of BCS, mastectomy rates in the early-stage breast malignancy population continue to rise [44]. The reason for this is likely multifactorial and includes the anxiety provoked by the need for prolonged surveillance, the perceived danger associated with a more conservative surgical approach, and prophylaxis required for patient populations at high risk for breast cancer development. In addition, surgical techniques have developed over the years, arming plastic and reconstructive surgeons with the ability to offer a variety of reconstructive options with excellent aesthetic results.

Skin-Sparing Mastectomy

The skin-sparing mastectomy (SSM) was developed in the early 1990s by Toth and Lappert and involves removal of the breast gland and nipple-areolar complex (NAC) while preserving the overlying skin envelope and inframammary fold (IMF) [45, 46]. Maintenance of these critical landmarks allows the breast to assume a more natural shape and contour and facilitates the process of immediate breast reconstruction with any technique [47]. Incision patterns employed in SSM are limited to the immediate periareolar skin and are easily concealed with completion of nipple reconstruction or areolar tattoo.

The goal of the breast surgeon in SSM is to secure negative margins and to provide optimal cosmetic results. The balance between the two depends on mastectomy skin flap thickness, which is recommended to be approximately 10 mm. The surgical literature has confirmed the oncologic safety of SSM, finding no significant difference in local recurrence or disease-free survival when compared to traditional mastectomy. The combination of SSM and immediate breast reconstruction is also safe in patients with advanced Stage IIB and III breast cancer [47].

Nipple-Sparing Mastectomy

First reported by Hinton in the 1980s, the nipple-sparing mastectomy (NSM) is more frequently used today and differs from the SSM by sparing the nipple-areolar complex (NAC). The NAC is a unique visual detail of a breast, and its preservation has proven to be a safe surgical option in a select group of patients, providing

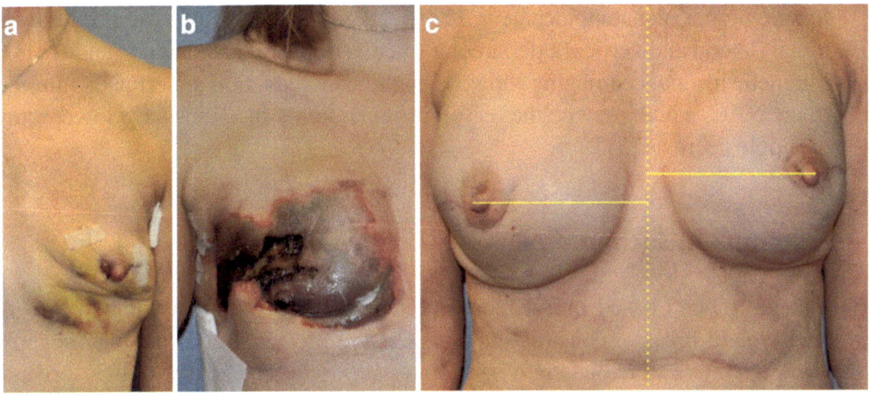

Fig. 7.3 Complications associated with nipple-sparing mastectomy (NSM). (**a**) Nipple ischemia demonstrated by inferior nipple mottling and desquamation. (**b**) Complete nipple and mastectomy skin flap necrosis. (**c**) Nipple areolar complex malposition

superior aesthetic outcomes and improved patient psychological well-being [48]. A recent systematic review highlights several factors that facilitate the process of appropriate patient selection to minimize breast cancer recurrence rates. These criteria include peripherally located tumors <5 cm in diameter, tumors located >2 cm from the NAC, lack of HER2 overexpression, and positive ER/PR status [49].

Common problems specific to NSM include nipple ischemia, partial or complete NAC loss, and nipple malposition (Fig. 7.3). Data regarding risk factors contributing to NSM complications are limited, conflicting, and variable, leading to a lack of consensus with respect to optimal surgical techniques. In light of this, Donovan et al. evaluated the effects of NSM incision location on rates of NAC ischemia, wound infection, and implant loss. There was an increased rate of NAC necrosis with use of periareolar incisions, while inframammary incisions had fewer ischemia-related compilations [50]. A retrospective review of 340 NSMs by a single surgeon over a 5-year period was completed to define specific and critical steps that should be utilized during NSM to reduce the risk of nipple necrosis and optimize cosmetic outcomes. The overall rate of nipple necrosis was reported to be 2.6%, with complete necrosis occurring in three cases (0.8%) and partial loss affecting six patients (1.8%) [51]. The authors recommend:

1. Preservation of major perforating vessels supplying the breast skin, specifically the second intercostal perforator off the internal mammary artery, which feeds the smaller vessels surrounding the nipple periphery.
2. Careful elevation of skin flaps in the plane between subcutaneous fat and breast glandular tissue, while keeping in mind that the thickness of the fat and of the skin flap changes with a tendency to become thicker as dissection proceeds away from the NAC. This subtle detail requires close attention to ensure dissection continues in the appropriate plane. Accidental deviation can lead to inadvertent thinning of the flap and ultimate vascular compromise.

3. Ensure proper incision placement. Three categories of incisions were described: radial (lateral and vertical), periareolar (medial or lateral extensions), and crease. Magnetic resonance imaging showed a significant reduction in perfusion inferior to the NAC, which may be the reason inframammary incisions have lower rates of nipple necrosis [51].

Breast Implant Technology

Two-stage implant-based breast reconstruction remains the most commonly performed type of breast reconstruction after mastectomy, as it does not significantly increase operative time or length of hospital stay, is a technically straightforward procedure performed through the mastectomy incision or scar, and may be performed in the outpatient setting (Fig. 7.4).

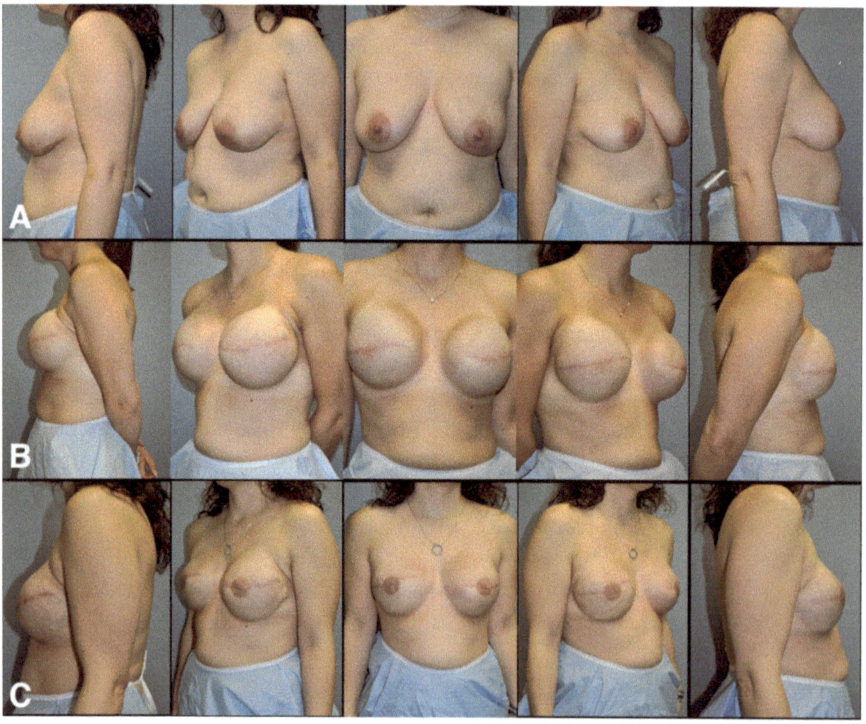

Fig. 7.4 Two-stage implant-based breast reconstruction. (**a**) 36-year-old female with left invasive ductal carcinoma managed with bilateral mastectomy and immediate submuscular tissue expander placement. (**b**) Fully inflated submuscular tissue expanders in preparation for exchange for final breast implants. (**c**) Patient at the completion of breast reconstruction with 500 cc smooth round moderate profile plus silicone gel breast implants, nipple reconstruction, and areolar tattoo

Tissue Expander Advances

The earliest of tissue expanders were designed by Dr. Chedomir Radovan and consisted of a silicone prosthesis with remotely placed valves/ports allowing for fluid injection in one port and its removal from the other [52]. Since then, breast tissue expanders have improved and have superior silicone shells and integrated filling ports. This type of expander is associated with lower infection rates and complications caused by using a remote valve/port such as valve flipping, tube kinking, and pain associated with repeated needle sticks for port access.

More recent technological advances in breast tissue expanders include changes in expander shape and the development of self-filling expanders. The round shape of initial expanders has been modified to a more anatomic or "tear-drop" shape, which allows for a more natural breast appearance as well as accommodation of shaped devices at the second stage. The geometry of this device allows for differential expansion and maximization of the lower pole of the breast. These expanders have produced lower complication rates with reported capsular contracture rate of 3%, infection rate of 1.2%, and no valve dysfunction [53]. Self-filling tissue expanders were introduced due to the theoretical benefit of fewer office visits for expansion, decreased number of needle sticks for implant access, and the potential for patient-controlled inflation of prostheses. They contain either an osmotic agent or gas to allow for progressive tissue expansion.

First-generation osmotic expanders were devised by Austed and Rose [54]. Rapid expansion of these expanders, which did not have an envelope, resulted in soft tissue ischemia at times. Modifications of early osmotic expanders, including integration of a silicone membrane, allow for safer, slower expansion speed. Vinyl pyrrolidone, an osmotic hydrogel, is the agent utilized within this type of expander producing migration of water through the silicone membrane of the device resulting in progressive expansion. This is in contrast to the self-inflating expander which use gas (CO2) for filling. This expander type includes a small cylinder which releases small amounts of gas into the expander allowing for progressive expansion. Gas-based self-filling expanders were introduced by Connell and have shown 100% expansion success rate with minor adverse events [55, 56].

Prosthesis Location Modifications

Recreation of the inframammary fold and maintenance of natural breast ptosis is the ultimate goal of breast reconstruction thus making expander shape and implant location of critical importance. Originally, breast tissue expanders were placed in the subcutaneous plane. This evolved to the preference of the subpectoral plane due to lower rates of capsular contracture which produced the firm, round, and unnatural appearance associated with subcutaneous placement. Subsequently, the partial submuscular plane was popularized due to the ability to place the prostheses lower on the chest wall augmenting lower pole expansion of the breast and accentuating the inframammary fold resulting in improved breast cosmesis. Currently, the inferolateral portions of the breast prosthesis are covered by the lateral inferior chest musculature (serratus anterior) or a form of dermal graft (see below).

Final Breast Implant Advances

The evolution of the contemporary breast prosthesis began with the "first-generation" silicone gel implant introduced by Cronin in 1962 and the first saline-filled breast implant by Arion in 1965. Since that time, both silicone gel and saline-filled implants have undergone several technical alterations and improvements to maximize safety and aesthetic results [57]. Saline implants are available as deflated devices which are to be filled with normal saline at the time of implantation. This allows for placement through a small incision as well as subtle size adjustments to be made at the time of surgery. These implants tend to be less popular than their silicone counterpart due to a less natural consistency similar to that of water compared to the more viscous natural breast tissue. In addition, overfilling may lead to a spherical shape and scalloping along the edge of the implant causing a firmer feel upon palpation.

Several versions of silicone gel implants have been developed since their introduction and differ with respect to the characteristics of the silicone gel filler, characteristics of the silicone shell surrounding the filler, and implant shape. Silicone is a mixture of polymeric molecules which can exhibit different physical properties depending on polymer chain length and degree of cross-linking between polymer chains [58]. There are two basic categories of silicone options available for use in breast implants, and they are termed "fluid form" and "form stable." The "fluid-form" liquid silicones are short polymers with very little cross-linking and have the consistency of oil [59]. They are usually used as surgical lubricants and are not cohesive enough to hold a given anatomic shape. When enough cross-linking is achieved, a more viscous "form-stable" silicone gel is created which allows the implant to maintain its dimensions and hold a given shape, affording the surgeon more control over the device. Technology exists to measure the cohesivity of silicone gel implants allowing measurement of implant stiffness. Form stability correlates with lower rates of capsular contracture, implant rupture, rippling, and improved patient satisfaction compared to low-cohesive fillings [60].

Extensive chemical cross-linking of the silicone gel polymers will create a solid form of silicone called an elastomer shell. Implant shell modifications, including barrier layers, have been introduced to protect the silicone gel filler. Shell characteristics, such as shell thickness, are important to consider as they contribute to the stability of implant shape. The maintenance of gel distribution within the implant shell helps to preserve this stability. The cohesivity of the gel and gel-shell fill ratio improves shape maintenance and varies among implant shapes. In addition to shell thickness, surface characteristics of the shell have undergone modifications with the ultimate goal of creating a surface texture that can minimize implant capsule formation [61]. The evolution of textured implants stemmed from the introduction of polyurethane-coated implants. These were foam-coated implants which were eventually dismissed due to concerns about possible carcinogenic conversion after chemical degradation of the foams. In the 1980s, a shift from foam-coated shells to textured silicone shells was made. Studies have shown that the pore size is critical to allow for tissue adherence leading to the adhesive effect of implant texturing and implant stabilization.

Round-shaped implants have been available for breast reconstruction since the 1980s and are described as having a "disk-like" shape. Several years later, anatomic or "tear-drop"-shaped implants were popularized outside of the United States and were subsequently approved by the FDA for use in the United States in 2013 [62]. Anatomic implants were developed to optimize the natural look of the reconstructed breast through implementation of a lower point of maximal projection resulting in a more prominent lower breast contour. They provide greater versatility and control of breast shape, which leads to a more "natural" aesthetic result. Although the anatomic, form-stable, silicone gel implants are gaining popularity, gel fracture and implant rotation are known risks associated with their use.

The "first-generation" prosthesis was anatomically shaped ("tear-drop"), filled with a viscous silicone gel, and covered with a smooth, thick outer silicone elastomer shell. In addition, they had Dacron fixation patches on their posterior aspect to maintain the proper position of the implant on the chest wall. The shell kept the liquid filler in one place creating a natural breast-like shape. Unfortunately, these devices had a high rate of capsular contracture due to the quality of the shells and the lack of cohesivity of the gel. Second-generation silicone gel implants were introduced about a decade later in attempts to address these complications. They were round in shape, had a thinner shell without Dacron patches, and were filled with a less viscous silicone gel. While these looked and felt more natural, the combination of the lower viscosity gel filler and permeable shell made them more likely to rupture and leak resulting in "gel bleed". The third-generation implants were developed in the 1980s to reduce the rate of implant rupture with subsequent gel migration by using a stronger multilayer silicone elastomer shell. Despite attempts to improve implant design, a moratorium on the use of third-generation silicone gel breast implants was issued by the FDA in 1992 in response to concern about the possible association between "gel bleed" and the development of connective tissue disorders. Subsequent studies and literature reviews failed to show this relationship, and restrictions on their use were lifted in 2006. The most recently designed silicone-filled breast implants are manufactured using the highest standards, concentrating on optimal shell thickness and gel cohesiveness to create a more natural feeling breast with reduced rates of complications [57]. Currently, fourth- and fifth-generation silicone implants are utilized. Fifth-generation implants have a more cohesive "form-stable" silicone gel and a textured surface and were manufactured with improved quality control allowing for several surface textures and implant shapes. Although they have been shown to be safe, a possible association between their use and anaplastic large-cell lymphoma (ALCL) was reported by the FDA in 2011. Although extremely rare, this finding must be reported to anyone considering having silicone breast implants.

Single-Stage Implant-Based Breast Reconstruction

Recently, single-stage implant-based breast reconstruction has been popularized [63]. This technique involves the insertion of the final breast implant at the time of the initial procedure (Fig. 7.5). The ability to perform single-stage

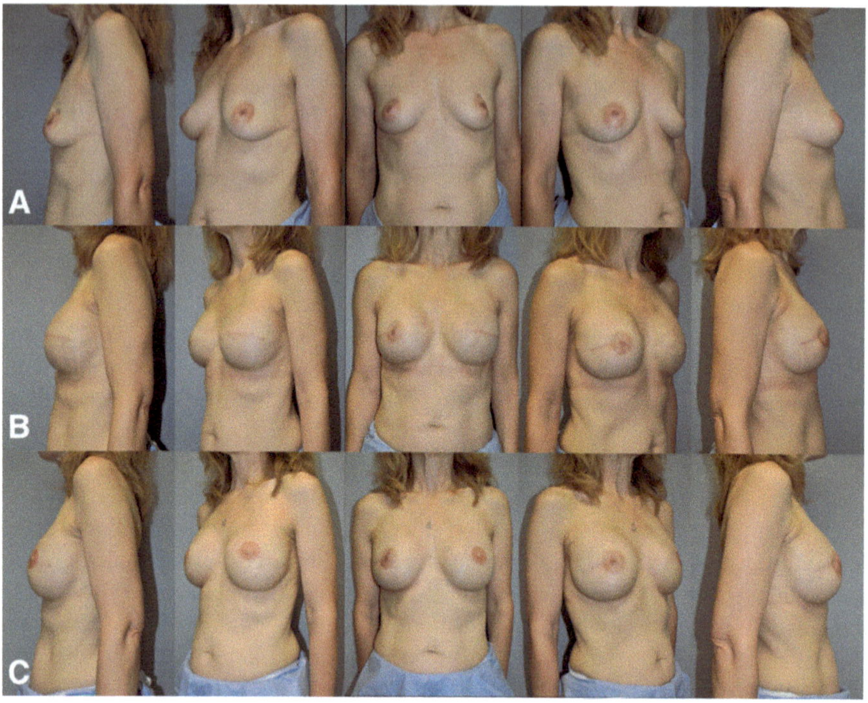

Fig. 7.5 Single-stage implant-based breast reconstruction. (**a**) 48-year-old female with left invasive ductal carcinoma managed with left skin sparing mastectomy, right prophylactic nipple-sparing mastectomy, and immediate bilateral submuscular 350 cc smooth round moderate profile plus silicone gel breast implants. (**b**) Postoperative appearance after single-stage implant-based breast reconstruction. (**c**) Patient at the completion of breast reconstruction with liposculpting (16 cc) of the right upper inner breast pole and left nipple reconstruction with C-V flaps and areolar tattoo

implant-based breast reconstruction depends on multiple factors. The amount and quality of the remaining mastectomy skin plays a large role in the ability to perform this operation safely in a single stage. To this end, the reconstructive surgeon must understand what surgical options the oncologic surgeon is willing to offer to each patient, as skin-sparing mastectomy, nipple-sparing mastectomy, and other advanced mastectomy techniques are not available at all institutions nor are they applicable to every individual. Likewise, the plan for adjuvant therapies, specifically any indications for PMRT, must be evaluated by the reconstructive surgeon due to the fact that radiotherapy significantly increases the risk of complications associated with prosthetic-based reconstruction. The immediate direct-to-implant reconstruction has been shown to reduce operating room time, cost, and potential added morbidity associated with a two-step expander/implant reconstruction and is ideal for certain patient populations allowing quicker return to normal daily activities [64].

Dermal Graft Utilization

The use of autologous dermal grafts in reconstructive surgery is not a new technique but one that has been recently applied in breast surgery. Implant-based breast reconstruction techniques have evolved from total submuscular coverage of the breast implant to a dual plane technique which leaves the lower third of the prosthesis/expander in a more superficial plane and only covered by mastectomy flaps. The use of autologous dermis or allogeneic acellular dermal matrices have been described to act as a "hammock" between the inferior border of the pectoralis major and inframammary fold. The benefits of autologous dermal tissue stem from the fact that it is not a foreign material, it is cheap, and it is readily available from common donor sites such as the abdomen.

The use of nonantigenic cadaveric human dermis or acellular dermal matrices (ADMs) to cover the lower pole of the implant expander was introduced in 2005 and has gained popularity due to an acceptable safety profile and improved breast aesthetics [65]. ADMs have provided a surgical option to address the previously reported challenges with two-staged breast reconstruction, including lack of total expander muscular coverage, low initial fill volumes, numerous outpatient visits, and poor inframammary fold definition, in addition to being available "off the shelf" obviating the need for a separate donor site. ADMs are soft tissue matrix grafts that are created by decellularization, leaving the extracellular matrix intact to function as a scaffold for cellular ingrowth and revascularization (Fig. 7.6). The tensile strength and low elasticity of acellular dermis allow tension to be applied preferentially to the graft during expansion instead of direct transmission to mastectomy flaps. The purpose of using ADMs in expander/implant reconstruction is to improve upon and maintain the goals of breast reconstruction including maintenance of inframammary fold and creation of breast ptosis. Inferior implant coverage with ADMs has the advantage of adding soft tissue thickness overlying the prosthesis reducing implant visibility, palpability, and increased initial fill volumes, therefore decreasing expansion duration. The use of ADMs may reduce the incidence of capsular contracture [66, 67].

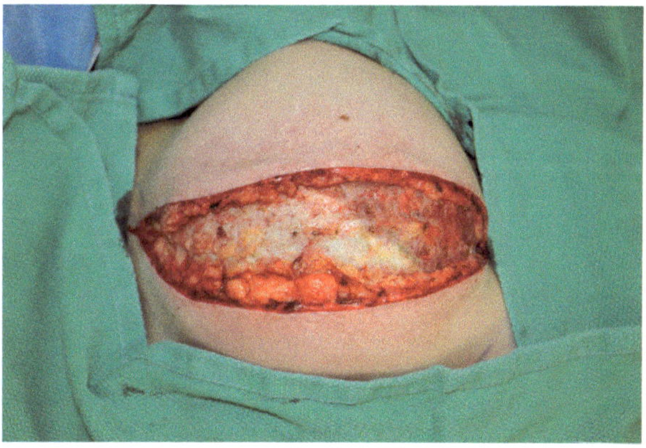

Fig. 7.6 Incorporated acellular dermal matrix interface with pectorals major musculature. Note the small blood vessels located on the superficial surface of the integrated ADM

Tissue Techniques

Oncoplastic Breast Surgery

Twenty to 30% of women who undergo BCS for breast cancer management will develop a breast contour irregularity that may require surgical correction. Oncoplastic breast surgery techniques were developed to address common deformities associated with BCS including segmental volume loss, nipple displacement, and breast asymmetry. In 1998, Dr. Werner Audretsch first coined the term "Oncoplastic Surgery" to describe a new surgical mindset in which the breast surgeon approaches the cancer patient with aesthetic principles guiding the surgical approach to the breast. Today, oncoplastic breast surgery is employed more frequently and combines the principles of oncologic and reconstructive surgery allowing partial breast reconstruction at the time of tumor resection and prior to breast irradiation, minimizing the potential for a BCS deformity. This type of surgery is most useful in candidates for lumpectomy who have large or ptotic breasts (Fig. 7.7).

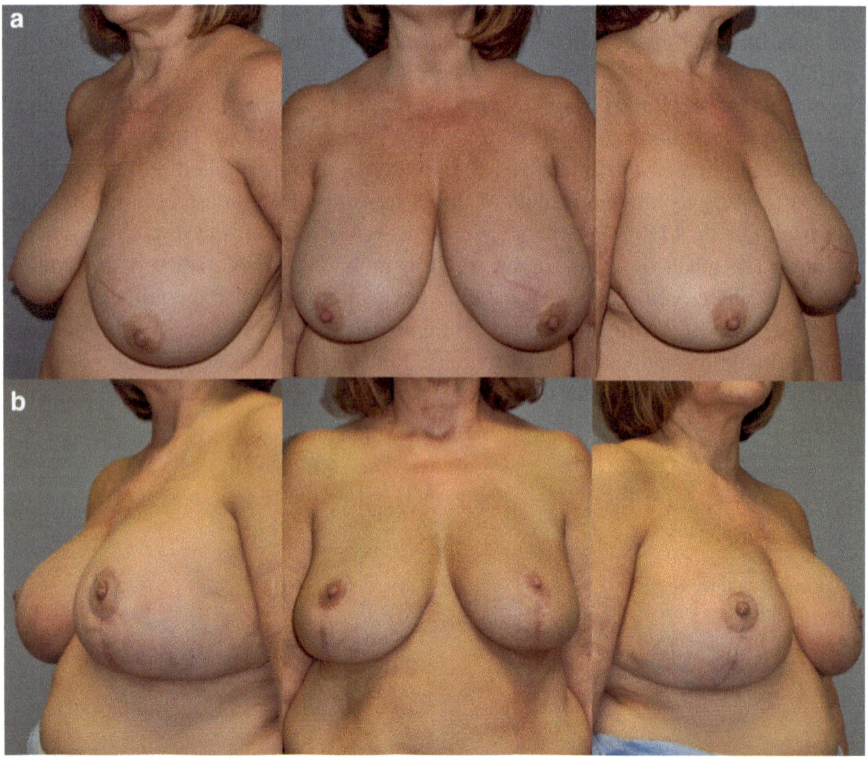

Fig. 7.7 (**a**) 50-year-old female with left invasive ductal carcinoma and bilateral symptomatic breast hypertrophy; note left breast upper inner pole healed breast biopsy site. (**b**) Patient with symmetrical and improved breast appearance after oncoplastic breast reduction. The nipple was transferred using the inferior pedicle located remotely from the upper inner quadrant malignancy extirpation zone

Oncoplastic breast interventions include a variety of accepted plastic surgical techniques which may be generally categorized into local tissue rearrangements, breast reduction/mastopexy techniques, and regional flaps. Local tissue rearrangement or breast remodeling techniques are frequently completed through circumareolar incisions providing surgical access to all regions of the underlying breast parenchyma. Once the tumor is resected, the surrounding soft tissues are plicated and the breast skin envelope is re-draped over the repaired breast mound. Breast reduction techniques utilize various designs of the dermoglandular vascular pedicle for nipple transposition as well as for tissue movement to fill in soft tissue defects created from lumpectomy. Finally, time-honored regional pedicled flaps such as the latissimus dorsi myocutaneous (LDMC) flap can be used when there is insufficient local breast tissue to reconstruct soft tissue deficits created by lumpectomy. Modification of the LDMC flap has been described such as partial LDMC flap, in which approximately half to one-third of the latissimus muscle is harvested along with overlying skin and subcutis and based on the distal branching pattern of the thoracodorsal pedicle. The thoracodorsal artery perforator (TDAP) flap is a further modification of this procedure to achieve similar volume-replacement goals. The TDAP flap is based on anatomic knowledge of the thoracodorsal artery perforosome and employment of microvascular techniques to dissect the thoracodorsal perforators from the surrounding latissimus musculature to the source thoracodorsal pedicle. The perforator flap provides similar adipocutaneous tissues as the muscle-containing flaps for breast volume replacement, and maintenance of the entire latissimus muscle with its motor innervation can help minimize upper extremity morbidity postoperatively.

Advances in Flap-Based Breast Reconstruction

The evolution of autogenous breast reconstruction is ongoing. Hartrampf and Dinner are considered the American forefathers of autologous breast reconstruction with the popularization of the pedicle transverse rectus abdominis myocutaneous (pTRAM) flap in the early 1980s [68]. Progress in angiosome and perforosome anatomic knowledge through preoperative imaging in conjunction with refinements in surgical technique have driven the ability of microvascular surgery to provide a variety of options for autologous breast reconstruction.

The TRAM flap can be transferred as either a pedicled flap, which is based on the superior epigastric system, or as a free flap, based on the deep inferior epigastric system. Still commonly used today, the pTRAM does not require microsurgery as the flap remains attached to the donor site using the rectus muscle as a vascular conduit to the recipient site. In contrast, the free TRAM (fTRAM) flap is completely detached from the abdomen and transferred to the mastectomy defect, requiring a microvascular anastomosis between the donor abdominal blood vessels and the recipient chest vascularity. Common recipient vessels utilized include the internal mammary or thoracodorsal vessels and, less frequently, the thoracoacromial and intercostal vessels.

The fTRAM is more technically challenging than its pedicled counterpart; however, for those experienced in microsurgery, the flap loss rate can be as low as 2% [69]. Free tissue transfer offers more predictable soft tissue perfusion with the ability to harvest smaller portions of muscle, translating to a decrease in abdominal donor site morbidity. The increasing interest to maximize muscle preservation led to the development of several "muscle-sparing" techniques, which differ with respect to the amount of rectus abdominis that is preserved [70]. Free tissue transferred from the abdominal donor site may be classified based upon the branching patterns of the deep inferior epigastric pedicle within the rectus abdominis, which is generally divided into three longitudinal segments – medial, lateral, and central. The MS-0 flap refers to the conventional fTRAM and involves harvesting the entire width of muscle. The MS-1 flap spares the medial or lateral segment of muscle, and the MS-2 flap includes only the portion of muscle lying between the medial and lateral row perforators. The MS-3, or deep inferior epigastric perforator (DIEP) flap, contains absolutely no muscle [70]. Nahabedian et al. compared the MS-2 and MS-3 (DIEP) fTRAMs and showed improved abdominal contour and strength with the DIEP flap [71, 72]. Additionally, the incidence of abdominal bulge was significantly lower after bilateral reconstruction with DIEP flaps (4.5%) when compared to the MS-2 flaps (21%). Studies continue to report favorable outcomes with muscle-sparing versions of abdominal free flaps, which has popularized the use of perforator-based free flaps in breast reconstruction [71, 72].

In certain cases, the abdominal adipocutaneous tissues may be predominantly supplied by the superficial inferior epigastric artery and vein (SIEAV) allowing harvest of the SIEAV flap. Benefits associated with the use of the SIEAV flap include less tedious operative dissection, and the abdominal wall does not require interruption. Although it is technically easier to harvest compared to DIEP or MS-TRAM, SIEAV flaps are associated with small caliber vessels for microvascular anastomosis, limited cutaneous territory perfused by this pedicle, increased rates of fat necrosis, and a higher rate of "redo" microvascular anastomoses.

Several studies have compared the MS-TRAM, SIEAV, and DIEP flaps in attempts to better understand the risks and benefits associated with each technique. Patient selection, anatomic considerations, harvesting techniques, and clinical outcomes should guide the ultimate decision on which method is best for the patient. Wu et al. compared donor site morbidity among the three using a patient questionnaire. The SIEAV flap received the highest scores with respect to improved postoperative lifting and shorter duration of abdominal pain. There was a significant increase in the ability to get out of bed following bilateral SIEAV flaps. The same group also investigated the incidence of total or partial flap loss and frequency of fat necrosis between the MS-TRAM, DIEP, and SIEAV flaps [73]. When techniques were compared, a marginal difference in flap loss was identified between techniques; however the MS-TRAM was noted to have a higher rate of abdominal wall hernias and a lower rate of fat necrosis when compared to the DIEP flap [73].

Breast volume replacement is usually achieved through abdominal-based free tissue transfer, exemplified by the TRAM, DIEP, and SIEAV flaps described above. However, a surgeon may consider an alternative donor site when the abdomen is not a suitable option, such as when a significant volume of soft tissue is required to recreate breasts or the presence of midline scars, which limit the ability to include contralateral zones. When the abdomen is not used as a donor site, the gluteal or thigh region can be considered. In comparison to the abdomen, these sites have smaller amounts of adipose tissue available for reconstruction making them ideal to use in patients who have small- to moderate-sized breasts.

The buttocks are usually a suitable alternative for reconstruction given that most women have sufficient gluteal adiposity available. Its location has the added benefit of minimal donor site morbidity and the ability to easily hide scars. This flap is known for being extremely durable and is recommended to women who lack sufficient abdominal soft tissue; however it is firmer than abdominal-based flaps due to the intrinsic quality of gluteal adipose tissue [74]. The superior gluteal artery perforator (SGAP) lies in the upper buttock above the piriformis muscle whereas the inferior gluteal artery perforator (IGAP) lies in the lower buttock, and both are commonly harvested without muscle. Both can pose a challenge technically due to short vascular pedicles and small arterial caliber.

The medial and posterior thigh regions have shown success as donor sites in the setting of microvascular breast reconstruction with benefits including the use of an expendable muscle and a well-hidden donor site. The transverse upper gracilis (TUG) flap is a medially based thigh flap and is ideal for reconstruction of small- to medium-sized breasts, given the limited volume of tissue in the area. It is based on the medial femoral circumflex branch of the profunda femoris artery. The medial thigh can be an advantageous donor site for patients with excess skin and fat (Fig. 7.8). In a report of 111 patients undergoing the TUG flap for breast reconstruction, Scholler et al. reported the ability to obtain a mean of 330 cc of adipose for breast volume replacement; however limitations of its use stem from concerns about short pedicle length and inadequate vessel caliber, similar to the gluteal flaps [75].

The profunda artery perforator (PAP) flap is based off the profunda femoris artery and vein and has several associated perforators within the posterior compartment of the thigh. It was first described by Hurwitz in 1980 and, after several modifications, eventually used as a form of breast reconstruction in 2010 [76]. Studies show the ability to consistently find a dominant perforator with sufficient length through use of preoperative imaging. Relative disadvantages of the PAP flap are due to size of the flap and inconvenience of donor site location, which may cause widening of the surgical scar and contour deformities of the lower buttock [76].

Flap Innervation

The sensory nerves supplying the breast are transected during mastectomy resulting in a reconstructed breast that is less sensitive than its native counterpart. Early priorities of breast surgery primarily focused on providing a safe oncologic surgery with acceptable cosmetic results. However, as surgical techniques continue to improve outcomes, patient demands and expectations continue to rise. It is clear that preservation of sensation to the new breast is becoming an increasingly important measure of patient quality of life and serves as the impetus behind recent investigations and efforts to neurotize flaps.

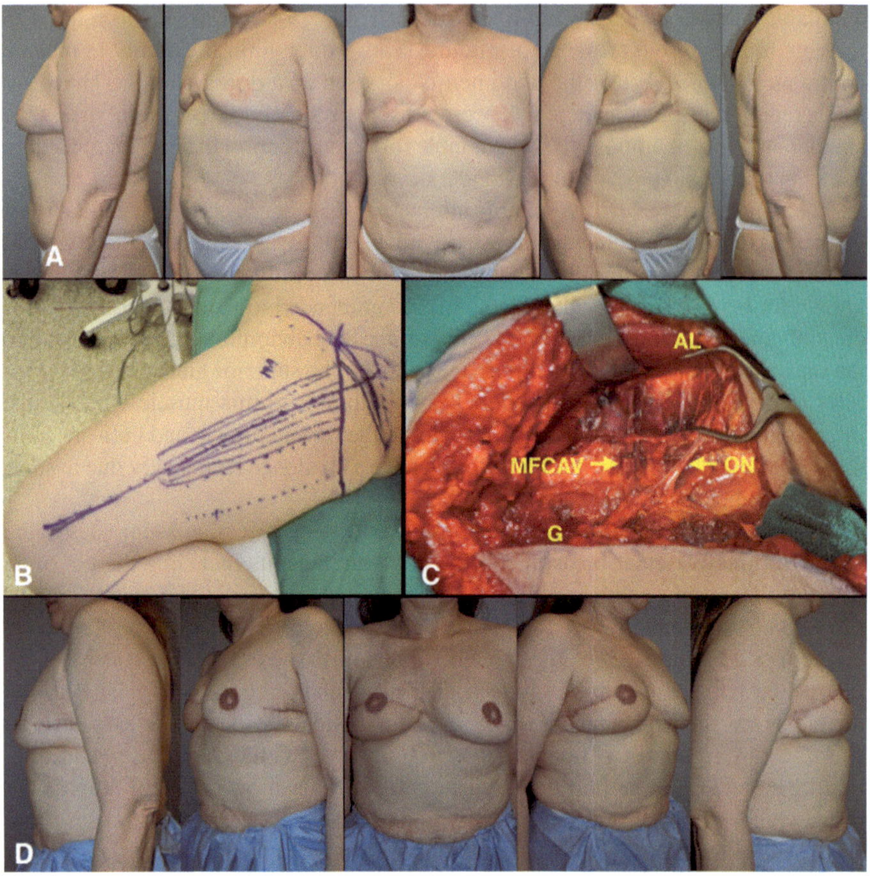

Fig. 7.8 (**a**) Female patient with a history of right breast cancer managed with bilateral mastectomy and autologous reconstruction from the abdominal donor site. The patient required postoperative radiotherapy of the right breast resulting in a contracted right breast reconstruction and patient dissatisfaction with the reconstruction result. Since the abdominal donor site had been previously utilized, the patient underwent transverse upper gracilis (TUG) free tissue transfer revision of her right breast reconstruction. (**b**) Preoperative markings for right TUG flap. (**c**). Intraoperative image of dissected flap. *AL* adductor longus, *G* gracilis, *ON* obturator nerve, *MFCAV* medial femoral circumflex artery and vein. (**d**) Postoperative outcome after free tissue transfer revision of autologous reconstruction and bilateral nipple and areolar revision with tattoo

Studies have documented the spontaneous return of sensation after reconstruction; however the timing and amount of recovery are highly variable and difficult to predict. In addition, the significant increase in operative time required to successfully achieve nerve transfer has been regarded as risky and inefficient. In general, nerve preservation and restoration are not routinely performed during breast reconstruction.

A pilot study done in 2013 by Margarakis et al. looked at the impact of different types of breast reconstruction (DIEP versus implants) and radiation therapy on the return of sensation. Their study concluded that, without irradiation, skin over an implant had better sensation; however, skin overlying a DIEP flap with irradiation recovered better than skin over implants [77].

Traditional attempts of neurotization during abdominal free tissue transfer used the lateral cutaneous branch of the fourth intercostal nerve, which is inconveniently located in a separate microsurgical field. Spiegal et al. proposed a new, more efficient method of neurotization during DIEP flaps using the anterior branch of the third intercostal nerve, which can reliably be found at the junction of the inferior portion of the third rib and sternum. It is located within the same microsurgical field during dissection of the internal mammary vessel and can easily be incorporated into the flap inset. Flap neurotization results in recovery of breast sensibility that is statistically better when compared to flaps without nerve coaptation as well as when compared to the mastectomy skin surrounding the flap [78]. This method may provide an experienced microsurgeon with a means to perform neurotization and contribute to patient satisfaction without significantly affecting time in the operating room.

Stacked Flaps

In some cases of breast reconstruction, a single-pedicle flap will not provide sufficient tissue required for adequate breast volume replacement [79]. A recently popularized technique for resolution of this problem is the use of "stacked" flaps consisting of multiple flap free tissue transfer configurations. Soft tissue flaps from well-accepted donor sites are raised on their individual vascular pedicles, and subsequently these pedicles are anastomosed producing blood flow through both flaps [80]. The flaps are then organized into a layered or folded configuration producing a more voluminous breast mound composed of multiple "stacked" flaps. These flaps are especially helpful in thin patients and those with abdominal scars. Several classification systems for pedicle arrangements have been developed and describe the different options for crossover anastomoses. When stacked DIEP flaps are not possible, the buttock and thigh flaps have been used as alternatives. Murray et al. used preoperative perforator mapping and created a classification system based on their experience with the technique. Although more technically demanding than the standard approach, stacked flaps can have good outcomes with proper preoperative planning with imaging, as well as knowledge about the vascular options available [81].

Fat Grafting

Fat grafting or "liposculpting" in breast reconstruction provides a versatile tool to further improve the shape, contour, and natural feel of a reconstructed breast. While fat grafting is becoming increasingly more popular, its use in breast reconstruction was initially discouraged due to concerns regarding the unknown risk of carcinogenesis and radiologic changes after the procedure. Since then, research has consistently demonstrated that fat grafting is not only safe but very durable. Furthermore, use of fat grafting in breast reconstruction has shown no long-term risk of cancer recurrence [82]. Although fat grafting has been demonstrated to be safe from an oncologic standpoint, minor abnormalities may be seen on breast imaging after breast reconstruction and fat grafting. These findings are commonly benign in nature and usually do not require further evaluation with biopsy [83]. A retrospective study by Kaoutzanis et al. found that only 2.4% of patients who underwent breast imaging after fat grafting required biopsy for suspicious findings [84]. The increasing body of evidence demonstrating the benefits of combining fat grafting and breast reconstruction led to the acceptance of this combination strategy in 2009.

The Coleman technique, pioneered and popularized by Dr. Sydney Coleman, is the most popular method of fat grafting and calls for meticulous, labor-intensive harvesting, processing, and injection of fat using small aliquots to maximize access to blood supply and improve graft viability [85]. The Coleman technique harvests 10-mL fat at a time using gentle, hand-applied low power suction (10-mL syringe) through a two-hole harvest cannula (17-gauge). Once the desired volume has been obtained, the syringe is replaced with a Luer-Lok cap. Lipoaspirate is then centrifuged at 3000 rpm for 3 minutes, yielding a mixture of oil, fat, and serum. The oil and serum are discarded, and the lipoaspirate is aliquoted to 1-mL or 3-mL syringes and injected into recipient sites gently upon withdrawal of the injection cannula. At least 3 months are required to complete fat engraftment, and during this period, graft volume is reduced by an amount ranging from 10 to 50%. The number of sessions required to achieve desired volume depends on the amount of adipose required for reconstruction, which can vary.

Graft survival is critical to the success of liposculpting. Several factors have been identified as potentially important determinants of graft viability including the cell type transferred (stem cells, adipocytes, stromal vascular fraction cells), prevention of trauma to adipocytes during harvest and application, graft preparation technique, and exclusion of noxious stimuli during preparation of the lipoaspirate [85].

Fat is a known reservoir of regenerative precursor cells termed adipose-derived regenerative cells (ADRC). These precursor cells have been identified in lipoaspirates and increase the survival of fat grafts by promotion of angiogenesis and a decrease in apoptosis as a response to released growth factors [86]. Rigotti et al. have demonstrated a benefit of applying fat containing adipose-derived stem cells beneath radiated tissue, which supports the healing process, improving quality of skin. The RESTORE-2 trial is the first prospective, multicenter clinical trial which evaluated the use of ADRC-enriched fat grafts to treat breast deformities following lumpectomy with or without radiation. In addition to using fat simply as a filler, the regenerative work of Rigotti et al. has demonstrated a significant reversal in radiation damage after fat grafting. Fat, not acting simply as a filler, may have a regenerative effect and may aid in the reversal of the radiation fibrosis and scarring [87].

Fat harvest is completed with the use of aspiration cannulas, a form of negative pressure creates the aspiration force, and with or without the use of tumescent solutions. Common cannula sizes for harvest range from 3 to 6 mm, and options for aspiration forces include syringe aspiration and the various forms of suction-assisted lipectomy (standard, power-assisted, ultrasound-assisted). Gravity separation, centrifugation, washing, and filtration are available fat graft processing/preparation methods. Fat graft application is accomplished with small-gauge application cannulas. Despite the expanding body of knowledge regarding the above factors, there remains a high degree of discordance on fat grafting techniques due to the inconsistent results from animal studies and human experiments. In clinical practice, one technique is clearly not superior to any other technique when all the data are considered [88].

The earliest application of breast reconstruction fat grafting was as an adjunct used to improve breast contour after implant-based reconstruction or to correct lumpectomy defects. Its initial success led to its use for increasing overall breast volume or focal breast volume deficits in patients who had already undergone autologous reconstruction [89]. Small to moderate volume fat transfers typically show good results and set the stage for the development of newer techniques to allowing transfer of large amounts of autologous fat. The BRAVA technique, pioneered by Dr. Roger Khouri, aims to establish a safe and efficient method of large volume ("mega-volume") autologous fat transfer for total breast reconstruction providing an alternative to implant and flap-based breast reconstruction [90]. BRAVA technique employs an external expansion device prior fat transfer into the breast. Proponents of the technique theorize that the mechanical forces caused by external expansion stimulate angiogenesis in addition to augmenting physical space for fat transfer. The concept of BRAVA expansion is similar to that employed by negative pressure wound therapy (NPWT) which exerts micromechanical forces to wound edges causing deformation of tissues. These deformational forces stimulate growth factor release which promote cell stretch, proliferation/division, and angiogenesis [91]. The authors postulate that the BRAVA technique enhances fat grafting through provision of *B*igger potential spaces available for the overall volume of the graft; *R*eduction of the demand on adipocytes to act as internal expanders, which may result in undue pressure; *A*ugmentation of the tension on internal constrictions and scars, to better address breast shape; elimination of *V*ariables that are time-consuming (i.e., centrifugation); and promotion of the *A*ngiogenesis effect, which may increase the oxygen supply to the recipient site and lead to better graft take.

In summary, fat transfer is a safe method and versatile tool for adding soft tissue volume in both implant-based and autologous reconstruction. Currently, mega-volume autologous fat grafting for breast reconstruction is being studied and may provide yet another option for total breast reconstruction.

Nipple Reconstruction

Recreation of the nipple and areola makes many women feel as though the journey through breast cancer management is complete and has significant psychological and emotional benefits [92]. Techniques for nipple reconstruction have remained relatively constant as breast reconstruction technology and techniques have evolved to their current status. The nipple is most commonly created using a variety of well-described local tissue rearrangements (Skate flap, star flap, C-V flap) and their modifications to produce a papule that projects 3–5 mm from the breast mound. The most recent advances in nipple reconstruction have developed from identification of

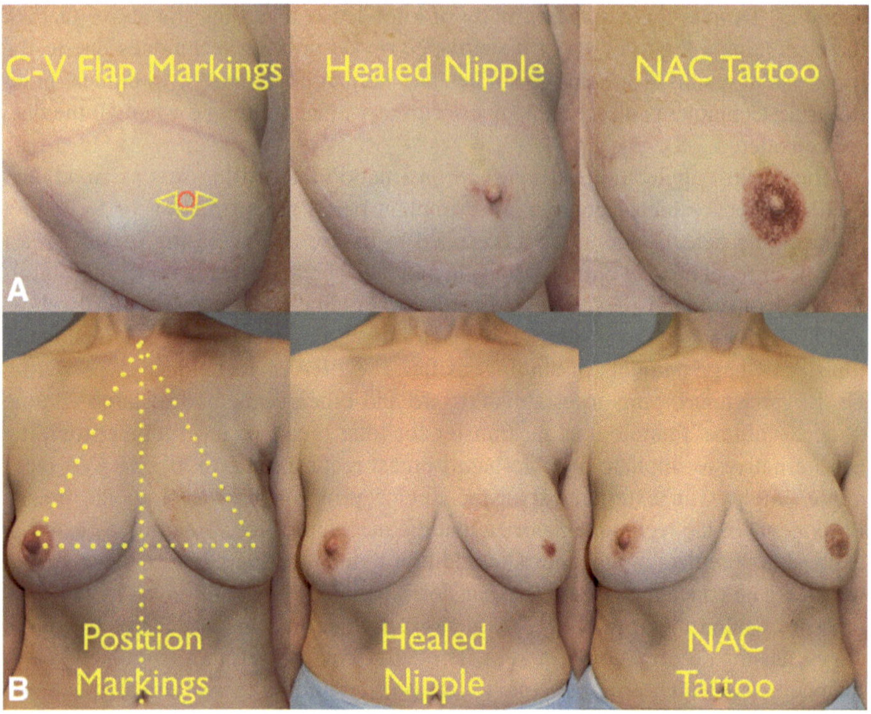

Fig. 7.9 (**a**) Sequence of nipple areolar reconstruction including markings for C-V flap technique. Note the use of various pigment hues to produce contrast which amplify nipple projection appearance as well as create a more natural appearance of the reconstruction. (**b**) Nipple-sharing technique markings and sequence of procedures completed with areolar tattoo. No secondary procedures were required for nipple projection and no pigment was needed for papule color

risk factors associated with poor outcomes in nipple areola complex (NAC) reconstruction, re-popularization of the nipple-sharing technique, and refinement in tattoo techniques (Fig. 7.9a).

A review of over 600 nipple reconstructions demonstrated higher rates of nipple projection problems with specific types of flaps such as the skate flap. Furthermore, the combination of radiotherapy and implant-based breast reconstruction translates to higher incidence of nipple reconstruction problems [93]. With the decreasing threshold for the use of post-mastectomy radiotherapy as well as an increase in reconstructions that have been radiated, the nipple-sharing technique has been re-popularized (Fig. 7.9b). Random pattern flap creation from thin irradiated skin overlying a prosthetic device is contraindicated. Nipple sharing allows the addition of contralateral nipple tissue with minimal manipulation of the reconstructed breast soft tissues and therefore should be especially considered an option in this patient population [94]. Finally, application of the artistic principles of contrast and shadowing has improved the aesthetic appearance of NAC reconstructions and improved patient satisfaction with the process [95].

Conclusion

Despite available techniques and federal support, there are patients who opt for no reconstruction or who are not surgical candidates. Preoperative patient assessment and stringent patient selection allow the identification of those patients who may be better served with a less complex reconstructive technique or those that should not be offered reconstructive interventions. Advances in breast reconstruction techniques, as well as the development of new ones, have led to decreased time to completion of reconstructive process, improved patient safety, excellent aesthetic outcomes, and higher patient satisfaction with the reconstructive process. Current techniques ensure that the vast majority of people who desire reconstruction after mastectomy will be able to be reconstructed with the goal of a balanced and aesthetic result.

References

1. Vandeweyer E, Deraemaecker R. Radiation therapy after immediate breast reconstruction with implants. Plast Reconstr Surg. 2000;106(1):56–8. discussion 9–60
2. Spear SL, Onyewu C. Staged breast reconstruction with saline-filled implants in the irradiated breast: recent trends and therapeutic implications. Plast Reconstr Surg. 2000;105(3):930–42.
3. Tran NV, Chang DW, Gupta A, Kroll SS, Robb GL. Comparison of immediate and delayed free TRAM flap breast reconstruction in patients receiving postmastectomy radiation therapy. Plast Reconstr Surg. 2001;108(1):78–82.
4. Shaikh-Naidu N, Preminger BA, Rogers K, Messina P, Gayle LB. Determinants of aesthetic satisfaction following TRAM and implant breast reconstruction. Ann Plast Surg. 2004;52(5):465–70. discussion 70
5. Ho AL, Klassen AF, Cano S, Scott AM, Pusic AL. Optimizing patient-centered care in breast reconstruction: the importance of preoperative information and patient-physician communication. Plast Reconstr Surg. 2013;132(2):212e–20e.
6. Zhong T, Hu J, Bagher S, O'Neill AC, Beber B, Hofer SO, et al. Decision regret following breast reconstruction: the role of self-efficacy and satisfaction with information in the preoperative period. Plast Reconstr Surg. 2013;132(5):724e–34e.
7. Morrow M, Mujahid M, Lantz PM, Janz NK, Fagerlin A, Schwartz K, et al. Correlates of breast reconstruction: results from a population-based study. Cancer. 2005;104(11):2340–6.
8. Alderman AK, Hawley ST, Janz NK, Mujahid MS, Morrow M, Hamilton AS, et al. Racial and ethnic disparities in the use of postmastectomy breast reconstruction: results from a population- based study. J Clin Oncol. 2009;27(32):5325–30.
9. Vargas CR, Kantak NA, Chuang DJ, Koolen PG, Lee BT. Assessment of online patient materials for breast reconstruction. J Surg Res. 2015;199(1):280–6.
10. Choban PS, Flancbaum L. The impact of obesity on surgical outcomes: a review. J Am Coll Surg. 1997;185(6):593–603.
11. Woerdeman LA, Hage JJ, Hofland MM, Rutgers EJ. A prospective assessment of surgical risk factors in 400 cases of skin-sparing mastectomy and immediate breast reconstruction with implants to establish selection criteria. Plast Reconstr Surg. 2007;119(2):455–63.
12. McCarthy CM, Mehrara BJ, Riedel E, Davidge K, Hinson A, Disa JJ, et al. Predicting complications following expander/implant breast reconstruction: an outcomes analysis based on preoperative clinical risk. Plast Reconstr Surg. 2008;121(6):1886–92.
13. Vyas RM, Dickinson BP, Fastekjian JH, Watson JP, Dalio AL, Crisera CA. Risk factors for abdominal donor-site morbidity in free flap breast reconstruction. Plast Reconstr Surg. 2008;121(5):1519–26.

14. Hanwright PJ, Davila AA, Hirsch EM, Khan SA, Fine NA, Bilimoria KY, et al. The differential effect of BMI on prosthetic versus autogenous breast reconstruction: a multivariate analysis of 12,986 patients. Breast. 2013;22(5):938–45.
15. Wolf AM, Kuhlmann HW. Reconstructive procedures after massive weight loss. Obes Surg. 2007;17(3):355–60.
16. Ozturk CN, Kundu N, Bernard S, Cooper K, Ozturk C, Djohan R. Breast reconstruction with abdominal-based free flaps in high body mass index population: postoperative complications and impact of weight loss. Ann Plast Surg. 2014;72(1):13–22.
17. Larson KE, Ozturk CN, Kundu N, Cooper KR, Bernard S, Djohan R. Achieving patient satisfaction in abdominally based free flap breast reconstruction: correlation with body mass index subgroups and weight loss. Plast Reconstr Surg. 2014;133(4):763–73.
18. Kearon C. Natural history of venous thromboembolism. Circulation. 2003;107(23 Suppl 1):I22–30.
19. Pannucci CJ, Chang EY, Wilkins EG. Venous thromboembolic disease in autogenous breast reconstruction. Ann Plast Surg. 2009;63(1):34–8.
20. Pannucci CJ, Bailey SH, Dreszer G, Fisher Wachtman C, Zumsteg JW, Jaber RM, et al. Validation of the Caprini risk assessment model in plastic and reconstructive surgery patients. J Am Coll Surg. 2011;212(1):105–12.
21. Chae MP, Hunter-Smith DJ, Rozen WM. Comparative analysis of fluorescent angiography, computed tomographic angiography and magnetic resonance angiography for planning autologous breast reconstruction. Gland Surg. 2015;4(2):164–78.
22. Pestana IA, Zenn MR. Correlation between abdominal perforator vessels identified with preoperative CT angiography and intraoperative fluorescent angiography in the microsurgical breast reconstruction patient. Ann Plast Surg. 2014;72(6):S144–9.
23. Giunta RE, Geisweid A, Feller AM. The value of preoperative Doppler sonography for planning free perforator flaps. Plast Reconstr Surg. 2000;105(7):2381–6.
24. Scott JR, Liu D, Said H, Neligan PC, Mathes DW. Computed tomographic angiography in planning abdomen-based microsurgical breast reconstruction: a comparison with color duplex ultrasound. Plast Reconstr Surg. 2010;125(2):446–53.
25. Masia J, Kosutic D, Cervelli D, Clavero JA, Monill JM, Pons G. In search of the ideal method in perforator mapping: noncontrast magnetic resonance imaging. J Reconstr Microsurg. 2010;26(1):29–35.
26. Rozen WM, Stella DL, Bowden J, Taylor GI, Ashton MW. Advances in the pre-operative planning of deep inferior epigastric artery perforator flaps: magnetic resonance angiography. Microsurgery. 2009;29(2):119–23.
27. Newman MI, Samson MC. The application of laser-assisted indocyanine green fluorescent dye angiography in microsurgical breast reconstruction. J Reconstr Microsurg. 2009;25(1):21–6.
28. Pestana IA, Coan B, Erdmann D, Marcus J, Levin LS, Zenn MR. Early experience with fluorescent angiography in free-tissue transfer reconstruction. Plast Reconstr Surg. 2009;123(4):1239–44.
29. Newman MI, Samson MC, Tamburrino JF, Swartz KA. Intraoperative laser-assisted indocyanine green angiography for the evaluation of mastectomy flaps in immediate breast reconstruction. J Reconstr Microsurg. 2010;26(7):487–92.
30. Duggal CS, Madni T, Losken A. An outcome analysis of intraoperative angiography for postmastectomy breast reconstruction. Aesthet Surg J. 2014;34(1):61–5.
31. Chang EI, Chang EI, Soto-Miranda MA, Zhang H, Nosrati N, Crosby MA, et al. Comprehensive evaluation of risk factors and management of impending flap loss in 2138 breast free flaps. Ann Plast Surg. 2016;77(1):67–71.
32. Swartz WM, Jones NF, Cherup L, Klein A. Direct monitoring of microvascular anastomoses with the 20-MHz ultrasonic Doppler probe: an experimental and clinical study. Plast Reconstr Surg. 1988;81(2):149–61.
33. Rozen WM, Chubb D, Whitaker IS, Acosta R. The efficacy of postoperative monitoring: a single surgeon comparison of clinical monitoring and the implantable Doppler probe in 547 consecutive free flaps. Microsurgery. 2010;30(2):105–10.

34. Kind GM, Buntic RF, Buncke GM, Cooper TM, Siko PP, Buncke HJ Jr. The effect of an implantable Doppler probe on the salvage of microvascular tissue transplants. Plast Reconstr Surg. 1998;101(5):1268–73. discussion 74–5
35. Um GT, Chang J, Louie O, Colohan SM, Said HK, Neligan PC, et al. Implantable Cook-Swartz Doppler probe versus Synovis Flow Coupler for the post-operative monitoring of free flap breast reconstruction. J Plast Reconstr Aesthet Surg. 2014;67(7):960–6.
36. Kempton SJ, Poore SO, Chen JT, Afifi AM. Free flap monitoring using an implantable anastomotic venous flow coupler: analysis of 119 consecutive abdominal-based free flaps for breast reconstruction. Microsurgery. 2015;35(5):337–44.
37. Hirigoyen MB, Blackwell KE, Zhang WX, Silver L, Weinberg H, Urken ML. Continuous tissue oxygen tension measurement as a monitor of free-flap viability. Plast Reconstr Surg. 1997;99(3):763–73.
38. Keller A. Noninvasive tissue oximetry for flap monitoring: an initial study. J Reconstr Microsurg. 2007;23(4):189–97.
39. Lin SJ, Nguyen MD, Chen C, Colakoglu S, Curtis MS, Tobias AM, et al. Tissue oximetry monitoring in microsurgical breast reconstruction decreases flap loss and improves rate of flap salvage. Plast Reconstr Surg. 2011;127(3):1080–5.
40. Halsted WS. I. The results of operations for the cure of cancer of the breast performed at the Johns Hopkins Hospital from June, 1889, to January, 1894. Ann Surg. 1894;20(5):497–555.
41. Fisher B, Redmond C, Fisher ER, Bauer M, Wolmark N, Wickerham DL, et al. Ten-year results of a randomized clinical trial comparing radical mastectomy and total mastectomy with or without radiation. N Engl J Med. 1985;312(11):674–81.
42. Veronesi U, Cascinelli N, Mariani L, Greco M, Saccozzi R, Luini A, et al. Twenty-year follow-up of a randomized study comparing breast-conserving surgery with radical mastectomy for early breast cancer. N Engl J Med. 2002;347(16):1227–32.
43. Fisher B, Anderson S, Bryan J. Twenty year follow up of a randomized trial comparing total mastectomy, lumpectomy and lumpectomy plus radiation for treatment of invasive breast cancer. N Engl J Med. 2002;347:1233–47.
44. Steiner CA, Weiss AJ, Barrett ML, Fingar KR, Davis PH. Trends in bilateral and unilateral mastectomies in hospital inpatient and ambulatory settings, 2005–2013: statistical brief #201. Healthcare Cost and Utilization Project (HCUP) Statistical Briefs. Rockville; 2006.
45. Toth BA, Lappert P. Modified skin incisions for mastectomy: the need for plastic surgical input in preoperative planning. Plast Reconstr Surg. 1991;87(6):1048–53.
46. Carlson GW, Bostwick J 3rd, Styblo TM, Moore B, Bried JT, Murray DR, et al. Skin-sparing mastectomy. Oncologic and reconstructive considerations. Ann Surg. 1997;225(5):570–5. discussion 5–8
47. Carlson GW. Technical advances in skin sparing mastectomy. Int J Surg Oncol. 2011;2011:7.
48. Agha RA, Wellstead G, Sagoo H, Al Omran Y, Barai I, Rajmohan S, et al. Nipple sparing versus skin sparing mastectomy: a systematic review protocol. BMJ Open. 2016;6(5):e010151
49. Zhang H, Li Y, Moran MS, Haffty BG, Yang Q. Predictive factors of nipple involvement in breast cancer: a systematic review and meta-analysis. Breast Cancer Res Treat. 2015;151(2):239–49.
50. Donovan CA, Harit AP, Chung A, Bao J, Giuliano AE, Amersi F. Oncological and surgical outcomes after nipple-sparing mastectomy: do incisions matter? Ann Surg Oncol. 2016;23(10):3226–31.
51. Stolier AJ, Levine EA. Reducing the risk of nipple necrosis: technical observations in 340 nipple-sparing mastectomies. Breast J. 2013;19(2):173–9.
52. Radovan C. Breast reconstruction after mastectomy using the temporary expander. Plast Reconstr Surg. 1982;69(2):195–208.
53. Spear SL, Majidian A. Immediate breast reconstruction in two stages using textured, integrated-valve tissue expanders and breast implants: a retrospective review of 171 consecutive breast reconstructions from 1989 to 1996. Plast Reconstr Surg. 1998;101(1):53–63.
54. Austad ED, Rose GL. A self-inflating tissue expander. Plast Reconstr Surg. 1982;70(5):588–94.
55. Connell AF. Patient-activated controlled expansion for breast reconstruction with controlled carbon dioxide inflation: a feasibility study. Plast Reconstr Surg. 2011;128(4):848–52.

56. Connell TF. Patient-activated controlled expansion for breast reconstruction using controlled carbon dioxide inflation: confirmation of a feasibility study. Plast Reconstr Surg. 2014;134(4):503e–11e.
57. Maxwell GP, Gabriel A. The evolution of breast implants. Plast Reconstr Surg. 2014;134(1 Suppl):12S–7S.
58. Heden P, Jernbeck J, Hober M. Breast augmentation with anatomical cohesive gel implants: the world's largest current experience. Clin Plast Surg. 2001;28(3):531–52.
59. Adams WP Jr, Potter J, Spear SL. Breast implants: materials and manufacturing past, present and future. In: Kluwer W, editor. Surger of the breast: principles and art. 3rd ed. Philadelphia: Lippincott Williams & Wilkins; 2011. p. 344–56.
60. Brown MH, Shenker R, Silver SA. Cohesive silicone gel breast implants in aesthetic and reconstructive breast surgery. Plast Reconstr Surg. 2005;116(3):768–79. discussion 80–1
61. Barnsley GP, Sigurdson LJ, Barnsley SE. Textured surface breast implants in the prevention of capsular contracture among breast augmentation patients: a meta-analysis of randomized controlled trials. Plast Reconstr Surg. 2006;117(7):2182–90.
62. Ersek RA, Salisbury AV. Textured surface, nonsilicone gel breast implants: four years' clinical outcome. Plast Reconstr Surg. 1997;100(7):1729–39.
63. Choi M, Frey JD, Alperovich M, Levine JP, Karp NS. "Breast in a Day": examining single-stage immediate, permanent implant reconstruction in nipple-sparing mastectomy. Plast Reconstr Surg. 2016;138(2):184e–91e.
64. Krishnan NM, Fischer JP, Basta MN, Nahabedian MY. Is single-stage prosthetic reconstruction cost effective? A cost-utility analysis for the use of direct-to-implant breast reconstruction relative to expander-implant reconstruction in postmastectomy patients. Plast Reconstr Surg. 2016;138(3):537–47.
65. Bindingnavele V, Gaon M, Ota KS, Kulber DA, Lee DJ. Use of acellular cadaveric dermis and tissue expansion in postmastectomy breast reconstruction. J Plast Reconstr Aesthet Surg. 2007;60(11):1214–8.
66. Leong M, Basu CB, Hicks MJ. Further evidence that human acellular dermal matrix decreases inflammatory markers of capsule formation in implant-based breast reconstruction. Aesthet Surg J. 2015;35(1):40–7.
67. Yu D, Hanna KR, LeGallo RD, Drake DB. Comparison of histological characteristics of acellular dermal matrix capsules to surrounding breast capsules in acellular dermal matrix-assisted breast reconstruction. Ann Plast Surg. 2016;76(5):485–8.
68. Hartrampf CR, Scheflan M, Black PW. Breast reconstruction with a transverse abdominal island flap. Plast Reconstr Surg. 1982;69(2):216–25.
69. Serletti JM. Breast reconstruction with the TRAM flap: pedicled and free. J Surg Oncol. 2006;94(6):532–7.
70. Nahabedian MY, Tsangaris T, Momen B. Breast reconstruction with the DIEP flap or the muscle-sparing (MS-2) free TRAM flap: is there a difference? Plast Reconstr Surg. 2005;115(2):436–44. discussion 45–6
71. Ulatowski L, Kaniewska A. The use of the diep flap in the modern reconstructive surgery. Pol Przegl Chir. 2015;87(9):472–81.
72. Blondeel PN. One hundred free DIEP flap breast reconstructions: a personal experience. Br J Plast Surg. 1999;52(2):104–11.
73. Wu LC, Bajaj A, Chang DW, Chevray PM. Comparison of donor-site morbidity of SIEA, DIEP, and muscle-sparing TRAM flaps for breast reconstruction. Plast Reconstr Surg. 2008;122(3):702–9.
74. Ahmadzadeh R, Bergeron L, Tang M, Morris SF. The superior and inferior gluteal artery perforator flaps. Plast Reconstr Surg. 2007;120(6):1551–6.
75. Schoeller T, Wechselberger G. Breast reconstruction by the free transverse gracilis (TUG) flap. Br J Plast Surg. 2004;57(5):481–2.
76. Allen RJ Jr, Lee ZH, Mayo JL, Levine J, Ahn C, Allen RJ Sr. The Profunda Artery Perforator (PAP) flap experience for breast reconstruction. Plast Reconstr Surg. 2016;138:968–75.

77. Magarakis M, Venkat R, Dellon AL, Shridharani SM, Bellamy J, Vaca EE, et al. Pilot study of breast sensation after breast reconstruction: evaluating the effects of radiation therapy and perforator flap neurotization on sensory recovery. Microsurgery. 2013;33(6):421–31.
78. Spiegel AJ, Menn ZK, Eldor L, Kaufman Y, Dellon AL. Breast reinnervation: DIEP neurotization using the third anterior intercostal nerve. Plast Reconstr Surg Glob Open. 2013;1(8):e72.
79. Hamdi M, Khuthaila DK, Van Landuyt K, Roche N, Monstrey S. Double-pedicle abdominal perforator free flaps for unilateral breast reconstruction: new horizons in microsurgical tissue transfer to the breast. J Plast Reconstr Aesthet Surg. 2007;60(8):904–12. discussion 13–4
80. Rozen WM, Patel NG, Ramakrishnan VV. Increasing options in autologous microsurgical breast reconstruction: four free flaps for 'stacked' bilateral breast reconstruction. Gland Surg. 2016;5(2):255–60.
81. Murray A, Wasiak J, Rozen WM, Ferris S, Grinsell D. Stacked abdominal flap for unilateral breast reconstruction. J Reconstr Microsurg. 2015;31(3):179–86.
82. Delay E, Garson S, Tousson G, Sinna R. Fat injection to the breast: technique, results, and indications based on 880 procedures over 10 years. Aesthet Surg J. 2009;29(5):360–76.
83. Gosset J, Guerin N, Toussoun G, Delaporte T, Delay E. Radiological evaluation after lipomodelling for correction of breast conservative treatment sequelae. Ann Chir Plast Esthet. 2008;53(2):178–89.
84. Kaoutzanis C, Xin M, Ballard TN, Welch KB, Momoh AO, Kozlow JH, et al. Autologous fat grafting after breast reconstruction in postmastectomy patients: complications, biopsy rates, and locoregional cancer recurrence rates. Ann Plast Surg. 2016;76(3):270–5.
85. Coleman SR, Saboeiro AP. Fat grafting to the breast revisited: safety and efficacy. Plast Reconstr Surg. 2007;119(3):775–85. discussion 86–7
86. Chen X, Yan L, Guo Z, Chen Z, Chen Y, Li M, et al. Adipose-derived mesenchymal stem cells promote the survival of fat grafts via crosstalk between the Nrf2 and TLR4 pathways. Cell Death Dis. 2016;7(9):e2369.
87. Rigotti G, Marchi A, Galie M, Baroni G, Benati D, Krampera M, et al. Clinical treatment of radiotherapy tissue damage by lipoaspirate transplant: a healing process mediated by adipose-derived adult stem cells. Plast Reconstr Surg. 2007;119(5):1409–22. discussion 23–4
88. Strong AL, Cederna PS, Rubin JP, Coleman SR, Levi B. The current state of fat grafting: a review of harvesting, processing, and injection techniques. Plast Reconstr Surg. 2015;136(4):897–912.
89. Kanchwala SK, Glatt BS, Conant EF, Bucky LP. Autologous fat grafting to the reconstructed breast: the management of acquired contour deformities. Plast Reconstr Surg. 2009;124(2):409–18.
90. Smith CJ, Khouri RK, Baker TJ. Initial experience with the Brava nonsurgical system of breast enhancement. Plast Reconstr Surg. 2002;110(6):1593–5. author reply 5–8
91. Saxena V, Hwang CW, Huang S, Eichbaum Q, Ingber D, Orgill DP. Vacuum-assisted closure: microdeformations of wounds and cell proliferation. Plast Reconstr Surg. 2004;114(5):1086–96. discussion 97–8
92. Didier F, Arnaboldi P, Gandini S, Maldifassi A, Goldhirsch A, Radice D, et al. Why do women accept to undergo a nipple sparing mastectomy or to reconstruct the nipple areola complex when nipple sparing mastectomy is not possible? Breast Cancer Res Treat. 2012;132(3):1177–84.
93. Satteson ES, Reynolds MF, Bond AM, Pestana IA. An analysis of complication risk factors in 641 nipple reconstructions. Breast J. 2016;22(4):379–83.
94. Zenn MR, Garofalo JA. Unilateral nipple reconstruction with nipple sharing: time for a second look. Plast Reconstr Surg. 2009;123(6):1648–53.
95. Halvorson EG, Cormican M, West ME, Myers V. Three-dimensional nipple-areola tattooing: a new technique with superior results. Plast Reconstr Surg. 2014;133(5):1073–5.

New Thoughts on Atypias of the Breast: Flat Epithelial Atypia, Atypical Ductal Hyperplasia, and Lobular Neoplasia

8

Megan E. Sullivan

Introduction

The widespread use of screening mammography as well as advances in imaging techniques has resulted in increased detection of high-risk breast lesions. Overall, high-risk lesions represent 7–8% of core biopsy diagnoses [1–3]. Benign breast lesions such as intraductal papillomas and radial scars are also considered high-risk lesions. However, the focus of this chapter will be on atypias of the breast: flat epithelial atypia (FEA), atypical ductal hyperplasia (ADH), and lobular neoplasia.

To complicate matters, breast atypias can be diagnosed in isolation, or multiple findings can be present in a single core biopsy, as these low-grade lesions are often associated with one another as well as with low-grade carcinomas, such as invasive tubular carcinoma, as part of the so-called "Rosen triad" [4].

The diagnosis of atypia in a core biopsy of the breast has traditionally led to surgical excision of that area, so a definitive assessment can be made as to whether the atypia was an isolated finding or the proverbial "tip of the iceberg" associated with a malignant lesion that was not sampled in the core biopsy. As advances have been made in imaging of the breast, radiologic findings that may not have been identified in the past are now getting biopsied, some resulting in an atypical diagnosis. These same imaging advances have also opened up the discussion regarding the necessity of routine surgical excisions for all types of atypia. In this chapter, the pathology of the various breast atypias will be discussed as well as the importance of pathologic-radiologic correlation in determining what patients are truly at high risk and should undergo surgical excision.

M.E. Sullivan, MD (✉)
Department of Pathology and Laboratory Medicine, Evanston Hospital, North Shore University Health System, 2650 Ridge Ave., Evanston, IL 60621, USA
e-mail: msullivan4@northshore.org

M. Howard-McNatt (ed.), *Changing Paradigms in the Management of Breast Cancer*, DOI 10.1007/978-3-319-60336-0_8

Flat Epithelial Atypia

Flat epithelial atypia (FEA) is an entity that has had many names in the pathology literature, ranging from "low-grade clinging carcinoma" to "columnar alteration with apical snouts and secretions". The current nomenclature of FEA is used in the WHO classification which defines it as a low-grade neoplastic process in which the native epithelial cells of the breast terminal duct lobular unit (TDLU) are replaced by a monomorphic population of cells in one or more layers that exhibit loss of nuclear polarity without architectural atypia. These dilated TDLUs often have central secretions which calcify and are therefore identified on mammography (Fig. 8.1a). Pure FEA is an uncommon diagnosis, with a reported incidence of about 3–4% of all core biopsies [5, 6]. FEA shares morphologic similarity as well as an immunoprofile similar to atypical ductal hyperplasia (ADH) and low-grade ductal carcinoma in situ (DCIS), suggesting that it may be a precursor lesion [7]. However, while the relative risk for subsequent development of breast cancer has been well defined for other categories of breast atypia, the risk associated with FEA is less clear. A Mayo cohort

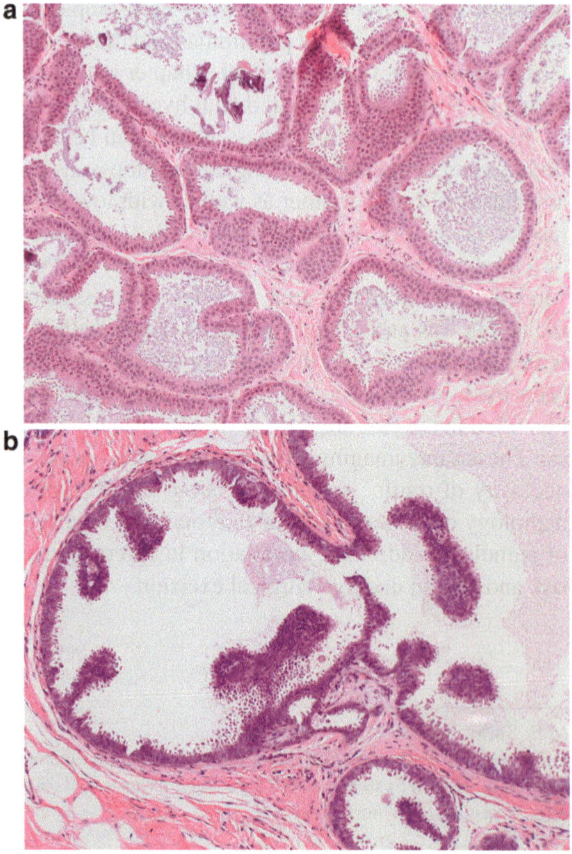

Fig. 8.1 (**a**) Flat epithelial atypia (FEA) (**b**) Atypical ductal hyperplasia (ADH)

study found that FEA had no independent elevation of risk beyond that conferred by the changes present in the background breast tissue [8].

The immediate question a clinician faces when a patient is diagnosed with pure FEA on core biopsy is whether surgical excision is necessary. In the literature, reported upgrade rates vary widely, ranging from 0 to 21% [6, 9–16] (Table 8.1). All

Table 8.1 Reported upgrade rates for FEA

Article	Number of pure FEA cases/number excised	Upgrades to DCIS or IC	Indication for biopsy	Residual lesion post-biopsy	Patients without excisions
Kunju and Kleer (2007)	14/14	3 (21%)	Calcifications	Unknown	N/A
Noel et al. (2009)	62/20	0	Calcifications	Present in the 20 excised cases	No changes in mammograms at 6–12 months post biopsy
Chivukula et al. (2009)	39/35	5 (14%)	Calcifications	Unknown	No follow-up provided
Lavoue et al. (2011)	60/60	8 (13%)	Calcifications, mass	Present in at least 42[a]	N/A
Uzoaru et al. (2012)	145/95	3 (3%)	Calcifications, mass	Unknown	No changes in mammograms with mean follow-up of 5 years
Peres et al. (2012)	128/95	9 (9%)[c]	Calcifications, mass	Unknown	No changes in mammograms with median follow-up of 13 months
Khoumanis et al. (2013)	104/94	10 (10%)	Calcifications, mass	Unknown	No changes in mammograms with mean follow-up of 36 months
Prowler et al. (2014)	24/24	0	Calcifications, mass, MRI enhancement	Unknown	N/A
Calhoun et al. (2015)	73/73	5 (7%)	Calcifications, mass, MRI enhancement	14 completely removed at biopsy[b]	N/A

[a]18 cases had >90% of the mammographic lesion removed at biopsy. One upgrade was from this category

[b]14 cases had all calcifications removed at biopsy, none of which were upgraded at excision. No other specifications about the residual lesions were provided

[c]An additional case with LCIS at excision was considered an "upgrade" in the original paper

the studies are limited by a retrospective design, and many also have a small sample size. The published recommendations for treatment are likewise variable. Some recommend routine excision for all FEA patients similar to when ADH is diagnosed on core biopsy. Alternatively, some argue for case-by-case decision-making that would factor in imaging findings (such as the presence of residual calcifications in the post-biopsy mammogram) as well as factors such as a personal history of breast cancer. This case-by-case process would allow for some patients to undergo imaging surveillance rather than immediate excision. Although no prospective, randomized data is available to definitively answer this question of excision vs. surveillance, there is some published data on patients who have not undergone immediate excision. These patients have not developed a subsequent breast cancer at the site of their FEA biopsy within the follow-up periods [6, 10, 13, 16].

Atypical Ductal Hyperplasia

Atypical ductal hyperplasia (ADH) morphologically resembles low-grade ductal carcinoma in situ (DCIS). Both are composed of a proliferation of monomorphic epithelial cells that are evenly spaced with distinct cell borders. Unlike FEA, the proliferating cells can be solid or have architecture and form bridges or micropapillae. Given the morphologic overlap, quantitative criteria are often used to distinguish ADH from low-grade DCIS. If the proliferation completely involves of at least two membrane-bound spaces or has a size greater than 2 mm, these lesions would be diagnosed as DCIS rather than ADH [17]. Some authors have suggested a conservative approach to low-grade ductal proliferations on core biopsy and will classify those measuring up to 3 mm as ADH [18]. This avoids overdiagnosing small lesions as low-grade DCIS by leaving the final determination of extent and therefore classification to the excision specimen rather than deciding based on the core biopsy findings alone.

Given the difficultly in accurately distinguishing ADH from low-grade DCIS on core biopsy alone, surgical excision is routinely recommended for ADH. The upgrade rates for ADH at excision are in the range of 10–20%.

Atypical Lobular Hyperplasia and Classic Lobular Carcinoma In Situ

Classic lobular neoplasia encompasses both atypical lobular hyperplasia (ALH) and lobular carcinoma in situ (LCIS). The cells in ALH and classic LCIS have identical morphology. Both lesions are composed of dyscohesive small, round cells with uniform nuclei that are often eccentrically placed. Cytoplasmic vacuoles are common. The difference between the two diagnoses comes with the degree of lobular involvement and/or distension by these cells. In comparison to ALH (Fig. 8.2a), classic LCIS shows greater distention of the acini within the TDLU as well as more complete involvement of the TDLU itself (Fig. 8.2b).

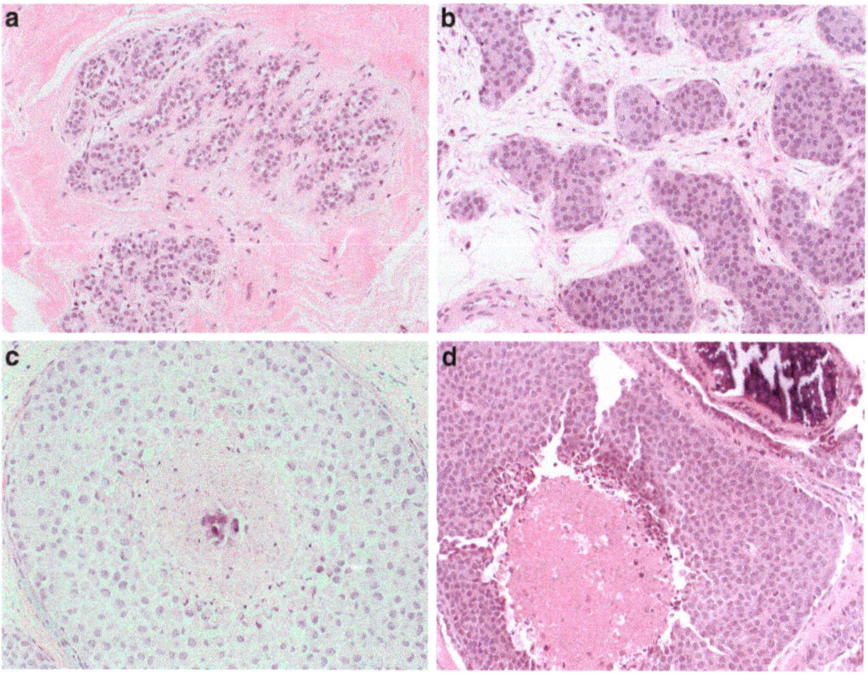

Fig. 8.2 (**a**) ALH (**b**) classic LCIS (**c**) pleomorphic LCIS (**d**) LCIS with necrosis

Lobular neoplasia is considered both a risk factor and a non-obligate precursor for developing invasive carcinoma in either breast. Cohort studies have shown that the relative risk of developing breast cancer for women with ALH or classic LCIS is estimated at 4 and 10×, respectively [19]. A minority of women with classic lobular neoplasia subsequently develops invasive breast cancer; no clinical or pathological features can accurately predict which women are at risk for progression.

ALH and classic LCIS are most often incidental findings in core biopsies, and the question of whether surgical excision of the biopsy site is necessary is still controversial. The reported upgrade rates in the literature are highly variable, and many studies have significant limitations including the selection bias inherent in their retrospective design. Many also fail to include crucial information about pathologic-radiologic concordance. Discordant cases such as classic LN associated with a mass on imaging should undergo excision to exclude an invasive component that was not sampled in the core biopsy. Unfortunately, discordant cases are sometimes reported as true "upgrades" in the literature, creating a falsely elevated upgrade rate. There is also the question of whether morphologic variants such as pleomorphic LCIS and necrotic LCIS were included for analysis in some studies. Retrospective studies that included pathologic review and imaging concordance had reported upgrade rates of 1.3–4% [20–22]. Prospective studies that included only women with classic lobular neoplasia (ALH and/or LCIS, no LCIS variants) diagnosed on core biopsy with

Table 8.2 Upgrade rates for prospectively excised classic lobular neoplasia in the recent literature

Study	Number of upgrades	Upgrade rate (%)
Rendi (2012)	3/68	4.4
Murray (2013)	2/72	3.0
Nakhlis (2016)	2/77	3.0
Susnik (2016)	7/180	3.9
Total	14/397	3.5

concordant imaging findings also show an upgrade rate of 3–4% [23–25] (Table 8.2). Therefore, when ALH or classic LCIS is an isolated incidental finding on core biopsy, radiologic-pathologic correlation is recommended to determine management. In contrast, patients with an associated mass, ductal atypia (such as ADH) with the same core biopsy, or a variant of LCIS should undergo excision.

Variants of Lobular Carcinoma In Situ

It is important to be aware of the morphologic variants of LCIS: pleomorphic and necrotic types. These are uncommon entities and in the past have likely been diagnosed and treated as DCIS [26]. Pleomorphic LCIS (P-LCIS) is composed of variably dyscohesive cells with nuclei 3–4× the size of a lymphocyte that are often eccentrically placed with prominent nucleoli [27] (Fig. 8.2c). Necrosis is sometimes present in P-LCIS but not required for the diagnosis. In contrast, identifying necrosis is necessary for the diagnosis of necrotic LCIS (N-LCIS) which is otherwise composed of cells with similar cytologic features to classic LCIS with more marked distension of the involved acini [28]. This necrosis can be puntate or comedo type. The presence of associated necrosis that undergoes calcification with either P-LCIS or N-LCIS leads to mammographic similarities with DCIS [29]. Although the aggressiveness of these variants is unknown, some studies have shown a higher association with invasive carcinoma. Therefore, in contrast to classic LCIS, the current recommendation for LCIS variants is surgical excision.

The Importance of Pathologic-Radiologic Concordance

Pathologic-radiologic concordance has been emphasized in the discussion of each category of atypia above, but how does one decide when it has been achieved? Multiple parameters come into making this assessment, and they vary from patient to patient. The most obvious question that needs to be answered after every core biopsy is: do the pathologic findings correlate with the imaging impression? Although the question itself is obvious, getting to the answer involves assessing multiple parameters. All the atypias discussed in this chapter are not by themselves mass-forming lesions, but they may secondarily involve a mass (such as when ALH is identified within a fibroadenoma).

FEA and ADH are often associated with the calcifications that were the target of the core biopsy. ALH and classic LCIS are most often a completely incidental finding, although they too can be associated with calcifications. When a core biopsy is performed targeting a mass seen on mammography and/or ultrasound and the resultant cores show only FEA, ALH/LCIS, or ADH, the pathologic-radiologic findings may be discordant. Not only the type of lesion identified on breast imaging but the level of suspicion assigned to that lesion by the radiologist should be taken into account. The imaging workup that precedes obtaining a core biopsy provides an overall assessment of the lesion using the Breast Imaging Reporting and Data System (BI-RADS). BI-RADS 4 lesions are considered suggestive of malignancy, and BI-RADS 5 lesions are highly suggestive of malignancy; biopsy is recommended for both categories (https://www.acr.org/). When a core biopsy is performed, targeting a finding categorized as BI-RADS 5 and the resultant cores show only atypia (ductal or lobular); the pathologic-radiologic findings may be discordant. The adequacy of the sample should also be considered, and can be evaluated by variables such as the number of cores obtained and the extent of the lesion removed by the core biopsy. Clinical variables such as age, breast cancer risk, and findings on physical examination may also factor into deciding whether or not surgical excision should be recommended.

Multidisciplinary conferences where radiologists, pathologists, and surgeons can discuss the management of patients with nonmalignant breast lesions are common at large academic centers. Although not possible in every practice setting, pathologic-radiologic correlation conferences provide a forum similar to breast cancer conferences in which management decisions can be discussed on a case-by-case basis. After instituting a correlation conference, one institution found that the case review and discussion that occurred resulted in significant changes in management for 5.3% of the patients presented at the conference [30]. The change in assessment from discordant to concordant enabled patients to avoid surgical excision and/or short-interval imaging. Importantly, in those that changed from concordant to discordant, three breast cancers were identified on the subsequent tissue sampling. MD Anderson utilized a "multidisciplinary clinical management conference" to separate patients with lobular neoplasia on core biopsy that needed surgical excision from those who could be adequately followed clinically and with imaging [31]. A pathologic-radiologic correlation conference has the potential to not only impact the care of individual patients but can impact a health care system financially by avoiding costly and unnecessary follow-up imaging and surgical intervention.

Breast MRI and Atypias

Breast magnetic resonance imaging (MRI) is being increasingly used to both diagnose and manage breast cancer. With its increased sensitivity, breast MRI can detect cancers that are not seen on mammography or ultrasound. However, with its low specificity, a variety of nonmalignant lesions will also enhance on MRI and findings with no mammogram or ultrasound correlate will lead to MRI-guided biopsy for tissue confirmation. The majority of the published literature regarding the risk of upgrade for breast atypia has focused on atypias detected using mammography and/or ultrasound; do atypias diagnosed on MRI-guided core biopsy carry the same risk? Reported upgrade rates for ADH and lobular neoplasia in this setting range from 15 to 32% and 0–29%, respectively [32–35]. Very little data is available for pure FEA diagnosed on MRI-guided core biopsy. No statistically significant difference was seen in the upgrade rate by lesion type (mass vs. non-mass enhancement) or size of the targeted lesion. It is important to remember that the patient population in these studies is also quite different as women getting a breast MRI are more often at high risk or already have breast cancer. In the aforementioned studies, 48–74% of the women had a history of past or concurrent breast cancer including in the same breast as their biopsy-proven atypia. Including patients with a recently diagnosed ipsilateral breast cancer could confound the finding of an "upgrade" at excision, and not all the studies included pathologic review to confirm that the areas were truly distinct. Given the limitations in the published literature, there are currently no different recommendations for atypias detected on MRI-guided biopsy.

It has been suggested that breast MRI may be able to help predict the risk of upgrade for high-risk lesions diagnosed using conventional image-guided biopsy techniques (MRI for "troubleshooting"). Londero et al. analyzed the subsequent breast MRI findings in women with high-risk lesions and no prior or concurrent history of ipsilateral breast cancer [36]. Biopsy-proven lobular neoplasia with enhancement has an upgrade rate of 46% compared to only 5% of non-enhancing cases. A similar pattern was seen with ADH: 44% of those with enhancement were upgraded, while none of the non-enhancing cases had invasive carcinoma or DCIS in the excision. However, other studies have found that the false-negative rate of MRI is too high to be used in management decisions for core biopsy-diagnosed lobular neoplasia or ADH [37]. Additional prospective studies are needed to more accurately determine the utility of breast MRI in this setting.

Conclusion

Flat epithelial atypia (FEA), atypical ductal hyperplasia (ADH), classic lobular neoplasia (atypical lobular hyperplasia (ALH), and classic lobular carcinoma in situ (LCIS) are all low-grade lesions that are considered non-obligate precursors as well as risk factors for the development of breast cancer. They can be diagnosed on breast core biopsies targeting calcifications, masses, or areas of enhancement. Given the morphologic overlap of ADH with low-grade DCIS, surgical excision is recommended in these cases, and about 10–20% of cases will be upgraded to invasive carcinoma or DCIS. Surgical excision is also recommended for the pleomorphic and necrotic variants of LCIS. In contrast, all patients with classic lobular neoplasia or FEA on core biopsy may not require excision when careful pathologic-radiologic concordance is assured. A uniform approach to all atypias of the breast may not be appropriate, and discussion of these cases in a multidisciplinary setting can be helpful in weighing the clinical, radiologic, and pathologic factors that can influence the decision on the best management for each individual patient.

References

1. Hayes BD, O'Doherty A, Quinn CM. Correlation of needle core biopsy with excision histology in screen-detected B3 lesions: the Merrion Breast Screening Unit experience. J Clin Pathol. 2009;62(12):1136–40.
2. El-Sayed ME, Rakha EA, Reed J, Lee AH, Evans AJ, Ellis IO. Predictive value of needle core biopsy diagnoses of lesions of uncertain malignant potential (B3) in abnormalities detected by mammographic screening. Histopathology. 2008;53(6):650–7.
3. M T, A P, F G, D S, S Z, M S. Positive predictive value of breast lesions of uncertain malignant potential (B3): can we identify high risk patients? The value of a multidisciplinary team and implications in the surgical treatment. Surg Oncol. 2016;25(2):119–22.
4. Brandt SM, Young GQ, Hoda SA. The "Rosen Triad": tubular carcinoma, lobular carcinoma in situ, and columnar cell lesions. Adv Anat Pathol. 2008;15(3):140–6.
5. Martel M, Barron-Rodriguez P, Tolgay Ocal I, Dotto J, Tavassoli FA. Flat DIN 1 (flat epithelial atypia) on core needle biopsy: 63 cases identified retrospectively among 1,751 core biopsies performed over an 8-year period (1992–1999). Virchows Arch. 2007;451(5):883–91.
6. Uzoaru I, Morgan BR, Liu ZG, Bellafiore FJ, Gaudier FS, Lo JV, et al. Flat epithelial atypia with and without atypical ductal hyperplasia: to re-excise or not. Results of a 5-year prospective study. Virchows Arch. 2012;461(4):419–23.
7. Abdel-Fatah TM, Powe DG, Hodi Z, Reis-Filho JS, Lee AH, Ellis IO. Morphologic and molecular evolutionary pathways of low nuclear grade invasive breast cancers and their putative precursor lesions: further evidence to support the concept of low nuclear grade breast neoplasia family. Am J Surg Pathol. 2008;32(4):513–23.
8. Said SM, Visscher DW, Nassar A, Frank RD, Vierkant RA, Frost MH, et al. Flat epithelial atypia and risk of breast cancer: a Mayo cohort study. Cancer. 2015;121(10):1548–55.
9. Kunju LP, Kleer CG. Significance of flat epithelial atypia on mammotome core needle biopsy: should it be excised? Hum Pathol. 2007;38(1):35–41.
10. Noel JC, Buxant F, Engohan-Aloghe C. Immediate surgical resection of residual microcalcifications after a diagnosis of pure flat epithelial atypia on core biopsy: a word of caution. Surg Oncol. 2010;19(4):243–6.
11. Chivukula M, Bhargava R, Tseng G, Dabbs DJ. Clinicopathologic implications of "flat epithelial atypia" in core needle biopsy specimens of the breast. Am J Clin Pathol. 2009;131(6):802–8.
12. Lavoue V, Roger CM, Poilblanc M, Proust N, Monghal-Verge C, Sagan C, et al. Pure flat epithelial atypia (DIN 1a) on core needle biopsy: study of 60 biopsies with follow-up surgical excision. Breast Cancer Res Treat. 2011;125(1):121–6.
13. Khoumais NA, Scaranelo AM, Moshonov H, Kulkarni SR, Miller N, McCready DR, et al. Incidence of breast cancer in patients with pure flat epithelial atypia diagnosed at core-needle biopsy of the breast. Ann Surg Oncol. 2013;20(1):133–8.
14. Prowler VL, Joh JE, Acs G, Kiluk JV, Laronga C, Khakpour N, et al. Surgical excision of pure flat epithelial atypia identified on core needle breast biopsy. Breast. 2014;23(4):352–6.
15. Calhoun BC, Sobel A, White RL, Gromet M, Flippo T, Sarantou T, et al. Management of flat epithelial atypia on breast core biopsy may be individualized based on correlation with imaging studies. Mod Pathol. 2015;28(5):670–6.
16. Peres A, Barranger E, Becette V, Boudinet A, Guinebretiere JM, Cherel P. Rates of upgrade to malignancy for 271 cases of flat epithelial atypia (FEA) diagnosed by breast core biopsy. Breast Cancer Res Treat. 2012;133(2):659–66.
17. Rosen PP, Hoda SA. Breast pathology: diagnosis by needle core biopsy. 3rd ed. Philadelphia: Wolters Kluwer/Lippincott Williams & Wilkins Health; 2010. p. xiv. 366 pp
18. Vandenbussche CJ, Khouri N, Sbaity E, Tsangaris TN, Vang R, Tatsas A, et al. Borderline atypical ductal hyperplasia/low-grade ductal carcinoma in situ on breast needle core biopsy should be managed conservatively. Am J Surg Pathol. 2013;37(6):913–23.
19. Hartmann LC, Sellers TA, Frost MH, Lingle WL, Degnim AC, Ghosh K, et al. Benign breast disease and the risk of breast cancer. N Engl J Med. 2005;353(3):229–37.

20. Hwang H, Barke LD, Mendelson EB, Susnik B. Atypical lobular hyperplasia and classic lobular carcinoma in situ in core biopsy specimens: routine excision is not necessary. Mod Pathol. 2008;21(10):1208–16.
21. Nagi CS, O'Donnell JE, Tismenetsky M, Bleiweiss IJ, Jaffer SM. Lobular neoplasia on core needle biopsy does not require excision. Cancer. 2008;112(10):2152–8.
22. Chaudhary S, Lawrence L, McGinty G, Kostroff K, Bhuiya T. Classic lobular neoplasia on core biopsy: a clinical and radio-pathologic correlation study with follow-up excision biopsy. Mod Pathol. 2013;26(6):762–71.
23. Nakhlis F, Gilmore L, Gelman R, Bedrosian I, Ludwig K, Hwang ES, et al. Incidence of adjacent synchronous invasive carcinoma and/or ductal carcinoma in-situ in patients with lobular neoplasia on Core biopsy: results from a prospective multi-institutional registry (TBCRC 020). Ann Surg Oncol. 2016;23(3):722–8.
24. Murray MP, Luedtke C, Liberman L, Nehhozina T, Akram M, Brogi E. Classic lobular carcinoma in situ and atypical lobular hyperplasia at percutaneous breast core biopsy: outcomes of prospective excision. Cancer. 2013;119(5):1073–9.
25. Susnik B, Day D, Abeln E, Bowman T, Krueger J, Swenson KK, et al. Surgical outcomes of lobular neoplasia diagnosed in core biopsy: prospective study of 316 cases. Clin Breast Cancer. 2016;16:507–13.
26. Sullivan ME, Khan SA, Sullu Y, Schiller C, Susnik B. Lobular carcinoma in situ variants in breast cores: potential for misdiagnosis, upgrade rates at surgical excision, and practical implications. Arch Pathol Lab Med. 2010;134(7):1024–8.
27. Sneige N, Wang J, Baker BA, Krishnamurthy S, Middleton LP. Clinical, histopathologic, and biologic features of pleomorphic lobular (ductal-lobular) carcinoma in situ of the breast: a report of 24 cases. Mod Pathol. 2002;15(10):1044–50.
28. Fadare O, Dadmanesh F, Alvarado-Cabrero I, Snyder R, Stephen Mitchell J, Tot T, et al. Lobular intraepithelial neoplasia [lobular carcinoma in situ] with comedo-type necrosis: a clinicopathologic study of 18 cases. Am J Surg Pathol. 2006;30(11):1445–53.
29. Georgian-Smith D, Lawton TJ. Calcifications of lobular carcinoma in situ of the breast: radiologic-pathologic correlation. AJR Am J Roentgenol. 2001;176(5):1255–9.
30. Prakash S, Venkataraman S, Slanetz PJ, Dialani V, Fein-Zachary V, Littlehale N, et al. Improving patient care by incorporation of multidisciplinary breast radiology-pathology correlation conference. Can Assoc Radiol J. 2016;67(2):122–9.
31. Middleton LP, Sneige N, Coyne R, Shen Y, Dong W, Dempsey P, et al. Most lobular carcinoma in situ and atypical lobular hyperplasia diagnosed on core needle biopsy can be managed clinically with radiologic follow-up in a multidisciplinary setting. Cancer Med. 2014;3(3):492–9.
32. Weinfurtner RJ, Patel B, Laronga C, Lee MC, Falcon SL, Mooney BP, et al. Magnetic resonance imaging-guided core needle breast biopsies resulting in high-risk histopathologic findings: upstage frequency and lesion characteristics. Clin Breast Cancer. 2015;15(3):234–9.
33. Strigel RM, Eby PR, Demartini WB, Gutierrez RL, Allison KH, Peacock S, et al. Frequency, upgrade rates, and characteristics of high-risk lesions initially identified with breast MRI. AJR Am J Roentgenol. 2010;195(3):792–8.
34. Khoury T, Kumar PR, Li Z, Karabakhtsian RG, Sanati S, Chen X, et al. Lobular neoplasia detected in MRI-guided core biopsy carries a high risk for upgrade: a study of 63 cases from four different institutions. Mod Pathol. 2016;29(1):25–33.
35. Lourenco AP, Khalil H, Sanford M, Donegan L. High-risk lesions at MRI-guided breast biopsy: frequency and rate of underestimation. AJR Am J Roentgenol. 2014;203(3):682–6.
36. Londero V, Zuiani C, Linda A, Girometti R, Bazzocchi M, Sardanelli F. High-risk breast lesions at imaging-guided needle biopsy: usefulness of MRI for treatment decision. AJR Am J Roentgenol. 2012;199(2):W240–50.
37. Linda A, Zuiani C, Furlan A, Lorenzon M, Londero V, Girometti R, et al. Nonsurgical management of high-risk lesions diagnosed at core needle biopsy: can malignancy be ruled out safely with breast MRI? AJR Am J Roentgenol. 2012;198(2):272–80.

New Techniques in Radiation Oncology

9

Ryan T. Hughes and Doris R. Brown

Introduction

The role of radiation therapy in the management of breast cancer has evolved significantly over the past several decades. In this modern era of improving surgical techniques and more effective chemotherapeutic, targeted biological agents and hormonal therapies, its use in patients with early stage as well as locally advanced breast cancer continues to be refined. Enhanced screening efforts have reduced the relative incidence of late-stage breast cancer with an associated increase in early-stage disease [1]. These trends highlight a need for clear guidelines in the management of early-stage breast cancer, which, given the heterogeneity of clinicopathologic risk factors, are sometimes difficult to elucidate. In the late twentieth century, breast-conserving surgery (BCS) followed by radiotherapy to the whole breast became an established standard of care in early-stage breast cancer with similar ipsilateral breast control rates relative to mastectomy alone [2, 3]. The addition of radiotherapy to breast-conserving surgery significantly reduced local recurrence rates at 5 years which translates into a 15-year breast cancer-specific mortality rate, irrespective of nodal status [4]. In locally advanced disease, radiation therapy to the chest wall and regional lymph node stations (supraclavicular, infraclavicular, axillary, and internal mammary) in addition to chemotherapy following mastectomy reduced locoregional recurrence (LRR) and improved disease-free and overall survival for patients with T3–T4 primary tumors or involved axillary lymph nodes [5–7]. High-risk patients with large tumors, high-grade histology, and increasing number of axillary lymph nodes involved at the time of mastectomy with axillary lymph node dissection (ALND) reaped the greatest benefit from adjuvant postmastectomy radiotherapy (PMRT). It has been generally accepted that patients with four

R.T. Hughes, MD • D.R. Brown, MD, PhD (✉)
Department of Radiation Oncology, Wake Forest Baptist Health,
Medical Center Boulevard, Winston-Salem, NC 27157, USA
e-mail: drbrown@wakehealth.edu

M. Howard-McNatt (ed.), *Changing Paradigms in the Management of Breast Cancer*, DOI 10.1007/978-3-319-60336-0_9

or more positive lymph nodes are at highest risk for LRR and thus would benefit most from PMRT to minimize that risk. These studies were limited by variability in axillary lymph node evaluation and less efficacious chemotherapy than that available in the present day. In this chapter, we will further discuss the radiotherapeutic management of the axilla and regional lymph nodes in the era of increasing surgical efficacy and sensitivity (via sentinel lymph node biopsy) and significantly improved adjuvant and neoadjuvant systemic treatment options.

Regional Nodal Irradiation for Patients with One to Three Lymph Nodes Involved

Since the aforementioned trials that initially defined the role of PMRT in node-positive breast cancer, there remains controversy regarding the optimal indications for regional nodal irradiation. The uncertainty lies mostly in the setting of less than four axillary lymph nodes involved. Previous trials designed to answer this question have closed without adequate accrual; current randomized controlled trial evidence remains forthcoming. Retrospective, single-institution analyses suggest that regional nodal irradiation for patients with one to three nodes involved does indeed reduce locoregional recurrence and improve disease-free survival, but despite a trend toward improvement in overall survival, a statistically significant survival benefit has not been demonstrated [8–10]. Furthermore, population-based analysis of T2N1 patients with one, two, and three lymph nodes positive at the time of mastectomy who did not receive radiation therapy revealed statistically significant differences in overall and cause-specific survival directly related to the number of LN involved [11]. Based on these results, the risk associated with involved axillary lymph nodes may be better considered as a continuous spectrum rather than on an ordinal scale. Upon subgroup analysis of patients with one to three positive lymph nodes after mastectomy with ALND, regional nodal radiotherapy resulted in a significant relative risk reduction of 87% (ARR 20%) for LRR and 17% (ARR 9%) for overall survival [12]. Meta-analysis of over 8000 patients undergoing mastectomy with axillary surgery randomized to chest wall/regional nodal irradiation vs. no radiotherapy assisted in further clarifying the role for regional nodal radiotherapy in patients with one to three positive lymph nodes after ALND [13]. This patient population experienced reductions in 10-year locoregional (20.3% vs. 3.8%, $2p < 0.00001$) and any recurrence rates (45.7% vs. 34.2%, $2p = 0.00006$), as well as 20-year breast cancer-specific mortality (50.2% vs. 42.3%, $2p = 0.01$). These risk reductions were similar to those experienced by the patients with four or more lymph nodes involved – the benefit of RT was not proportional to the number of lymph nodes involved. The benefits also remained irrespective of the use of systemic therapy, though approximately 90% of patients received at least one form of chemotherapy or hormonal therapy. These data regarding the benefit of postmastectomy RNI are, however, limited by the age of the comprising trials and do not evaluate the potential toxicities of additional radiotherapy to the regional nodes, including increased risk of pulmonary, cardiac, skin/soft tissue, and lymphatics.

A recent randomized trial (EORTC 22922/10925) compared the addition of regional nodal (internal mammary and medial supraclavicular fossa) irradiation to either whole breast or chest wall irradiation versus no RNI in patients with externally located tumors and axillary nodal involvement or medially located tumors regardless of nodal involvement [14]. The majority (76%) of patients underwent BCS; the others received mastectomy (24%). Both groups underwent ALND; SLNB was allowed in the later years of the trial to be followed by completion ALND if pathologically node positive. The addition of IMN and supraclavicular RNI to either whole breast or chest wall radiotherapy resulted in reduced disease-free (HR 0.89, CI 0.80–1.00, $p = 0.04$) and breast cancer-specific mortality (HR 0.82, CI 0.70–0.97, $p = 0.02$). Overall survival at 10 years was 82.3% in the RNI group and 80.7% in the control group with a trend toward statistical significance ($p = 0.05$). Analysis of 3- and 10-year toxicity rates revealed elevated risks of pulmonary fibrosis with the addition of RNI (4.4% vs. 1.7%) but no difference in cardiac fibrosis or heart disease ($p = 0.06$ and $p = 0.25$, respectively) or skin toxicity [15].

Recent consensus guidelines published by a joint American Society of Clinical Oncology, American Society for Radiation Oncology, and Society of Surgical Oncology panel regarding the use of PMRT in this setting "unanimously agreed that the available evidence shows that PMRT reduces the risks of locoregional failure (LRF), any recurrence, and breast cancer mortality for patients with T1-2 breast cancer and one to three positive lymph nodes [16]." This panel did, however, caution that patients may exist with such an inherently low risk of LRF that the potential toxicity may outweigh the benefits of PMRT. There is no validated predictive model to aid in identification of patients within this particular subgroup. As such, careful consideration of clinical (advanced age, short life expectancy, comorbidities, or coincident conditions that may increase radiation toxicity) and pathologic factors (T1 tumor size, absence of LVSI, single LN positive, small size of nodal metastases, or good response to NAC) for each individual patient is necessary to evaluate each patient's risk of recurrence which may then be compared to their risk of toxicity from PMRT.

Regional Nodal Irradiation After Breast-Conserving Surgery

The results of an international randomized controlled trial (NCIC-CTG MA.20) comparing the addition of RNI to whole breast irradiation (WBI) after breast-conserving surgery in node-positive or high-risk node-negative (primary tumor size ≥5 cm or size ≥2 cm with <10 axillary nodes dissected and either grade 3 histology, ER negativity, or the presence of LVSI) patients allow for the comparison of clinical outcomes as well as toxicity rates for WBI with or without RNI in early-stage breast cancer patients [17]. All patients underwent BCS with either axillary lymph node dissection or sentinel lymph node biopsy, 91% received adjuvant chemotherapy based on institutional practice, and 76% received hormonal therapy. Radiation to the whole breast and internal mammary nodes (IMN) was delivered to 50 Gy in 25 fractions using opposed tangents using either wide tangents to include the IMN or standard tangents with a matched IMN field. High axillary, supraclavicular and infraclavicular nodal regions were covered with an anteroposterior beam alignment; posteroanterior field was recommended but not required. A 10–16 Gy boost in 2 Gy fractions to the lumpectomy cavity was allowed per institutional policy. At 10 years, locoregional disease-free survival was significantly higher in the RNI group compared to the control (95.2% vs. 92.2%, $p = 0.009$). Overall 10-year disease-free survival was also improved in the RNI group (82% vs. 77%, $p = 0.01$; HR 0.76, CI 0.61–0.94, $p = 0.01$). These differences were comprised mostly by a reduction in regional recurrence rates; the regions at highest risk were the axillary and supraclavicular areas. This translated into an improvement in distant disease-free survival (HR 0.76, CI 0.60–0.97, $p = 0.03$) but not in overall survival (HR 0.91, CI 0.72–1.13) at 10 years.

Upon comparison of adverse outcomes following WBI alone versus WBI + RNI, significant increases in acute toxicities such as Grade 2–3 radiation dermatitis (40.1% vs. 49.5%, $p < 0.001$) and Grade 2 pneumonitis (0.2% vs 1.2%, $p = 0.01$) were observed. Significantly more frequent delayed toxicities included moderate to severe lymphedema (4.5% vs. 8.4%, $p = 0.001$) and late skin and subcutaneous tissue changes such as telangiectasia, atrophy, or fibrosis (skin, 4.3% vs. 6.9%, $p = 0.02$; subcutaneous tissue 2.0% vs. 4.1%, $p = 0.01$). There were no differences in the rates of fatigue, pain, delayed cardiotoxicity, neuropathy, late pneumonitis, or second cancers between the two groups. Grade 4 toxicity was rare and occurred in only 3 of the 893 patients in the WBI + RNI group. These results suggest that for carefully selected patients with node positive or high-risk node negative disease, the addition of regional nodal irradiation to whole breast irradiation improves locoregional and disease-free survival with a modestly increased risk of few acute and delayed toxicities.

Regional Nodal Irradiation by Extent of Axillary Surgery

The twenty-first century has witnessed a growing body of evidence in support of a novel approach to limited axillary surgery in the form of sentinel lymph node biopsy for the clinically negative axilla. Multiple randomized trials have demonstrated equivalent clinical outcomes when ALND is foregone after a negative SLNB [18, 19]. In the NSABP B-32 control group, which underwent SLNB followed by completion ALND, accuracy was high (97%), and false-negative rates were relatively low (approximately 10%) [20]. Additionally, SLNB alone is significantly better tolerated in comparison to ALND with respect to ipsilateral arm function, lymphedema, and ipsilateral arm paresthesias [21, 22]. These findings suggest that modern breast surgeons may avoid relatively high-risk axillary procedures without significantly sacrificing staging and therapeutic efficacy. However, in this nascent era of limited axillary dissections, the indications for postoperative regional nodal irradiation must simultaneously adapt.

The American College of Surgeons Oncology Group (ACOSOG) Z0011 trial aimed to identify the optimal axillary therapy with regard to overall and disease-free survival for early-stage, clinically node-negative (cT1–2N0) patients found with positive sentinel lymph nodes [23]. All patients underwent lumpectomy followed by adjuvant whole breast radiotherapy; no third-field axillary directed radiation was permitted. Despite the difference in median number of nodes obtained by SNLB and ALND (2, IQR 1–4 and 17, IQR 13–22, respectively), the number of positive nodes was equal in both groups (1, IQR 1–2). The majority of both groups received adjuvant systemic therapy: 97% in the SLNB arm and 96% in the ALND arm. Long-term follow-up has revealed 10-year locoregional recurrence rates of 6.2% in the ALND arm vs. 5.3% in the SLNB arm ($p = 0.36$). Specific ipsilateral axillary regional recurrence rates at 10 years in the ALND and SLNB groups were low: 0.5% vs. 1.5%, respectively [24]. It should be noted that at the time this trial was ongoing, many radiation oncologists would consider RNI as the standard of care for patients with positive lymph nodes, especially in the setting of incomplete axillary evaluation such as SLNB. The fact that no further axillary directed therapy was permitted was controversial, prompting concerns regarding deviations from protocol by the participating radiation oncologists. Of the radiotherapy records obtained by Jagsi and colleagues, high tangential fields (covering the low axilla) were used for at least one-half of the patients in both groups and 18.9% received RNI using at least three fields [25]. Further review of patients with radiation field deviations revealed that no RT resulted in statistically significant increases in LRR but that the addition of high tangents or supraclavicular fields to the standard breast tangents did not significantly affect this risk [24].

A modern European trial comparing axillary lymph node dissection versus axillary nodal radiotherapy in patients with positive sentinel lymph nodes was also recently published [26]. Women with primary tumors <3 cm who were clinically node negative were randomized prior to SLNB to either ALND or axillary RT in the setting of SLN-positive disease. Patients randomized to the RT arm received 50 Gy in 25 fractions to all three axillary levels as well as the medial supraclavicular region. Adjuvant nodal RT was allowed in the setting of >4 lymph nodes positive in the ALND arm. Representative of a common breast cancer patient today, the majority (82%) underwent BCS, and 90% received systemic treatment (hormonal and/or chemotherapeutic). Five-year axillary recurrence rates were low in both arms: 0.43% (CI 0.00–0.92) after ALND and 1.19% (CI 0.31–2.08) after axillary RT. The SLN-negative group experienced a similar 5-year axillary recurrence rate of 0.72% (CI 0.39–1.04). There was no difference in overall or disease-free survival between the groups, but rates of clinically significant lymphedema were significantly higher after ALND than after RT at 1, 3, and 5 years. This trial puts forth compelling evidence that, in the setting of sentinel lymph node-positive disease, axillary radiotherapy may be comparable to axillary dissection with regard to outcome. As expected, RNI was better tolerated with regard to ipsilateral arm lymphedema. Nonetheless, due to the low rates of axillary recurrence (consistent with the aforementioned ACOSOG study), this study was underpowered to detect noninferiority of axillary RT. These findings do, however, stand testament to the improving efficacy of systemic therapy in reducing regional recurrence compared to historical trials in which no systemic therapy was given and more aggressive surgical interventions were performed [27].

There is growing evidence in support of axillary radiotherapy after sentinel lymph node biopsy in lieu of axillary lymph node dissection in patients undergoing mastectomy, though this practice remains controversial. This is in part related to modern trials as described above which included proportionally more patients receiving breast-conserving surgery than mastectomy. Based on the available data, if the patient and the multidisciplinary team decide to omit axillary lymph node dissection after SLNB alone, patients determined to be at high risk of locoregional recurrence based on primary tumor and SLNB data alone may warrant adjuvant PMRT irrespective of the prognostic and therapeutic effect of ALND. This is reflected in recent guidelines which recommend PMRT after mastectomy and SLNB "only if there is already sufficient information to justify its use without needing to know that additional axillary lymph nodes are involved [16]."

Internal Mammary Nodal Irradiation

The internal mammary nodes (IMN) have been a suspected harbor for regional spread in patients with central-medial tumors [28, 29]. In multiple previous trials, IMN irradiation (IMNI) has been considered a standard component of complete regional nodal irradiation, despite recent controversy over its utility [5, 6, 14, 17, 30]. Further evidence regarding radiation-induced cardiotoxicity has emerged as impetus to further evaluate the risks and benefits of IMNI [31, 32].

In order to assess the benefit for IMNI in early-stage breast cancer, a French phase 3 trial randomized over 1400 women with stage I–II breast cancer with either positive axillary nodes or a medial/central primary tumor to modified radical mastectomy and ALND followed by adjuvant chest wall radiotherapy with or without IMNI [33]. No internal mammary dissection was allowed. Radiation was delivered via mixed photon-electron beam to the ipsilateral parasternal region in the first five intercostal spaces. This study demonstrated no significant difference in disease control or survival between the two groups. There was no significant increase in cardiac toxicity in the IMNI group within a relatively limited median follow-up of approximately 8 years.

Conversely, a prospective analysis of a Danish population with early-stage, node-positive disease demonstrated a small survival benefit for a very specific subset of patients [34]. Over 3300 patients were treated with adjuvant radiotherapy to the breast/chest wall and regional nodes after BCS or mastectomy to 48 Gy in 24 fractions. Patients with right-sided tumors received IMNI via either an en face electron field or tangential photons. In left-sided disease the risk of cardiac toxicity precluded IMNI. Eight-year breast-cancer specific mortality with and without IMNI was 20.9% vs. 23.4% ($p = 0.03$). Subgroup analysis of patients with medial/central tumors or ≥4 LN involved revealed a significant survival benefit (aHR 0.76, CI 0.66–0.89, $p = 0.001$). These data are difficult to interpret given the study's nonrandomized nature and unilateral treatment paradigm, but they may suggest that there exist certain cohorts of patients that may benefit from IMNI.

In general, it may be reasonable to include the IMN as a component of RNI when technically feasible with respect to heart dose constraints (i.e., right-sided and select left-sided tumors), especially for patients with medial or central primary tumors. While there are likely undefined groups of low-risk patients that would not benefit from IMNI, this general treatment paradigm is discussed in recent guidelines advocating the use of IMNI along with supraclavicular and axillary RNI for patients with positive axillary lymph nodes [16].

Neoadjuvant Chemotherapy and Its Implications on Regional Nodal Irradiation

Over the last two decades, the use of neoadjuvant chemotherapy (NAC) has become more commonly administered to patients with operable breast cancer as a result of two large randomized clinical trials through the National Surgical Adjuvant Breast and Bowel Project (NSABP). NSABP B-18 compared neoadjuvant AC (doxorubicin 60 mg/m2, cyclophosphamide 600 mg/m2, every 21 days for four cycles) followed by either lumpectomy/ALND or modified radical mastectomy versus the same chemotherapy postoperatively [35]. NSABP B-27 randomized patients to four cycles of neoadjuvant AC plus 5 years of tamoxifen (receptor status was not required at registration) followed by four cycles of docetaxel (100 mg/m2 every 21 days) before or after surgery [36]. Patients enrolled included operable breast cancer with T1–T3, N0–N1 primary disease; the majority of patients were clinical stage I–II. In a long-term analysis of both studies, neoadjuvant AC resulted in a clinical response in 79% of patients (partial clinical response 43%, complete clinical response 36%) but a pathologic complete response (pCR) rate of only 13% [37]. With the addition of docetaxel to the neoadjuvant regimen, the pCR rate increased to 26% ($p < 0.001$). Additionally, patients undergoing NAC had higher rates of BCS (68% vs. 60%, $p < 0.001$). There were no differences in disease-free, relapse-free, or overall survival between the groups in either study, but there were significant overall survival benefits for patients achieving pCR (B-18: HR 0.32, $p < 0.0001$; B-27: HR 0.36, $p < 0.0001$). Notably, locoregional recurrence rates were low in comparison to the distant metastasis rate in the more modern NSABP B-27 study: overall rates of IBTR, regional, and distant recurrence were 6%, 2%, and 18%, respectively.

This new paradigm, especially in the setting of a pathologic complete response, complicates the role of radiotherapy in the adjuvant setting. When clinicopathologic status prior to receiving chemotherapy had previously predicted the benefit of radiotherapy, we must now consider these prechemotherapy factors as well as each patient's particular response to neoadjuvant chemotherapy. The majority of data regarding the benefit of adjuvant radiotherapy after NAC remains retrospective in nature. Analysis of 150 patients that received NAC prior to mastectomy from 1974 to 2000 revealed high rates of locoregional recurrence (27%) even after pathologic complete response (19%), suggesting a response to neoadjuvant chemotherapy did not obviate the need for adjuvant radiotherapy [38]. Further retrospective analysis of a larger population comprising multiple prospective institutional clinical trials found that PMRT after NAC reduced the 10-year LRR rates from 22% to 11% ($p = 0.0001$) [39]. Generally, patients with more advanced primary tumors (cT3–T4) and nodal involvement (cN2–3) also experienced a statistically significant benefit in locoregional control from PMRT. Of the 676 patients, 86 (13%) achieved a complete response to neoadjuvant chemotherapy. In clinical stage I–II patients, 10-year LRR rates were similar with or without PMRT ($p = 0.22$), but LRR was significantly lower for patients with stage III–IV disease that underwent PMRT (3% vs. 33%, $p = 0.006$). These findings were again demonstrated in a larger analysis of 106 patients with stage II–III disease achieving a pCR; PMRT was associated with significantly improved overall survival rates for the patients with stage III disease (77% with PMRT vs. 33% without, $p = 0.0016$) [40].

Analysis of the aforementioned NSABP trials provides insight into which patients are at highest risk for locoregional recurrence in this setting [41]. In these trials, adjuvant radiotherapy was specifically regulated: all patients who underwent mastectomy did not receive radiotherapy, all patients undergoing lumpectomy received WBI only, and no patients received RNI. This allows for the specific evaluation of locoregional recurrence risks in the absence of PMRT or post-BCS RNI. Upon multivariate analysis, the extent of pathologic response after NAC significantly predicted for locoregional recurrence at 10 years: conversion to node-negative disease (ypN0) with residual disease in the breast was associated with increased risk when compared to pCR in both the breast and axilla (HR 1.55, $p < 0.001$). Additionally, pathologically positive nodes after NAC (ypN+) versus a breast/nodal pCR carried a proportionally higher risk of LRR (HR 2.71, $p < 0.001$). Expected clinical factors such as younger age, larger tumor size, and clinical nodal status also significantly predicted for LRR. One caveat when applying these data in the clinical setting is the relatively small numbers of patients in some of the comparison groups (i.e., ypT0/ypN0 and ypT+/ypN0).

When evaluating the role for RNI in patients receiving neoadjuvant chemotherapy followed by breast-conserving surgery, it is helpful to specifically consider regional recurrence rates, especially in the setting of a clinically positive axilla. In the 506 clinically node-positive patients that underwent BCS + WBI in these two trials, 10-year regional recurrence was less likely in pathologically node negative when compared to patients with persistently positive nodes (0–2.4% vs. 7.5–8.7%). Similarly, in the postmastectomy setting, the risk of chest wall and/or regional recurrence is the predominant consideration. Patients with clinically T3, node-negative disease had 10-year chest wall recurrence rates of 0–8.6% and regional recurrence rates of 3.2–6.2%. With clinically positive but pathologically negative nodes, regardless of primary tumor size, chest wall recurrence rates were 0–9.2%, regional recurrence rates were 0–8.1%, and combined LRR rates were 0–10.8%. As such, the relative benefit of adjuvant RNI (in addition to WBI) or PMRT may not be enough to warrant exposure to potential treatment toxicities in these patients, especially for left-sided cancers. Recent consensus guidelines indicate that, while current studies suggest patients with axillary pCR may have a low risk of LRR, these is insufficient evidence regarding the use of PMRT in this setting [16].

In order to answer this complex question, two randomized clinical trials are currently ongoing. For stage II–III patients with biopsy-proven node-positive disease that convert to pathologically node negative after neoadjuvant chemotherapy, the NSABP B-51/RTOG 1304 trial evaluates the impact of regional nodal irradiation to the undissected axilla, ipsilateral supraclavicular fossa, and first three intercostal IMN in addition to either WBI or chest wall RT on local/regional/distant recurrence and breast cancer mortality rates [42]. Sentinel lymph node biopsy, axillary lymph node dissection, or both are allowed at the time of BCS/mastectomy. Similar patients undergoing SLNB found with persistent node-positive disease after NAC are eligible for the Alliance A011202 trial, an alternate study with compatible baseline inclusion criteria. This trial randomizes ypN+ patients to either completion ALND followed by RNI as outlined above versus RNI alone. Measured outcomes will include invasive breast cancer recurrence-free survival, overall survival, locoregional control, and rates of arm/breast lymphedema. These two studies will assist in clarifying the role for regional nodal irradiation in the management of breast cancer treated with neoadjuvant chemotherapy.

References

1. Helvie MA, Chang JT, Hendrick RE, Banerjee M. Reduction in late-stage breast cancer incidence in the mammography era: implications for overdiagnosis of invasive cancer. Cancer. 2014;120:2649–56.
2. Fisher B, Anderson S, Bryant J, Margolese RG, Deutsch M, Fisher ER, Jeong J-H, Wolmark N. Twenty-year follow up of a randomized trial comparing total mastectomy, lumpectomy, and lumpectomy plus irradiation for the treatment of invasive breast cancer. N Engl J Med. 2002;347:1233–41.
3. Veronesi U, Cascinelli N, Mariani L, Greco M, Saccozzi R, Luini A, Aguilar M, Marubini E. Twenty-year follow-up of a randomized study comparing breast-conserving surgery with radical mastectomy for early breast cancer. N Engl J Med. 2002;347:1227–32.
4. Clarke M, Collins R, Darby S, et al. Effects of radiotherapy and of differences in the extent of surgery for early breast cancer on local recurrence and 15-year survival: an overview of the randomised trials. Lancet. 2005;366:2087–106.
5. Overgaard M, Hansen PS, Overgaard J, et al. Postoperative radiotherapy in high-risk premenopausal women with breast cancer who receive adjuvant chemotherapy. Danish Breast Cancer Cooperative Group 82b trial. N Engl J Med. 1997;337:949–55.
6. Overgaard M, Jensen MB, Overgaard J, et al. Postoperative radiotherapy in high-risk postmenopausal breast-cancer patients given adjuvant tamoxifen: Danish Breast Cancer Cooperative Group DBCG 82c randomised trial. Lancet. 1999;353:1641–8.
7. Ragaz J, Olivotto IA, Spinelli JJ, et al. Locoregional radiation therapy in patients with high-risk breast cancer receiving adjuvant chemotherapy: 20-year results of the British Columbia randomized trial. J Natl Cancer Inst. 2005;97:116–26.
8. Macdonald SM, Abi-Raad RF, Alm El-Din MA, Niemierko A, Kobayashi W, McGrath JJ, Goldberg SI, Powell S, Smith B, Taghian AG. Chest wall radiotherapy: middle ground for treatment of patients with one to three positive lymph nodes after mastectomy. Int J Radiat Oncol Biol Phys. 2009;75:1297–303.
9. Truong PT, Jones SO, Kader HA, Wai ES, Speers CH, Alexander AS, Olivotto IA. Patients with t1 to t2 breast cancer with one to three positive nodes have higher local and regional recurrence risks compared with node-negative patients after breast-conserving surgery and whole-breast radiotherapy. Int J Radiat Oncol Biol Phys. 2009;73:357–64.

10. Cosar R, Uzal C, Tokatli F, et al. Postmastectomy irradiation in breast in breast cancer patients with T1-2 and 1-3 positive axillary lymph nodes: is there a role for radiation therapy? Radiat Oncol. 2011;6:28.
11. Dai Kubicky C, Mongoue-Tchokote S. Prognostic significance of the number of positive lymph nodes in women with T1-2N1 breast cancer treated with mastectomy: should patients with 1, 2, and 3 positive lymph nodes be grouped together? Int J Radiat Oncol Biol Phys. 2013;85:1200–5.
12. Overgaard M, Nielsen HM, Overgaard J. Is the benefit of postmastectomy irradiation limited to patients with four or more positive nodes, as recommended in international consensus reports? A subgroup analysis of the DBCG 82 b&c randomized trials. Radiother Oncol. 2007;82:247–53.
13. EBCTCG (Early Breast Cancer Trialists' Collaborative Group), Mc Gale P, Taylor C, et al. Effect of radiotherapy after mastectomy and axillary surgery on 10-year recurrence and 20-year breast cancer mortality: meta-analysis of individual patient data for 8135 women in 22 randomised trials. Lancet. 2014;383:2127–35.
14. Poortmans PM, Collette S, Kirkove C, et al. Internal mammary and medial supraclavicular irradiation in breast cancer. N Engl J Med. 2015;373:317–27.
15. Matzinger O, Heimsoth I, Poortmans P, et al. Toxicity at three years with and without irradiation of the internal mammary and medial supraclavicular lymph node chain in stage I to III breast cancer (EORTC trial 22922/10925). Acta Oncol. 2010;49:24–34.
16. Recht A, Comen EA, Fine RE, et al. Postmastectomy radiotherapy: an American Society of Clinical Oncology, American Society for Radiation Oncology, and Society of Surgical Oncology focused guideline update. J Clin Oncol. 2016; doi:10.1200/JCO.2016.69.1188.
17. Whelan TJ, Olivotto IA, Parulekar WR, et al. Regional nodal irradiation in early-stage breast cancer. N Engl J Med. 2015;373:307–16.
18. Veronesi U, Paganelli G, Viale G, et al. Sentinel-lymph-node biopsy as a staging procedure in breast cancer: update of a randomised controlled study. Lancet Oncol. 2006;7:983–90.
19. Krag DN, Anderson SJ, Julian TB, et al. Sentinel-lymph-node resection compared with conventional axillary-lymph-node dissection in clinically node-negative patients with breast cancer: overall survival findings from the NSABP B-32 randomised phase 3 trial. Lancet Oncol. 2010;11:927–33.
20. Krag DN, Anderson SJ, Julian TB, et al. Technical outcomes of sentinel-lymph-node resection and conventional axillary-lymph-node dissection in patients with clinically node-negative breast cancer: results from the NSABP B-32 randomised phase III trial. Lancet Oncol. 2007;8:881–8.
21. Ashikaga T, Krag DN, Land SR, et al. Morbidity results from the NSABP B-32 trial comparing sentinel lymph node dissection versus axillary dissection. J Surg Oncol. 2010;102:111–8.
22. Mansel RE, Fallowfield L, Kissin M, et al. Randomized multicenter trial of sentinel node biopsy versus standard axillary treatment in operable breast cancer: the ALMANAC trial. J Natl Cancer Inst. 2006;98:599–609.
23. Giuliano AE, Hunt KK, Ballman KV, Beitsch PD, Whitworth PW, Blumencranz PW, Leitch AM, Saha S, McCall LM, Morrow M. Axillary dissection vs no axillary dissection in women with invasive breast cancer and sentinel node metastasis: a randomized clinical trial. JAMA. 2011;305:569–75.
24. Giuliano AE, Ballman K, McCall L, Beitsch P, Whitworth PW, Blumencranz P, Leitch AM, Saha S, Morrow M, Hunt KK. Locoregional recurrence after sentinel lymph node dissection with or without axillary dissection in patients with sentinel lymph node metastases: long-term follow-up from the American College of Surgeons Oncology Group (Alliance) ACOSOG Z0011 randomized trial. Ann Surg. 2016;264:413–20.
25. Jagsi R, Ballman K, Chadha M, Moni J, Laurie F, Buchholz TA, Haffty BG, Giuliano A (2013) Radiation field design on the ACOSOG Z0011 trial 32:3600.
26. Donker M, van Tienhoven G, Straver ME, et al. Radiotherapy or surgery of the axilla after a positive sentinel node in breast cancer (EORTC 10981-22023 AMAROS): a randomised, multicentre, open-label, phase 3 non-inferiority trial. Lancet Oncol. 2014;15:1303–10.

27. Fisher B, Jeong J-H, Anderson S, Bryant J, Fisher ER, Wolmark N. Twenty-five-year follow-up of a randomized trial comparing radical mastectomy, total mastectomy, and total mastectomy followed by irradiation. N Engl J Med. 2002;347:567–75.
28. Lacour J, Bucalossi P, Cacers E, Jacobelli G, Koszarowski T, Le M, Rumeau-Rouquette C, Veronesi U. Radical mastectomy versus radical mastectomy plus internal mammary dissection. Five-year results of an international cooperative study. Cancer. 1976;37:206–14.
29. Huang O, Wang L, Shen K, et al. Breast cancer subpopulation with high risk of internal mammary lymph nodes metastasis: analysis of 2269 Chinese breast cancer patients treated with extended radical mastectomy. Breast Cancer Res Treat. 2008;107:379–87.
30. Ragaz J, Jackson SM, Le N, et al. Adjuvant radiotherapy and chemotherapy in node-positive premenopausal women with breast cancer. N Engl J Med. 1997;337:956–62.
31. Darby SC, Ewertz M, McGale P, et al. Risk of ischemic heart disease in women after radiotherapy for breast cancer. N Engl J Med. 2013;368:987–98.
32. Taylor CW, Wang Z, Macaulay E, Jagsi R, Duane F, Darby SC. Exposure of the heart in breast cancer radiation therapy: a systematic review of heart doses published during 2003 to 2013. Int J Radiat Oncol Biol Phys. 2015;93:845–53.
33. Hennequin C, Bossard N, Servagi-Vernat S, et al. Ten-year survival results of a randomized trial of irradiation of internal mammary nodes after mastectomy. Int J Radiat Oncol Biol Phys. 2013;86:860–6.
34. Thorsen LBJ, Offersen BV, Danø H, Berg M, Jensen I, Pedersen AN, Zimmermann SJ, Brodersen H-J, Overgaard M, Overgaard J. DBCG-IMN: a population-based cohort study on the effect of internal mammary node irradiation in early node-positive breast cancer. J Clin Oncol. 2016;34:314–20.
35. Fisher B, Brown A, Mamounas E, et al. Effect of preoperative chemotherapy on local-regional disease in women with operable breast cancer: findings from National Surgical Adjuvant Breast and Bowel Project B-18. J Clin Oncol. 1997;15:2483–93.
36. Bear HD, Anderson S, Brown A, et al. The effect on tumor response of adding sequential preoperative docetaxel to preoperative doxorubicin and cyclophosphamide: preliminary results from National Surgical Adjuvant Breast and Bowel Project Protocol B-27. J Clin Oncol. 2003;21:4165–74.
37. Rastogi P, Anderson SJ, Bear HD, et al. Preoperative chemotherapy: updates of National Surgical Adjuvant Breast and Bowel Project Protocols B-18 and B-27. J Clin Oncol. 2008;26:778–85.
38. Buchholz TA, Tucker SL, Masullo L, et al. Predictors of local-regional recurrence after neoadjuvant chemotherapy and mastectomy without radiation. J Clin Oncol. 2002;20:17–23.
39. Huang EH, Tucker SL, Strom EA, et al. Postmastectomy radiation improves local-regional control and survival for selected patients with locally advanced breast cancer treated with neoadjuvant chemotherapy and mastectomy. J Clin Oncol. 2004;22:4691–9.
40. McGuire SE, Gonzalez-Angulo AM, Huang EH, et al. Postmastectomy radiation improves the outcome of patients with locally advanced breast cancer who achieve a pathologic complete response to neoadjuvant chemotherapy. Int J Radiat Oncol Biol Phys. 2007;68:1004–9.
41. Mamounas EP, Anderson SJ, Dignam JJ, Bear HD, Julian TB, Geyer CE Jr, Taghian A, Wickerham DL, Wolmark N. Predictors of locoregional recurrence after neoadjuvant chemotherapy: results from combined analysis of National Surgical Adjuvant Breast and Bowel Project B-18 and B-27. J Clin Oncol. 2012;30:3960–6.
42. NSABP Foundation, Inc: NCT01872975: standard or comprehensive radiation therapy in treating patients with early-stage breast cancer previously treated with chemotherapy and surgery. https://clinicaltrials.gov/ct2/show/NCT01872975 (2016). Accessed 21 Aug 2016.

Radiotherapy and Regional Nodes 10

Andrew Zhang, Bruce G. Haffty, and Sharad Goyal

Axillary Management

Routine axillary management involves either axillary lymph node dissection (ALND), sentinel lymph node biopsy (SLNB), radiation therapy (RT), or a combination of both. Patients that are clinically node negative (cN0) can be treated with either therapy alone. An Italian trial randomized cT1N0 patients aged 18–65 years to either whole breast irradiation (WBI) with ALND or radiation, showing that the later arm experienced 9% nodal involvement with a median follow-up of 10.6 years [1]. In elderly patients, Martelli et al. showed that in 238 cN0 patients aged 65–80 who were initially treated with quadrantectomy and similarly randomized, the 15-year cumulative incidence of overt axillary disease in the radiation alone arm was only 6% [2]. The NSABP B-04 also trial demonstrated that among cN0 patients treated with axillary dissection, axillary radiation, and no axillary treatment, nodal recurrence as the first recurrence event was seen in 4%, 4%, and 6% of the randomized arms, respectively.

This suggests that certain patient populations with cN0 have acceptably low risk of recurrence with or without ALND. Specifically in elderly T1N0 and estrogen receptor-positive (ER+) patients, axillary treatment can be omitted altogether. Hughes et al. showed that women with early-stage breast cancer and favorable receptor profiles who are 70 years of age or older can be treated with tamoxifen alone. Ipsilateral breast recurrence was 8% with tamoxifen alone and 2% with tamoxifen and radiation, while axillary recurrence was 1% and 0%, respectively [3]. Other studies have also found similar results in elderly patients [4].

A. Zhang, MD • B.G. Haffty, MD • S. Goyal, MD, MS (✉)
Department of Radiation Oncology, Rutgers Cancer Institute of New Jersey and Rutgers Robert Wood Johnson Medical School, 195 Little Albany Street, New Brunswick, NJ 08903, USA
e-mail: az106@cinj.rutgers.edu; hafftybg@cinj.rutgers.edu; goyalsh@rutgers.edu

M. Howard-McNatt (ed.), *Changing Paradigms in the Management of Breast Cancer*, DOI 10.1007/978-3-319-60336-0_10

NSABP B-06 randomized women with stage I and II breast tumors less than 4 cm in greatest diameter to either simple mastectomy, lumpectomy, or lumpectomy followed by WBI. Axillary dissection of the lower two levels of lymph nodes was performed regardless of the treatment assignment. Radiation was delivered 50 Gy with tangents alone, not including supraclavicular or internal mammary fields. Despite 38% of patients having pathologically positive lymph (pN+) nodes, nodal recurrence was only 5%. This is in part attributable to both the ALND as well as the tangential radiation fields incidentally sterilizing microscopic disease in the axillary levels I and II lymph node basins.

Conversely, patients who are clinically node positive (cN+) in the axilla should be treated primarily with ALND instead of upfront RT since 46–50 Gy of radiation alone cannot fully eliminate gross axillary disease. NSABP B-04 showed that 1% of cN+ patients treated with radical mastectomy and ALND had axillary recurrence compared to 11% of those treated with total mastectomy and radiation [5]. Strom et al. demonstrated that in their cohort of 1031 patients treated with mastectomy and doxorubicin-based chemotherapy, only 21 patients experienced recurrence in the low-mid axilla. While 90% of patients received an ALND of ten or more LNs, among the 100 patients (10%) who received an ALND fewer than ten nodes (1% of patients received an ALND of fewer than five nodes), only three patients experienced an axillary recurrence. The risk of failure in the low-mid axilla was not significantly increased based on number of involved nodes, percentage of involved nodes, nodal size, or gross extra-nodal extension (ECE) [6].

While ALND serves both a therapeutic and diagnostic role, it also has been associated with surgical complications and arm lymphedema in 12–20% of the cases [7]. With the introduction of the less morbid sentinel lymph node biopsy (SLNB), rates of lymphedema, shoulder dysfunction, loss of sensation in the distribution of the intercostobrachial nerve, infection, length of hospital stay, time to resumption of normal day-to-day activities after surgery, and quality of life have dramatically improved [8]. Thus, ALND is typically reserved for patients who present with high nodal burden, fixed or matted nodes, when an SLNB reveals extensive ECE or when SLNs cannot be identified.

SLNB represents a strategy for directed sampling that increases the probability of identifying positive nodes, thus allowing fewer nodes to be removed without increasing the axillary failure rate. SLNBs have been validated showing a low false-negative rate (FNR) of <10% and a low axillary recurrence rate of <5% [9, 10]. Consequently, treatment decisions based on a negative SLNB are considered equivalent to those based on negative ALND. This is supported by the NSABP B-32 study, which demonstrated that SLNB in patients achieves the same survival and regional control as ALND with acceptable side effects [11]. Five thousand six hundred eleven patients with invasive breast cancer and cN0 axilla were identified and randomized to either SLNB with ALND ($N = 2807$) or SLNB alone ($N = 2804$). Although the FNR was 9.7% for the SLNB alone arm, which was corroborated by a large meta-analysis of 69 trials and 8059 patients also showing a FNR of about 7.3% [12], 8-year follow-up shows no statistical benefit in overall survival (92.9% vs. 91.6%), disease-free survival (75.1% vs. 76.1%), or local-regional control between either arms. The authors concluded that when SLNB is negative, there is no further need for ALND and that SLN surgery alone is an appropriate, safe, and effective therapy for breast cancer patients with clinically negative lymph nodes. Although previous B-32 results did show that ALND was associated with high patient-reported morbidity in terms of arm range of motion and sensory defects compared to SLNB alone, SLNB does however increase the risk of lymphedema and functional and neurological deficits [13].

Recently, the standard of care that mandated performing an ALND in node-positive patients was reexamined after the publication of International Breast Cancer Study Group (IBCSG) 23-01 and the American College of Surgeons Oncology Group (ACOSOG) Z11 studies [14, 15]. The IBCSG 23-01 study randomized 931 patients with micrometastatic (<2 mm) deposit in the SLNB to ALND or no additional surgery [16]. The majority of the patients (97%) received adjuvant RT without regional nodal irradiation (RNI). In the ALND arm, additional axillary nodal involvement was detected in 13% of the patients. There was no difference in the overall survival or disease-free survival between the two study arms. Although the study closed before meeting target accrual, the authors concluded that breast cancer patients with limited SLN involvement could be spared from the morbidity of an ALND.

In contrast to the IBCSG 23-01, the ACOSOG Z11 study randomized 856 patients out of a planned 1900 patients with clinically T1-2N0 breast cancer after lumpectomy and a pathologically positive SLNB, which included one or two macrometastatic SLNs, to either ALND or no further treatment [17]. Patients were excluded if they received neoadjuvant chemotherapy or hormonal therapy, were bilateral or multicentric breast cancers, had matted nodes, or had ≥3 LN with disease. Z11 did not reveal a significant difference in OS (91.8% vs. 92.5%) and DFS (82.2% vs. 83.9%) between the study arms. In ALND group, axillary dissection revealed additional metastases in 27.3% of the patients. Assuming an equal percentage of positive nodes is left untreated in the no dissection arm, a higher regional failure would be expected. However, 5-year breast recurrences were 3.1% in the ALND arm vs. 1.6% in the SLNB-alone arm (NS) while axilla recurrences were 0.5% vs. 0.9% (NS), respectively.

This nonsignificance could be explained in part due to favorable patient population selection. The majority of the patients in the above trial had ER-positive (80%), T1 (69%), single-positive SLN (65%) disease. Adjuvant systemic therapy was given to 97% of the patients (hormones 46%, chemotherapy 58%). Despite adjuvant RT given with tangents alone without dedicated axillary treatment, the lower lymphatic regions I–II would still receive some dose. Of note, a third field directed to the supraclavicular and axillary region was used in up to 18% of the patients whose radiation data were available [18].

Additionally, the use of fine needle biopsy over ALND has also been substantiated among node-positive patients with clinically high nodal burdens of disease who receive neoadjuvant chemotherapy. ACOSOG Z1071 showed that FNB resulted in a FNR of 12.6% in cN1 disease and an FNR of 0% in cN2 disease [19]. FNRs were also lower when three or more SLNs were evaluated compared to only two

SLNs being evaluated (9.1% vs. 21.1%, $p = 0.007$) and when dual-agent mapping was implemented rather than single-agent mapping (10.8% vs. 20.3%, $p = 0.05$).

The risk of local-regional recurrences in breast cancer patients with clinically negative nodes and the role of radiation instead of an ALND dissection have also been examined in the EORTC 10981-22023 AMAROS trial. Four thousand eight hundred six patients were randomized to receive either ALND alone or RT alone following a positive SLNB. Five-year axillary recurrence rates were nonsignificant: 0.43% after ALND vs. 1.19% after RT. However, lymphedema rates were 23.2% vs. 10.8% ($p < 0.0001$) in favor of the RT arm. Notably, the EORTC/AMAROS trial provides additional data contributing to the low regional failure rates in the Z11 study by restating the regional nodal irradiation ability to eradicate subclinical disease remaining after excision of the positive SLNs.

When patients do receive conservative therapy and axillary LN dissection, however, Mehta and Haffty showed that patients may forgo radiation to the dissected region despite node-positive disease [20]. In 51 of 1040 patients treated with conservative surgery and radiation therapy and found with four or more positive lymph nodes, only 2 patients of the 51 patients experienced LN failures (one supraclavicular and one axillary/supraclavicular) and both failed within the irradiated volume. Of the 51 patients, 40 patients received RT to the supraclavicular region without axilla to a median dose of 46 Gy, 10 patients received radiation to the supraclavicular region and axilla to a median dose of 46 Gy, and 1 patient received tangents alone. Forty nine of the 51 patients (96%) received adjuvant therapy. Of the 40 patients treated to the supraclavicular fossa (omitting complete axillary radiation), none failed in the dissected axilla, suggesting that conservative therapy with ALND and radiation therapy is acceptable. Actuarial statistics reveal a 10-year distant metastases-free rate of 65%, 10-year nodal recurrence-free rate of 96%, and a 10-year breast recurrence-free rate of 82%. Patients who require irradiation to the dissected axilla include those patients with ECE, >9 positive lymph nodes, or those with fixed or matted nodes upon presentation.

Supraclavicular and Internal Mammary Management

NSABP B-06 demonstrated that for patients with either positive or negative axillary LNs found on ALND treated by lumpectomy and radiation compared to lumpectomy alone, local-regional nodal control was improved with the addition of radiation, with 17 (2.7%) vs. 56 (8.8%) of patients first failing locally and 34 (5.4%) vs. 55 (8.7%) patients first failing in the regional nodes, respectively [21]. This suggests that while radiation after lumpectomy is effective in controlling local-regional post-surgical microscopic disease, the regional LN failures are rare even without radiation. Other studies have shown that in patients with one to three axillary LN that are positive on dissection, supraclavicular failures (1–2%) are low with tangential radiation alone without intentional nodal irradiation [22, 23]. Patient with four or more axillary LN positive for disease may experience slightly higher rates of supraclavicular failures (3–5%) [24].

In pathologic N1 (pN1) breast cancer patients treated with mastectomy or breast-conserving treatment, but without supraclavicular RT, retrospective analysis has shown that statistically significant prognostic factors for supraclavicular node recurrence included lymphovascular invasion ($p < 0.0001$), ECE ($p < 0.0001$), the number of involved axillary nodes ($p = 0.0003$), and the level of involved axillary nodes ($p = 0.012$). Five-year supraclavicular RFS showed that patients with two or more factors showed a significantly higher recurrence rate than did patients with fewer than two factors (96.8% and 72.9%, respectively; $p < 0.0001$). Of the 448 patients included in this review, treatment failed in 101 patients (22.5%), and only 39 patients (8.7%) had supraclavicular node recurrence [25].

The management of IM nodes is controversial. Sentinel lymph node (SLN) mapping often identifies nonaxillary nodes, although the ability to identify these nodes does not imply a clinical benefit for biopsy or removal. Four early randomized trials showed no survival benefit from IM nodal dissection as compared in the absence of chemotherapy [26–29]. Furthermore, given the advent and usage of adjuvant systemic therapy (both chemotherapy and hormonal therapy), the importance of IM management has diminished over time. However, several recently published studies have demonstrated a survival benefit to chest wall or WBI with RNI by addressing postsurgical axillary residual microscopic disease subclinical disease in the supraclavicular (SCV) and internal mammary nodes (IMN) not accessible to surgery.

The Canadian MA.20 intergroup study showed the benefit for RNI in node-positive or high-risk node-negative disease [30]. One thousand eight hundred thirty-two women were randomized after lumpectomy, ALND, and adjuvant therapy (91% of patients received adjuvant chemotherapy and 71% received hormonal therapy) to either WBI with or without regional nodal coverage (axillary, SCV, and ipsilateral IMN in the upper three intercostal spaces). Eighty-five percent of patients had one to three positive nodes. Regional nodal irradiation improved 10-year DFS (82% vs. 77%, HR 0.76, $p = 0.01$), distant DFS (86.3% vs. 82.4%, HR 0.76, $p = 0.03$), and isolated local-regional DFS (95.2% vs. 92.2%, HR 0.59, $p = 0.009$). Certain high-risk patient populations on subgroup analysis (especially those with negative estrogen and progesterone receptor statuses) benefited from RNI. Overall survival was not significant.

Similarly, the EORTC 22922/10925 study randomized 4004 node-positive or node-negative breast cancer with central or medial tumors after lumpectomy or mastectomy and adjuvant therapy (85% of patients received either chemotherapy, hormonal therapy, or both) to either RNI or observation [31]. At a median follow-up of 11 years, RNI improved DFS (72.1% vs. 69.1%, HR 0.89, $p = 0.04$), distant DFS (78% vs. 75%, HR 0.86, $p = 0.02$), and breast cancer mortality (12.5% vs. 14.4%, HR 0.82, $p = 0.02$).

The relative reduction of 24% of distant metastasis seen in the MA.20 study was substantiated in the EORTC study and is probably due to the reduction in regional nodal recurrence and subclinical regional nodal disease [32, 33]. Interestingly, OS was nonsignificant in both studies. However, a meta-analysis of both studies showed a significant improvement of OS (HR 0.88, CL 0.78–0.99) with absolute benefits at 10 years of 1% in the MA.20 trial and 1.6% in the EORTC trial [34]. Subgroup analysis suggests that patient with N0 disease and a complete ALND (>10 nodes) has a larger OS advantage from RNI than N1-3 disease or an incomplete ALND. Further investigation remains necessary to identify patients who benefit the most from RNI.

Recently, a prospective Danish study reported the results of 3089 early-stage breast cancer patients treated according to the national guidelines that directed RNI (including IM nodes) of all right-sided disease but RNI (excluding IM nodes) of all left-sided disease [35]. RT was given 48 Gy in 24 fractions regardless of cancer laterality. With a median follow-up of 8.9 years, the overall survival rates (75.9% vs. 72.2%, HR 0.82, $p = 0.005$), breast cancer mortality (20.9% vs. 23.4%, HR 0.85, $p = 0.03$), and risk of distant recurrence (27.4% vs. 29.7%, HR 0.89, $p = 0.07$) all favored internal mammary irradiation. Subgroup analysis suggested that tumor size ≥51 mm and ≥4 axillary nodes positive (especially if the primary cancer was in the lateral quadrants) predicted an overall survival benefit for internal mammary irradiation.

The Danish study suggested that the effect of treating the internal mammary nodes depended on risk of IM node metastasis. In contrast, an older study examining the dissection of internal mammary nodes in T1-3, N0-1 invasive breast cancer patients who underwent either Halsted mastectomy or extended mastectomy with regional node dissection without postoperative RT showed that, in 30 years, the dissection of internal mammary nodes does not improve the survival of patients. However, the prognostic value of axillary and internal mammary nodal positivity is high as it impacts overall survival. Annual death rates were 0.163 with both sites positive, 0.077 with axillary LNs positive, 0.055 with internal mammary nodes positive, and 0.031 with neither site positive for disease [29].

Post-mastectomy Radiation Therapy

Locally advanced breast cancer was initially treated with aggressive surgery before chemotherapy was available. Patients who underwent radical mastectomy performed poorly, with 5-year survival rates around 25% [36]. The majority of these patients unfortunately developed and succumbed to metastatic disease. With the advent of trimodality therapy including chemo/endocrine therapy, radiation, and new surgical procedures, 5-year survival rates increased to 80% with patients with stage IIIA disease and 45% with stage IIB disease [37]. Local-regional control, distant disease-free survival also dramatically improved [38].

Patients treated with upfront surgery (usually lumpectomy, total mastectomy, or modified radical mastectomy) are at risk for recurrence either in the chest wall or regional lymphatics [39]. Among patients who recur, major risk factors include the gross extent of tumor and local-regional LNs involved. Earlier studies have suggested that local-regional irradiation improves survival by reducing these recurrences not prevented by systemic therapy [40, 41]. Overall, the majority of trials have demonstrated benefit for patients with T4 disease and at least four lymph nodes pathologically positive for disease on sentinel lymph node biopsy or axillary lymph node dissection. Small breast cancers (T1-2) and lymph node-negative patients have not experienced significant benefit from post-mastectomy radiation therapy (PMRT).

An earlier study NSABP B-04 aimed to determine whether patients with either clinically negative or clinically positive axillary nodes who received local or regional treatments other than radical mastectomy would have similar outcomes with radical mastectomy. The first cohort with clinically positive LNs was randomized to either radical mastectomy or total mastectomy with PMRT and the second with clinically negative LNs was randomized to either radical mastectomy and ALND, total mastectomy and ALND if evidence of nodal recurrence, or total mastectomy with PMRT. Radiation was delivered 50 Gy to the chest wall and axilla with a 10–20 Gy boost if patients were clinically lymph node positive and 45 Gy to internal mammary and supraclavicular lymph nodes.

At 25-years follow-up, no overall survival difference or local-regional recurrence was seen among the clinically lymph node-positive (cN+) group [42]. However, among the clinically lymph node-negative (cN0) group, total mastectomy with PMRT showed a substantial improvement in terms of local-regional control compared to total mastectomy alone. Of note, a total of 40% of patients with cN0 treated with radical mastectomy had pN+, suggesting that probably a substantial percentage of patients in the cN0 total mastectomy with PMRT arm were also pN+. Therefore, the local control benefit probably was derived from these N+ patients that were initially thought to be cN0. Interestingly, the local control was similar in both arms of the cN+ patients. Most likely, this suggests that while the total mastectomy arm with RT recurred more likely in the axilla, the radical mastectomy arm occurred more often in the supraclavicular region, where surgeons were unable to dissect. Overall, B-04 suggested that PMRT may very well have a benefit in patients with pN+ disease, regardless if lymph nodes are suspected on physical exam. This study did not include patients who received systemic therapy and did not examine exactly how many LN needs to be involved to benefit from PMRT in subgroup analysis.

Both of these concerns were in part answered by the Danish group who examined both premenopausal and postmenopausal high-risk post-mastectomy patients. In both the Danish 82B premenopausal and Danish 82C postmenopausal studies, high risk was defined by either positive axillary LNs (≥N1), tumor size >5 cm (T3), or invasion of skin or pectoral fascia (T4) [43, 44]. All patients received total mastectomy and ALND with a median of seven LN removed followed by a randomization to receive systemic therapy alone (CMF in 82B or tamoxifen in 82C) or concurrent systemic therapy and RT (CMF in 82B or tamoxifen in 82C). Radiation was prescribed either 50 Gy in 25 fractions in 5 weeks or 48 Gy in 22 fractions in 5.5 weeks of chest wall with electrons and regional lymph node including the supraclavicular, infraclavicular, and axillary lymph nodes with anterior photon field and IMNs with electron field (to first four intercostal spaces).

The Danish 82B and the 82C studies both found that the addition of radiation to the systemic therapy significantly improved disease-free survival at 10 years, with an increase from 34% to 48% and 24–36%, respectively. When patients were analyzed based on the number of LNs positive, patients who were N0 did not experience a 10-year actuarial disease-free survival benefit in either study. But patients who were 1–3 LN+ did experience a 13–14% actuarial DFS benefit in both studies and a substantially larger DFS benefit of they had ≥4 LN+ (14–27% and 6–18%, respectively).

The number of LNs involved also translated to a modest overall survival benefit in both studies. The Danish 82B study showed an improvement in 10-year OS of around 10% regardless of whether patients were node positive or negative. 82C however only showed a benefit in LN+ patients, from 44 to 55% if 1–3 LN+, or 17–24% in patients with ≥4 LN+ disease. The 82B subset analysis of patients who had 0–3 LN removed had the largest OS benefit compared to patients with 4–9 LN removed or >9 LNs removed, suggesting that adjuvant chemoradiation therapy, regardless of the number of lymph nodes positive, cannot compensate for inadequate surgical dissection. Other factors that influenced DFS and OS include age, tumor size, malignancy grade, and skin or deep fascia invasion. Of note, tamoxifen was only given 1 year in the 82 C trial, whereas newer studies have found that 5-year treatment may improve survival outcomes [45].

When then patient population of 82B and 82C were combined examining patients with only eight or more LN removed, Overgaard et al. reported that radiation therapy decreased LRR from 51 to 10% in patients with ≥4 LN+ and from 27 to 4% in patients with 1–3 LN+ in their 15-year follow-up [46]. Four patients were required to be treated to avoid one LRR in the ≥4 LN+ subgroup and five patients in the 1–3 LN+ group. Overall survival was also statistically significant in both subsets.

Although it is standard treatment to treat PM patients with ≥4 LN+ with PMRT, studies have not all been consistent to recommend treating 1–3 LN+ patients with PMRT [47–49]. The British Columbia trial randomized 318 premenopausal women with LN+ breast cancer s/p modified radical mastectomy to either observation vs. hypofractionated radiation (37.5 Gy in 16 fractions) [50, 51]. While every outcome including overall survival, breast cancer-specific survival, systemic breast cancer-free survival, and event-free survival were statistically significant for all 318 patients showing that approximately a third of systemic breast cancer events and breast cancer deaths were mitigated by PMRT, subset analysis by the number of positive LNs showed that the majority of these benefits did not persist either in patients with 1–3 LN+ or ≥4 LN+. Other studies also raised concerns about potential cardiac risk in especially younger patients which may offset the relatively modest survival benefits in patients with less LN disease burden [52].

The British Columbia trial did, however, describe that treating the chest wall can effectively eradicate the source of metastasis in more than 30% of patients who otherwise would be at risk of systemic dissemination. Local-regional control with RT having a systemic effect was seen only after 3–4 years of follow-up regardless of whether the patient had 1–3 LN+ or ≥4 LN+ suggesting that perhaps the abscopal effect of radiation benefits patients receiving chemotherapy additively.

In 2014, the EBCTCG published a meta-analysis of 8135 patients over 22 trials from 1964 to 1986 to ascertain the benefit of PMRT of patients with 1–3 LN+ [53]. Of all 3131 patients who are pN+, PMRT significantly decreased the risk of

Table 10.1 EBCTCG meta-analysis data on the effect of radiotherapy (RT) after mastectomy and axillary lymph node (ALN) dissection on risk of local-regional recurrence (LRR), any first recurrence, and breast cancer mortality by number of lymph nodes involved. Values are all statistically significant ($p < 0.05$)

	LRR (10 years)			Any first recurrence (10 years)			Breast cancer mortality (20 years)		
	No RT	RT	Abs	No RT	RT	Abs	No RT	RT	Abs
$N = 1314$, 1–3+ ALN	20.3	3.8	16.5	45.7	42.3	3.4	50.2	42.3	7.9
$N = 1133$, 1–3+ ALN	21.0	4.3	16.7	45.5	33.8	11.7	49.4	41.5	7.9
$N = 177$, ≥ 4+ ALN	32.1	13	19	75.1	66.3	8.8	80.0	70.7	9.3

local-regional recurrence at 10 years (26–8%), any first recurrence at 10 years (62.5–51.9%), and breast cancer mortality at 20 years (66.4–58.3%). When patient subsets were analyzed based on positive LNs, 1314 women with 1–3 pN+ and 1772 women with ≥4 pN+ statistically benefited similarly. Among 1133 women with 1–3 pN+ who received mastectomy and ALND along with chemotherapy, the benefits of radiation were more pronounced (Table 10.1).

The absolute difference of any first recurrence that radiation provides in case of these patients with chemotherapy was larger than the larger subset of 1–3 pN+ patients, also suggesting that the effect of local-regional radiation impacting distant disease may work in conjunction with patients receiving chemotherapy. Although the data for PMRT in 1–3 LN+ patients is convincing, there is currently no consensus statement to recommend radiation treatment for all patients who fall within this subset, especially patients with solitary micrometastatic disease (Table 10.2).

However, patients who have high-risk features, especially triple negative disease, have been shown by prospective randomized evidence to have a substantial RFS and OS benefit with adjuvant therapy and regional nodal radiation therapy after mastectomy compared with adjuvant chemotherapy after mastectomy alone without a significant change in the toxicity profile [54]. After a median follow-up of 86.5 months, 5-year RFS rates were 88.3% vs. 74.6% for adjuvant chemotherapy plus radiation and adjuvant chemotherapy alone, respectively (HR 0.77, $p = 0.02$). Five-year OS also improved 90.4% vs. 78.7% in favor of radiation (HR 0.79, $p = 0.03$).

Neoadjuvant Chemotherapy and Adjuvant Radiation

For patients with non-resectable and advanced primary tumors, neoadjuvant chemotherapy use has increased in the recent years because of the potential to downstage disease. Nearly 80% of patients on neoadjuvant chemotherapy experience a decrease in tumor size [55]. Further, the subset of these patients who obtain a complete pathological response also experiences the lowest risk of local-regional failure, substantiating the idea that pathologic response to chemotherapy can also influence the use of adjuvant and regional nodal irradiation.

Table 10.2 Anatomic borders of breast nodal volumes

–	Superior	Inferior	Anterior	Posterior	Lateral	Medial
Supraclavicular	Inferior border of the cricoid cartilage	Head of the clavicle	Sternocleidomastoid (SCM) muscle	Anterior aspect of the scalene muscle	Superior: lateral edge of SCM inferior: junction of the first rib and clavicle	Lateral border of thyroid and trachea
Axillary Lv. III	Insertion of pec. minor in the coracoid process of scapula	Axillary artery crosses medial edge of pec. minor	Posterior surface of pec. major	Ribs and intercostal muscles	Medial border of pec. minor	Thoracic inlet
Axillary Lv. II	Axillary artery crosses medial edge of pec. minor	Axillary artery crosses lateral edge of pec. minor	Posterior surface of pec. major (volume includes all of pec. minor)	Ribs and intercostal muscles	Lateral border of pec. minor	Medial border of pec. minor
Axillary Lv. I	Axillary artery crosses lateral edge of pec. minor	Insertion of pec. major into ribs	Plane defined by the anterior surface of pec. major and lat. dorsi	Anterior surface of subscapularis m	Medial border of lat. dorsi m	Lateral border of pec. minor m
Internal mammary	Superior aspect of the 1st rib	Superior aspect of the 4th rib	Encompasses both IM artery and vein			

Two NSABP trials (B-18 and B-27) addressed these issues by randomizing patients with stages T1-3 and N0-1 breast cancer to either neoadjuvant or postoperative chemotherapy [56]. In NSABP B-18, neoadjuvant doxorubicin and cyclophosphamide (AC) demonstrated an objective clinical response in 79% of patients, of which 43% was a clinical partial response (cPR) and 36% was a clinical complete response (cCR). Thirteen percent had a pathologic complete response (pCR). Preoperative chemotherapy patients also experienced an increased incidence of pathologically negative axillary nodes compared with postoperative chemotherapy patients (58% vs. 42%, respectively; $p < 0.0001$). NSABP B-27 showed that the addition of docetaxel to AC preoperatively increased clinical response rates from 86 to 91% ($p < 0.001$), cCR from 40 to 63% ($p < 0.001$), and pCR from 13 to 26% ($p < 0.001$) [57].

Although neither study showed a statistically significant survival advantage with either arms, certain subsets of patients benefit from neoadjuvant chemotherapy. Patients who experience a pCR, for example, experience significant OS (HR = 0.32, $p < 0.0001$) and DFS (HR = 0.47, $p < 0.0001$) benefits compared to those who have a partial or no response. This is in part due to cPR patients having the lowest risk of local-regional recurrence. Similarly, pathologic nodal status by number of lymph nodes involved at the time of surgery was also an excellent indicator of OS and DFS. Node-positive patients who received neoadjuvant chemotherapy followed by mastectomy and found have residual disease exhibit recurrence rates from 11 to 22%. Node-positive patients who have a cPR have a local-regional recurrence rate of 0%.

Regarding age, women less than 50 years of age seemed to benefit the most from preoperative chemotherapy. This is likely because younger women are more likely to have receptor-negative disease, which has been shown to have a better pathologic response to early initiation of adjuvant systemic therapy than receptor-positive tumors [58]. A small series has shown that patients whose tumors were ER negative were more likely to achieve a pCR than patients who were ER positive (21.6% vs. 8.1%, $p < 0.001$) [59]. Women who are 50 years of age or older, however, had better outcomes with postoperative chemotherapy. This is most likely because the delay in delivering hormonal therapy with receptor positive tumors negatively impacts survival (Figs. 10.1 and 10.2).

Unfortunately, the data that are available for treating locally advanced breast cancer after neoadjuvant chemotherapy are mostly small single-arm institutional analyses. Huang et al. conducted a pooled analysis of 542 patients treated on six consecutive institutional prospective trials with neoadjuvant chemotherapy and showed that PMRT reduced local-regional recurrence for patients with clinical T3 or T4 tumors, pathological tumor size >2 cm, or four or more positive LNs [60]. Similarly, PMRT improved cause-specific survival (CSS) patients with stage ≥ IIIB disease, clinical T4 tumors, and seven or more positive nodes. Among the 20% of patients who achieved a pCR, PMRT still had a significant impact on LRR rates, with 10-year LRR rates improving from 33 to 3% ($p = 0.006$). On multivariate analysis, the lack of radiation had the largest 10-year LRR hazard of 4.68 ($p < 0.0001$), more so than stage ≥IIIB (HR = 2.38, $p = 0.001$) or minimal or worse clinical response to chemotherapy (HR = 1.88, $p = 0.021$).

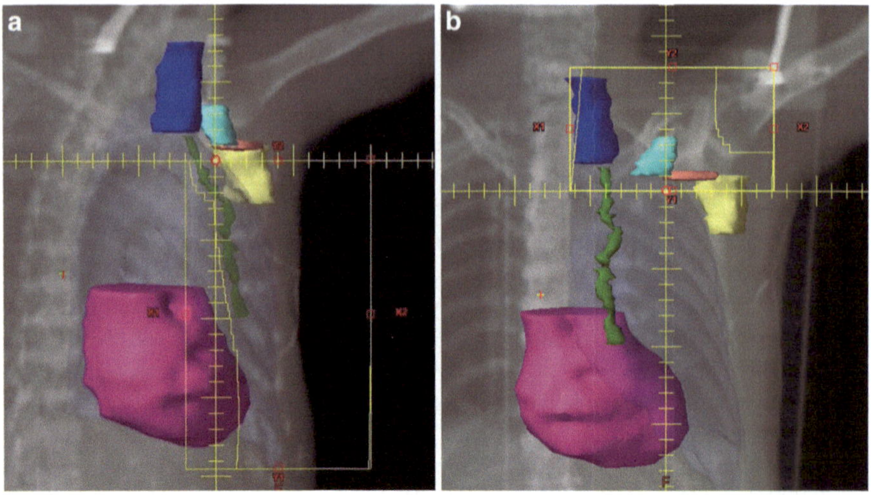

Fig. 10.1 (**a**, **b**) Comprehensive nodal irradiation involves coverage of the axillary level I (*yellow*), level II (*pink*), level III (*teal*), supraclavicular (*dark blue*), and internal mammary (*green*) lymph nodes typically with a three-field technique. The first two tangential fields are half beam blocked to avoid overlap with the third supraclavicular field. Field angling and multi-leaf collimators are used to minimize heart (*magenta*), lung (*pale blue*), spinal cord, and humeral head doses

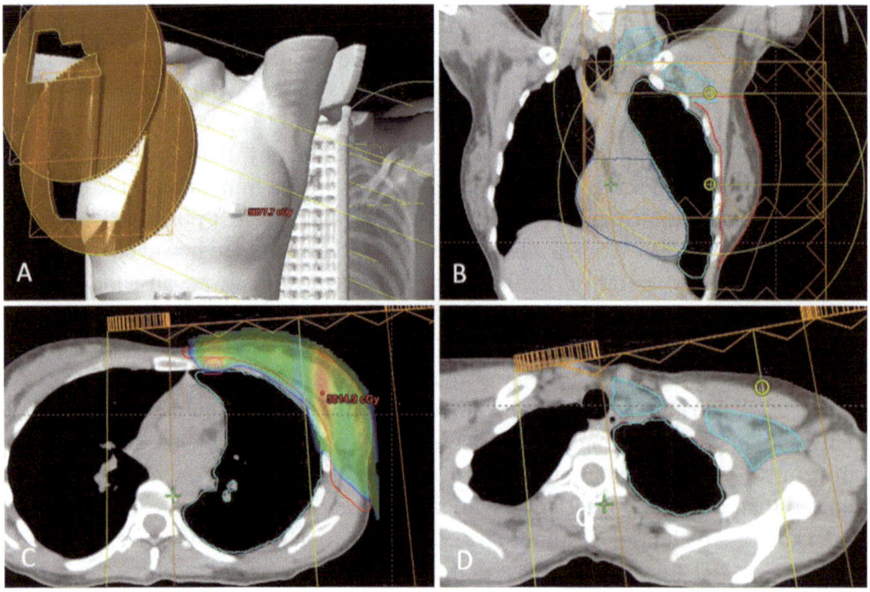

Fig. 10.2 Comprehensive nodal irradiation with proton therapy involves a supraclavicular field and a primary field (**a**, **b**), which cover the PTV breast (*red*), internal mammary nodes (*magenta*) (**c**), and supraclavicular and axillary lymph nodes I–III (*teal*) (**d**). The dose delivered spares the majority of the lung and heart while providing adequate PTV coverage. The dose wash border represents 95% of total dose

Therefore, adjuvant radiation may be beneficial especially for locally advanced tumors with high nodal burden. Currently, randomized phase III studies are being conducted to determine the need for PMRT and regional nodal irradiation specifically in early-stage pathologic node-positive breast cancers. NSABP B-51 is currently enrolling those with a complete nodal response to neoadjuvant chemotherapy to either WBI with RNI vs. WBI without RNI if patients underwent a lumpectomy or PMRT with RNI vs. no additional radiation if patients underwent a mastectomy. In patients who remain node positive on intraoperative SLNB, the Alliance A011202 trial randomizes similar patients to either ALND and RNI (without RT to the dissected axilla) or RNI covering all lymph node basins. Both trials are currently enrolling patients and the data is not currently available.

Conclusion

Nodal management in breast cancer patients has rapidly evolved over the last decade to include minimally invasive diagnostic procedures such as SLNB instead of the more morbid ALND as well as comprehensive nodal irradiation. While nodal irradiation in patients with 1-3 lymph nodes is controversial in the post-mastectomy, high-risk node-positive patients have been shown to benefit from comprehensive nodal irradiation including the internal mammary nodes.

References

1. Agresti R, Martelli G, Sandri M, Tagliabue E, Carcangiu ML, Maugeri I, et al. Axillary lymph node dissection versus no dissection in patients with T1N0 breast cancer: a randomized clinical trial (INT09/98). Cancer. 2014;120(6):885–93.
2. Martelli G, Boracchi P, Ardoino I, Lozza L, Bohm S, Vetrella G, et al. Axillary dissection versus no axillary dissection in older patients with T1N0 breast cancer: 15-year results of a randomized controlled trial. Ann Surg. 2012;256(6):920–4.
3. Hughes KS, Schnaper LA, Bellon JR, Cirrincione CT, Berry DA, McCormick B, et al. Lumpectomy plus tamoxifen with or without irradiation in women age 70 years or older with early breast cancer: long-term follow up of CALGB 9343. J Clin Oncol. 2013;31(19):2382–7.
4. Martelli G, Miceli R, Costa A, Coradini D, Zurrida S, Piromalli D, et al. Elderly breast cancer patients treated by conservative surgery alone plus adjuvant tamoxifen: fifteen-year results of a prospective study. Cancer. 2008;112(3):481–8.
5. Fisher B, Redmond C, Fisher ER, Bauer M, Wolmark N, Wickerham DL, et al. Ten-year results of a randomized clinical trial comparing radical mastectomy and total mastectomy with or without radiation. N Engl J Med. 1985;312(11):674–81.
6. Strom EA, Woodward WA, Katz A, Buchholz TA, Perkins GH, Jhingran A, et al. Clinical investigation: regional nodal failure patterns in breast cancer patients treated with mastectomy without radiotherapy. Int J Radiat Oncol Biol Phys. 2005;63(5):1508–13.
7. Veronesi U, Paganelli G, Viale G, Luini A, Zurrida S, Galimberti V, et al. A randomized comparison of sentinel-node biopsy with routine axillary dissection in breast cancer. N Engl J Med. 2003;349(6):546–53.
8. Mansel RE, Fallowfield L, Kissin M, Goyal A, Newcombe RG, Dixon JM, et al. Randomized multicenter trial of sentinel node biopsy versus standard axillary treatment in operable breast cancer: the ALMANAC Trial. J Natl Cancer Inst. 2006;98(9):599–609.

9. Andersson Y, de Boniface J, Jonsson PE, Ingvar C, Liljegren G, Bergkvist L, et al. Axillary recurrence rate 5 years after negative sentinel node biopsy for breast cancer. Br J Surg. 2012;99(2):226–31.
10. Veronesi U, Viale G, Paganelli G, Zurrida S, Luini A, Galimberti V, et al. Sentinel lymph node biopsy in breast cancer: ten-year results of a randomized controlled study. Ann Surg. 2010;251(4):595–600.
11. Krag DN, Anderson SJ, Julian TB, Brown AM, Harlow SP, Costantino JP, et al. Sentinel-lymph-node resection compared with conventional axillary-lymph-node dissection in clinically node-negative patients with breast cancer: overall survival findings from the NSABP B-32 randomised phase 3 trial. Lancet Oncol. 2010;11(10):927–33.
12. Kim T, Giuliano AE, Lyman GH. Lymphatic mapping and sentinel lymph node biopsy in early-stage breast carcinoma: a metaanalysis. Cancer. 2006;106(1):4–16.
13. Fleissig A, Fallowfield LJ, Langridge CI, Johnson L, Newcombe RG, Dixon JM, et al. Post-operative arm morbidity and quality of life. Results of the ALMANAC randomised trial comparing sentinel node biopsy with standard axillary treatment in the management of patients with early breast cancer. Breast Cancer Res Treat. 2006;95(3):279–93.
14. Lyman GH, Giuliano AE, Somerfield MR, Benson AB 3rd, Bodurka DC, Burstein HJ, et al. American Society of Clinical Oncology guideline recommendations for sentinel lymph node biopsy in early-stage breast cancer. J Clin Oncol. 2005;23(30):7703–20.
15. Lyman GH, Temin S, Edge SB, Newman LA, Turner RR, Weaver DL, Benson AB III, Bosserman LD, Burstein HJ, Cody H III, Hayman J, Perkins CL, Podoloff DA, Giuliano AE. Sentinel lymph node biopsy for patients with early-stage breast cancer: American Society of Clinical Oncology clinical practice guideline update. J Clin Oncol. 2013;54:1177.
16. Galimberti V, Cole BF, Zurrida S, Viale G, Luini A, Veronesi P, et al. Axillary dissection versus no axillary dissection in patients with sentinel-node micrometastases (IBCSG 23-01): a phase 3 randomised controlled trial. Lancet Oncol. 2013;14(4):297–305.
17. Giuliano AE, Hunt KK, Ballman KV, Beitsch PD, Whitworth PW, Blumencranz PW, et al. Axillary dissection vs no axillary dissection in women with invasive breast cancer and sentinel node metastasis: a randomized clinical trial. JAMA. 2011;305(6):569–75.
18. Jagsi R, Chadha M, Moni J, Ballman K, Laurie F, Buchholz TA, et al. Radiation field design in the ACOSOG Z0011 (Alliance) Trial. J Clin Oncol. 2014;32(32):3600–6.
19. Boughey JC, Suman VJ, Mittendorf EA, Ahrendt GM, Wilke LG, Taback B, et al. Sentinel lymph node surgery after neoadjuvant chemotherapy in patients with node-positive breast cancer: the ACOSOG Z1071 (Alliance) clinical trial. JAMA. 2013;310(14):1455–61.
20. Mehta K, Haffty BG. Long-term outcome in patients with four or more positive lymph nodes treated with conservative surgery and radiation therapy. Int J Radiat Oncol Biol Phys. 1996;35(4):679–85.
21. Fisher B, Anderson S, Bryant J, Margolese RG, Deutsch M, Fisher ER, et al. Twenty-year follow-up of a randomized trial comparing total mastectomy, lumpectomy, and lumpectomy plus irradiation for the treatment of invasive breast cancer. N Engl J Med. 2002;347(16):1233–41.
22. Galper S, Recht A, Silver B, Manola J, Gelman R, Schnitt SJ, et al. Factors associated with regional nodal failure in patients with early stage breast cancer with 0–3 positive axillary nodes following tangential irradiation alone. Int J Radiat Oncol Biol Phys. 1999;45(5):1157–66.
23. Reddy SG, Kiel KD. Supraclavicular nodal failure in patients with one to three positive axillary lymph nodes treated with breast conserving surgery and breast irradiation, without supraclavicular node radiation. Breast J. 2007;13(1):12–8.
24. Livi L, Paiar F, Simontacchi G, Barca R, Detti B, Fondelli S, et al. Loco regional failure pattern after lumpectomy and breast irradiation in 4185 patients with T1 and T2 breast cancer. Implications for nodal irradiation. Acta Oncol. 2006;45(5):564–70.
25. Yu JI, Park W, Huh SJ, Choi DH, Lim YH, Ahn JS, et al. Determining which patients require irradiation of the supraclavicular nodal area after surgery for N1 breast cancer. Int J Radiat Oncol Biol Phys. 2010;78(4):1135–41.
26. Meier P, Ferguson DJ, Karrison T. A controlled trial of extended radical versus radical mastectomy. Ten-year results. Cancer. 1989;63(1):188–95.

27. Lacour J, Le M, Caceres E, Koszarowski T, Veronesi U, Hill C. Radical mastectomy versus radical mastectomy plus internal mammary dissection. Ten year results of an international cooperative trial in breast cancer. Cancer. 1983;51(10):1941–3.
28. Morimoto T, Monden Y, Takashima S, Itoh S, Kimura T, Yamamoto H, et al. Five-year results of a randomized clinical trial comparing modified radical mastectomy and extended radical mastectomy for stage II breast cancer. Surg Today. 1994;24(3):210–4.
29. Veronesi U, Marubini E, Mariani L, Valagussa P, Zucali R. The dissection of internal mammary nodes does not improve the survival of breast cancer patients. 30-year results of a randomised trial. Eur J Cancer. 1999;35(9):1320–5.
30. Whelan TJ, Olivotto IA, Parulekar WR, Ackerman I, Chua BH, Nabid A, et al. Regional nodal irradiation in early-stage breast cancer. N Engl J Med. 2015;373(4):307–16.
31. Poortmans PM, Collette S, Kirkove C, Van Limbergen E, Budach V, Struikmans H, et al. Internal mammary and medial supraclavicular irradiation in breast cancer. N Engl J Med. 2015;373(4):317–27.
32. Huang O, Wang L, Shen K, Lin H, Hu Z, Liu G, et al. Breast cancer subpopulation with high risk of internal mammary lymph nodes metastasis: analysis of 2269 Chinese breast cancer patients treated with extended radical mastectomy. Breast Cancer Res Treat. 2008;107(3):379–87.
33. Veronesi U, Arnone P, Veronesi P, Galimberti V, Luini A, Rotmensz N, et al. The value of radiotherapy on metastatic internal mammary nodes in breast cancer. Results on a large series. Ann Oncol. 2008;19(9):1553–60.
34. Budach W, Kammers K, Boelke E, Matuschek C. Adjuvant radiotherapy of regional lymph nodes in breast cancer – a meta-analysis of randomized trials. Radiat Oncol. 2013;8:267.
35. Thorsen LB, Offersen BV, Dano H, Berg M, Jensen I, Pedersen AN, et al. DBCG-IMN: a population-based cohort study on the effect of internal mammary node irradiation in early node-positive breast cancer. J Clin Oncol. 2016;34(4):314–20.
36. Fracchia AA, Evans JF, Eisenberg BL. Stage III carcinoma of the breast: a detailed analysis. Ann Surg. 1980;192(6):705–10.
37. Hortobagyi GN, Strom EA, Buchholz TA. Locally advanced breast cancer. In: Singletary SER, Hortobagyi GN, editors. Advanced therapy of breast disease. 2nd ed. Hamilton: B.C. Decker; 2004. p. 498–508.
38. Smith BD, Jiang J, McLaughlin SS, Hurria A, Smith GL, Giordano SH, et al. Improvement in breast cancer outcomes over time: are older women missing out? J Clin Oncol. 2011;29(35):4647–53.
39. Overgaard M, Christensen JJ, Johansen H, Nybo-Rasmussen A, Brincker H, van der Kooy P, et al. Postmastectomy irradiation in high-risk breast cancer patients. Present status of the Danish Breast Cancer Cooperative Group trials. Acta Oncol. 1988;27(6A):707–14.
40. Harris JR, Halpin-Murphy P, McNeese M, Mendenhall NP, Morrow M, Robert NJ. Consensus statement on postmastectomy radiation therapy. Int J Radiat Oncol Biol Phys. 1999;44(5):989–90.
41. Recht A, Edge SB, Solin LJ, Robinson DS, Estabrook A, Fine RE, et al. Postmastectomy radiotherapy: clinical practice guidelines of the American Society of Clinical Oncology. J Clin Oncol. 2001;19(5):1539–69.
42. Fisher B, Jeong JH, Anderson S, Bryant J, Fisher ER, Wolmark N. Twenty-five-year follow-up of a randomized trial comparing radical mastectomy, total mastectomy, and total mastectomy followed by irradiation. N Engl J Med. 2002;347(8):567–75.
43. Overgaard M, Hansen PS, Overgaard J, Rose C, Andersson M, Bach F, et al. Postoperative radiotherapy in high-risk premenopausal women with breast cancer who receive adjuvant chemotherapy. Danish Breast Cancer Cooperative Group 82b trial. N Engl J Med. 1997;337(14):949–55.
44. Overgaard M, Jensen MB, Overgaard J, Hansen PS, Rose C, Andersson M, et al. Postoperative radiotherapy in high-risk postmenopausal breast-cancer patients given adjuvant tamoxifen: Danish Breast Cancer Cooperative Group DBCG 82c randomised trial. Lancet. 1999;353(9165):1641–8.

45. Whelan T, Levine M. More evidence that locoregional radiation therapy improves survival: what should we do? J Natl Cancer Inst. 2005;97(2):82–4.
46. Overgaard M, Nielsen HM, Overgaard J. Is the benefit of postmastectomy irradiation limited to patients with four or more positive nodes, as recommended in international consensus reports? A subgroup analysis of the DBCG 82 b&c randomized trials. Radiother Oncol. 2007;82(3):247–53.
47. Goldhirsch A, Glick JH, Gelber RD, Coates AS, Thurlimann B, Senn HJ, et al. Meeting highlights: international expert consensus on the primary therapy of early breast cancer 2005. Ann Oncol. 2005;16(10):1569–83.
48. Overgaard J, Bartelink H. Breast cancer survival advantage with radiotherapy. Lancet. 2000;356(9237):1269–70. author reply 71
49. Overgaard M. Radiotherapy as part of a multidisciplinary treatment strategy in early breast cancer. Eur J Cancer. 2001;37:33–43.
50. Ragaz J, Jackson SM, Le N, Plenderleith IH, Spinelli JJ, Basco VE, et al. Adjuvant radiotherapy and chemotherapy in node-positive premenopausal women with breast cancer. N Engl J Med. 1997;337(14):956–62.
51. Ragaz J, Olivotto IA, Spinelli JJ, Phillips N, Jackson SM, Wilson KS, et al. Locoregional radiation therapy in patients with high-risk breast cancer receiving adjuvant chemotherapy: 20-year results of the British Columbia randomized trial. J Natl Cancer Inst. 2005;97(2):116–26.
52. Kurtz J, Party EW. The curative role of radiotherapy in the treatment of operable breast cancer. Eur J Cancer. 2002;38(15):1961–74.
53. Ebctcg, McGale P, Taylor C, Correa C, Cutter D, Duane F, et al. Effect of radiotherapy after mastectomy and axillary surgery on 10-year recurrence and 20-year breast cancer mortality: meta-analysis of individual patient data for 8135 women in 22 randomised trials. Lancet. 2014;383(9935):2127–35.
54. Wang J, Shi M, Ling R, Xia Y, Luo S, Fu X, et al. Adjuvant chemotherapy and radiotherapy in triple-negative breast carcinoma: a prospective randomized controlled multi-center trial. Radiother Oncol. 2011;100(2):200–4.
55. Fisher B, Brown A, Mamounas E, Wieand S, Robidoux A, Margolese RG, et al. Effect of preoperative chemotherapy on local-regional disease in women with operable breast cancer: findings from National Surgical Adjuvant Breast and Bowel Project B-18. J Clin Oncol. 1997;15(7):2483–93.
56. Bear HD, Anderson S, Smith RE, Geyer CE Jr, Mamounas EP, Fisher B, et al. Sequential preoperative or postoperative docetaxel added to preoperative doxorubicin plus cyclophosphamide for operable breast cancer: National Surgical Adjuvant Breast and Bowel Project Protocol B-27. J Clin Oncol. 2006;24(13):2019–27.
57. Bear HD, Anderson S, Brown A, Smith R, Mamounas EP, Fisher B, et al. The effect on tumor response of adding sequential preoperative docetaxel to preoperative doxorubicin and cyclophosphamide: preliminary results from National Surgical Adjuvant Breast and Bowel Project Protocol B-27. J Clin Oncol. 2003;21(22):4165–74.
58. Colleoni M, Viale G, Zahrieh D, Pruneri G, Gentilini O, Veronesi P, et al. Chemotherapy is more effective in patients with breast cancer not expressing steroid hormone receptors: a study of preoperative treatment. Clin Cancer Res. 2004;10(19):6622–8.
59. Ring AE, Smith IE, Ashley S, Fulford LG, Lakhani SR. Oestrogen receptor status, pathological complete response and prognosis in patients receiving neoadjuvant chemotherapy for early breast cancer. Br J Cancer. 2004;91(12):2012–7.
60. Huang EH, Tucker SL, Strom EA, McNeese MD, Kuerer HM, Buzdar AU, et al. Postmastectomy radiation improves local-regional control and survival for selected patients with locally advanced breast cancer treated with neoadjuvant chemotherapy and mastectomy. J Clin Oncol. 2004;22(23):4691–9.

Triple-Negative Breast Cancer

11

Tiffany P. Avery

Introduction

Triple-negative breast cancer (TNBC) lacks expression of the three markers that define breast cancer subtypes and treatment: estrogen receptor (ER), progesterone receptor (PR), and *Her-2/neu*. The clinical features, relapse patterns, and treatment of TNBC differ from other types of breast cancer. Compared to other breast cancer subtypes, triple-negative breast cancer tends to be a higher grade, more aggressive tumor that presents at later stages among younger women [1]. Interval tumors, which develop rapidly and are detected within 12 months of a normal screening exam, tend to be TNBC [2]. Compared to endocrine-responsive tumors, TNBC tends to relapse earlier after an initial early stage diagnosis, with the highest risk of relapse in the first 3 years. While ER-positive cancer tends to relapse several years later, TNBC relapse is rare after 10 years [2]. When distant relapse recurs, TNBC tends to relapse in visceral organs, rather than the bone. Overall survival is shorter among metastatic patients with TNBC compared to other breast cancer subtypes. Systemic treatment of TNBC is limited to chemotherapy for early stage and metastatic patients. In contrast to ER/PR+ and Her-2-overexpressed types of breast cancer, there are no targeted agents for TNBC. Current research efforts are focused on identifying treatable targets in TNBC to impact prognosis and survival, just as endocrine therapies and Her-2-directed therapies have impacted ER/PR + and Her-2-overexpressed breast cancers. Different molecular subtypes of TNBC have been identified. Identifying molecular targets by subtypes and tailoring treatments according to subtype is a promising emerging approach to TNBC tailored therapy.

T.P. Avery, MD (✉)
Department of Hematology and Oncology, Wake Forest Baptist Health,
One Medical Center Boulevard, Winston-Salem, NC 27157, USA
e-mail: tavery@wakehealth.edu

M. Howard-McNatt (ed.), *Changing Paradigms in the Management of Breast Cancer*, DOI 10.1007/978-3-319-60336-0_11

Epidemiology and Risk Factors

Epidemiologic studies have shown that the incidence of TNBC is highest among African-American women compared to other racial and ethnic groups within the USA. In the Carolina Breast Cancer study, 42% of women with TNBC were African-American, and 20% were White women [3]. In a study of the California Cancer Registry, which included over 6,000 TNBC patients, 25% of the TNBC patients were African-American compared to 10.8% who were White and 17% who were Hispanic [4]. In the Nashville Breast Health Study, Cui et al. reported that among 1,866 breast cancer cases, African-American women were more likely to have TNBC and to be diagnosed at a younger age than the White patients in this cohort [5]. Similarly, in cohort studies of TNBC patients in several US cities., including Washington D.C., Philadelphia, Atlanta, and Boston, African-American women represented from 21 to 46% of TNBC patients compared to White women who represented 10–20% [6]. Patients diagnosed with triple-negative breast cancer also tend to be younger at diagnosis than patients with other types of breast cancer. In the California Cancer Registry study, 63% of the patients with triple-negative tumors were diagnosed before the age of 60 compared with less than half among patients of other tumor types [4, 6]. In the Carolina breast study, patients with triple-negative breast cancer were five times as likely to be younger than 40 compared to those patients with ER/PR-positive tumors [4, 6].

A few possible risk factors for developing triple-negative breast cancer have emerged, particularly in African-American women. The Women's Circle of Health Study which included 786 African-American women with breast cancer showed that having children increased the risk of triple-negative breast cancer but that breast-feeding reduced the risk of ER-negative cancer associated with parity [7]. Results from the African-American Breast Cancer Epidemiology and Risk (Amber) Consortium had similar findings. This study included 567 African-American women with triple-negative breast cancer and found that compared to women with other types of breast cancer, lactation was associated with a reduced risk of developing ER-negative cancer. Additionally ER-negative cancer risk increased with each additional birth among women who had not breastfed [8]. It has been estimated that breastfeeding for at least 4–6 months decreases the risk of triple-negative breast cancer by 25–50% among parous women [9].

Obesity in premenopausal women has been implicated as a risk factor for the development of TNBC. In a study of 620 patients in a rural population with high rates of obesity, there was an association of TNBC among younger women who were obese [10]. Similarly, a study by Kwan et al. confirmed that among cases of TNBC, women who were premenopausal and developed breast cancer were more likely to be overweight or obese [11]. In the North Carolina Breast study, higher weight-to-hip ratio was associated with increased risk of developing TNBC [3]. In a population-based study of 2,659 women with invasive breast cancer, premenopausal women with body mass index (BMI) >30 kg/m^2 were found to have an 82% increased risk of TNBC compared to women with BMI measurements that were less than 25 kg/m^2. Women in the highest quartile of weight had a 79% increased risk of

TNBC compared to those in the lowest quartile for weight [12]. A meta-analysis of the association between obesity and risk of developing TNBC also confirmed an association of obesity among premenopausal woman with development of TNBC [13]. Changes in BMI and obesity over time are also associated with development of TNBC. In a study by Kawai et al., women who had experienced a greater than or equal to 10 kg/m^2 increase in body weight from age 18 to their current age had a twofold increase risk of developing TNBC compared to women who had less of a weight change over time [14]. In postmenopausal women, the impact of obesity is different than among premenopausal women. Studies of obesity among postmenopausal women have shown an association between obesity and the development of ER-positive breast cancers. It appears, then, that the risk of obesity and development of different types of breast cancer varies by age.

Genetics is also associated with development of TNBC. In particular, *BRCA1* mutations are associated with TNBC. A meta-analysis of over 2,500 breast cancer patients showed that patients who developed TNBC were more likely to be *BRCA1* mutation carriers compared to women with other types of breast cancer [15]. *BRCA1* mutation carriers tend to be younger at diagnosis then non-mutation carriers. A study of 400 patients found that the median age of diagnosis among *BRCA1* carriers was 39 years old and that the prevalence of *BRCA1* mutations among women diagnosed younger than 40 was 36% [16]. The association of *BRCA2* mutations with TNBC has also been reported, with prevalence of mutations ranging from 4 to 16%, depending on the patient population studied [17, 18]. Due to the association of *BRCA* mutations and TNBC, genetic testing for *BRCA* mutations in all patients diagnosed with TNBC before the age of 60 is recommended in clinical practice [19].

Treatment of TNBC

Because triple-negative breast tumors do not express ER/PR receptors and do not overexpress *Her-2/neu*, current targeted strategies for breast cancer are ineffective. Chemotherapy remains the only treatment option for these tumors. Among patients with lymph node-positive disease, the addition of a taxane to a regimen of doxorubicin and cyclophosphamide decreased recurrence and improved progression-free and overall survival compared to doxorubicin and cyclophosphamide alone [20, 21]. Among women with lymph node-positive or high-risk breast cancer, a regimen of doxorubicin and cyclophosphamide followed by either every 3 week docetaxel or weekly paclitaxel resulted in improvement in disease-free and overall survival, respectively [22].

In the neoadjuvant setting, trials using combinations of anthracycline and taxanes have shown that pathologic complete response (the absence of invasive breast cancer in the surgical specimen) is higher with these regimens among patients with TNBC compared to other types of breast cancer. A retrospective analysis of 1,118 breast cancer patients, Stage I–III, treated with neoadjuvant chemotherapy (NACT) showed that the patients with TNBC had significantly higher pathologic complete response (pCR) rates compared with all other subtypes of breast cancer. Three-year progression-free survival (PFS) rates and overall survival (OS) rates were significantly less among the TNBC group. However, if pCR was attained, there was no difference in OS. The most commonly used regimens included anthracyclines and taxanes in this analysis [23]. In a similar study, molecular classifications were performed on 82 patients prior to undergoing NACT with paclitaxel followed by doxorubicin and cyclophosphamide (AC) with 5-fluorouracil. Basal-like subtypes had the highest rates of pCR compared to tumors expressing hormone receptors [24]. In a study that retrospectively evaluated pCR and disease-free survival (DFS) of 151 breast cancer patients who had been treated with neoadjuvant anthracycline and taxane regimens, the highest pCR rates were observed among the patients with TNBC (38% v 12%). Overall, patients with TNBC had worse DFS if they did not attain pCR. If pCR was obtained, there was no difference in DFS [25]. In a similar analysis, among 107 patients treated with neoadjuvant, anthracycline-based chemotherapy, clinical response was highest among the basal-like, TNBC subtype, and pCR was higher among basal-like TNBC compared to ER/PR + cancers [26]. Patients with basal-like subtypes had worse DFS and OS if pCR was not achieved.

Neoadjuvant chemotherapy trials performed in TNBC patients have shown that the addition of platinum agents to anthracycline- and taxane-containing regimens results in increased pCR among TNBC patients. The mechanism of action of platinum agents, which causes inhibition of DNA transcription and replication, exploits the sensitivity of TNBC to agents that involve DNA repair [27]. CALBG 40603 demonstrated a statistically significant improvement in pCR among TNBC patients when carboplatin was added to a standard anthracycline- and taxane-containing regimen with bevacizumab. PCR rates improved from 41 to 54% with the addition of carboplatin [28]. The GeparSixto trial similarly demonstrated an improvement among TNBC patients in pCR with the addition of carboplatin to anthracycline, taxane, and bevacizumab. PCR rates improved from 36.9 to 53.2% with carboplatin. Further, DFS was also improved with carboplatin [29]. In a neoadjuvant study of cisplatin, epirubicin, and paclitaxel, 62% achieved pCR. Additional trials have examined the addition of carboplatin to standard anthracycline and taxane regimens. The pCR rates range from 30 to 54% with the addition of carboplatin [30].

In the metastatic setting, sequential, single-agent chemotherapy is a standard approach. A study of 69 patients with metastatic TNBC showed response rates of 35% to single-agent cisplatin and 23% to single-agent carboplatin with some durable responses of several years in the patients treated with cisplatin [31]. Among clinical trials of single-agent carboplatin or cisplatin, response rates range from 18 to 68% [32]. In addition to platinum agents, standard single agents include anthracyclines, taxane, antimetabolites, and microtubule inhibitors. In patients with a high burden of visceral disease and good performance status, combination therapy may be undertaken for a faster reduction in tumor volume. Efficacious combinations in this setting include gemcitabine and paclitaxel, capecitabine and docetaxel, capecitabine and ixabepilone, and gemcitabine and carboplatin [33].

Targeted Therapies for TNBC

One of the challenges in treating TNBC lies in finding a suitable target for therapeutic options. Much of the progress in breast cancer outcomes and survival has been made due to targeted therapies, such as endocrine treatments for ER + disease and trastuzumab for *Her-2*-overexpressed cancer. Targets that have been studied to tailor TNBC therapy include poly-ADP-ribose polymerase (*PARP*) inhibition, tyrosine kinase inhibitors, anti-angiogenic agents, and androgen receptor antagonists (Table 11.1).

PARP inhibitors are targeted agents that inhibit the activity of the PARP polymerase family of enzymes. These enzymes are essential in repairing DNA damage, particularly single-strand breaks through the base excision repair pathway [34]. In cells that are deficient in alternate DNA repair pathways, inhibiting the activity of PARP enzymes leads to cell death through synthetic lethality [34]. An example of synthetic lethality is illustrated by the use of PARP inhibitors in *BRCA*-mutated cancers. *BRCA*-mutated cells are deficient in the homologous recombination (HR) pathway for repair of DNA double-strand breaks. By inhibiting the activity of the PARP enzymes, the base excision repair pathway is also eliminated as a potential mechanism for DNA repair. Single-strand breaks can then accumulate, due to inefficient base excision repair, and lead to double-strand breaks at replication forks. In this way, cell death can occur through synthetic lethality [35]. This concept has been tested clinically in populations of *BRCA*-mutated carriers and shown to be active in

Table 11.1 Current clinical trials of targeted therapies in TNBC

Agent	Target	Stage	Phase	NCI number
Glembatumumab vedotin	gpNMB	Metastatic	I	NCT01997333
Panitumumab + chemotherapy	EGFR	Neoadjuvant	II	NCT02593175
Selumetinib	MEK	Neoadjuvant	II	NCT02685657
Veliparib + lapatinib	PARP, EGFR/Her-2	Metastatic	Pilot study	NCT02158507
Afatinib + paclitaxel	EGFR	Neoadjuvant	II	NCT02511847
Everolimus + eribulin	PI3K/mTOR	Metastatic	II	NCT02616848
Everolimus + cisplatin	PI3K/mTOR	Neoadjuvant	II	NCT1931163
Pemetrexed + sorafenib	Multikinase inhibitor	Metastatic	II	NCT02624700
Sacituzumab govitecan	Trop-2	Metastatic	III	NCT02574455
Trametinib + GSK2141795	AKT, MEK	Metastatic	II	NCT01964924
Ipatasertib + paclitaxel	AKT	Metastatic	II	NCT02162719
BKM120, BYL719 + olaparib	PI3 kinase, PARP	Metastatic	I	NCT01623349
Enzalutamide	AR	Adjuvant	Feasibility study	NCT02750358
GTx-024	AR	Metastatic	II	NCT02368691

BRCA-mutated cancers [35]. A phase II trial of the PARP inhibitor, olaparib, in *BRCA*-mutated metastatic breast cancer patients showed objective response rates ranging from 21 to 44%. Over 50% of these patients had TNBC. Objective response rates ranged from 21 to 44% [35]. Since *BRCA*-mutated breast cancers and TNBC share clinical and pathologic characteristics, such as sensitivity to DNA-damaging agents, high pathologic grade, and high rate of p53 mutations, it is proposed that TNBC, which is most like *BRCA*-mutated breast cancer, is also deficient in the HR pathway [34]. This characteristic would render TNBC vulnerable to PARP inhibition in the same way as *BRCA*-mutated breast cancer. The use of PARP inhibitors in TNBC is an area of active research. A phase II trial of the intravenous PARP inhibitor, iniparib (BSI-201), in combination with gemcitabine and carboplatin was performed in a population of 120 women with metastatic, pretreated TNBC [36]. Clinical benefit rates were 62% in patients who had received BSI-208 versus 21% with chemotherapy alone. Progression-free and overall survival were also improved with the addition of BSI-201 [36]. A phase III follow-up study compared iniparib in combination with gemcitabine and carboplatin to gemcitabine and carboplatin alone in 519 women with metastatic, pretreated TNBC. The primary endpoints of overall survival and progression-free survival were not met. Subgroup analysis showed that there was a survival benefit in the group of women who had received two or more prior lines of treatment [37]. In vitro data has shown, however, that iniparib demonstrates little or no ability to inhibit formation of PARP polymers or induce apoptosis in cell lines which are deficit in homologous repair pathway, such as *BRCA*-mutated cells [38, 39]. Further studies of agents with true PARP inhibition have shown promising results. A neoadjuvant study of the PARP inhibitor, veliparib, in combination with paclitaxel and carboplatin showed pCR rates that improved from 26 to 51% with the addition of veliparib in TNBC. Potential biomarker candidates to predict pCR were also evaluated [40, 41]. This combination will be evaluated in a phase III trial.

The PI3K/AKT/mTOR pathway is frequently activated in breast cancer and is another area of active research. This pathway leads to cell survival through activation of a series of proteins, including AKT kinase and mTOR (mammalian target of rapamycin inhibitors) [42]. The pathway is activated by binding of a ligand to various tyrosine kinase receptors, including HER proteins, EGFR, and IGF-1 (insulin growth factor) receptors [42]. This rich pathway presents a number of options for drug targets. A neoadjuvant study of an AKT inhibitor, MK-2206, in combination with standard chemotherapy showed a pCR rate of 40% [43]. The PI3K/AKT/mTOR pathway provides stability of the homologous recombination repair pathway, which is deficient among *BRCA*-mutated cells. Inhibition of AKT has been shown to render TNBC more sensitive to PARP inhibitors by inducing deficiencies in the HR pathway [42]. In an in vitro study of TNBC, the AKT inhibitor, buparlisib, was shown to sensitize TNBC cells to the PARP inhibitor, olaparib [44]. The tyrosine kinase inhibitor, neratinib, which inhibits binding of the ligand for ErbB and Her family of receptors, was evaluated in the neoadjuvant setting in all subtypes of breast cancer. While neratinib was found to be most efficacious in ER-, Her-2 + breast cancers, there was a subset of TNBC which showed pCR rates of up to 66%

with neratinib in combination with anthracycline and taxane. Molecular signatures of these responders show that these tumors showed phosphorylation of EGFR or Her-2/neu [45].

Antibody-drug conjugates are being tested in the treatment of TNBC. Sacituzumab govitecan is a humanized anti-Trop-2 antibody linked to a high concentration of SN-38, which is the active metabolite of irinotecan. Trophoblast cell-surface antigen, Trop-2, is a target that is expressed in multiple solid tumors. The *Trop-2* gene encodes a transmembrane calcium signal transducer, which is linked to cell migration. The gene is also referred to as tumor-associated calcium signal transducer 2 (*TACSTD2*) [46]. Among breast cancer patients, increased expression of Trop-2 is linked to shorter survival [47]. Expression of *TACSTD2* is active among TNBC cell lines [48]. A phase II trial of sacituzumab govitecan conducted in 58 TNBC patients, with a median of 4 prior therapies, demonstrated an overall response rate (CR + PR) of 31% and clinical benefit rate (CR+PR+SD) of 49%. Given that this study was conducted among a heavily pretreated population, these outcomes are very promising in patients with refractory TNBC [49]. Glembatumumab vedotin is an antibody-drug conjugate of the cytotoxin, monomethyl auristatin E, that targets glycoprotein NMB (gpNMB). gpNMB is overexpressed in a multiple tumor types and is a poor prognostic factor among breast cancer patients. A phase I trial glembatumumab vedotin among metastatic breast cancer showed response rates of up to 40% among TNBC patients with gpNMB overexpression [50].

Targeted Therapies by TNBC Subtype

Different molecular subtypes of TNBC have been identified through gene expression profiling. Six molecular subtypes have been identified: two types of basal-like (BL1 and BL2), mesenchymal (M), mesenchymal stemlike (MSL), luminal androgen receptor (LAR), and an immunomodulatory subtype (IM) [51]. These subtypes have been further refined in four subtypes (BL1, BL2, M, and LAR) [52]. The responses to neoadjuvant chemotherapy have been correlated by different subtypes and suggest varying responses to treatment among the different subtypes.

The luminal androgen receptor (LAR) type is characterized by hormonally regulated pathways, expression of androgen receptors and display positivity for phosphatidylinositol-4,5-bisphosphae 3-kinase subunit PIK3CA-α activating mutations with less responsiveness to chemotherapy. This type of TNBC has the lowest responsiveness to chemotherapy, which is estimated to be about 10% pathologic complete response rates in the neoadjuvant setting [53]. Preclinical models have suggested the utility of androgen receptor antagonist in the androgen receptor (AR)-positive TNBC. One study combined PI3K kinase inhibitors with an AR antagonist and showed inhibitory effects in laboratory models [51]. In a study of 50 metastatic TNBC patients with IHC >10% for AR, a 19% 6-month clinical benefit rate was achieved with single-agent bicalutamide, an AR antagonist, [54]. Enzalutamide is an androgen receptor inhibitor that is approved for use in metastatic prostate cancer patients. Because of the mechanism of action, it is also a potential treatment for the AR subtype. A phase II study of enzalutamide was conducted among TNBC patients with advanced disease. AR expression was measured by immunohistochemistry, and an androgen-driven gene signature was constructed by genomic profiling of tumors. Results were measured by those patients with tumors that displayed the androgen-driven signature (AR+) and those that did not (AR−). Of 118 patients enrolled, 47% of patients were AR+. Patients in this group had better outcomes, with a clinical benefit rate (CBR) of 39% and 36% at 16 and 24 weeks of follow-up, respectively. Among AR− patients, CBR was 11% and 7%, respectively. Among the AR+ group, progression-free survival was 16 weeks, compared to 8 weeks among the AR− group [55]. Median PFS extended to 32 weeks among patients who received enzalutamide in the first- or second-line setting.

The mesenchymal type of TNBC tends to be enriched in cell motility and interactions of the extracellular matrix receptors. The IM subtype is represented by enrichment in genes related to immune cell processes and may be a viable target for immunotherapies. The basal-like type shows enrichment in cell cycle pathways, increased expression of DNA damage response genes, and high Ki-67 expression [32].

Immunotherapy in TNBC

Immunotherapy has changed the treatment landscape for several solid tumors, including melanoma and lung cancer. Approved drugs, such as pembrolizumab, act by disrupting binding of programmed death ligand 1 (PD-L1) expressed on tumor cells to PD-1 receptors on T-cells. Binding of PD-L1 to PD-1 results in T-cell inhibition. Blocking this interaction results in T-cell activation. There is evidence to suggest that immunotherapy may be a viable option in the treatment of TNBC patients and several clinical trials are ongoing (Table 11.2). The presence of tumor-infiltrating lymphocytes (TILs) is associated with better prognosis in TNBC. Higher numbers of TILS in patients with TNBC showed a strong correlation with prognosis in the GeparSixto neoadjuvant trial of TNBC patients. Higher levels of TILs in the tumor specimen

Table 11.2 Current clinical trial of immunotherapy in TNBC

Agents	Target	Stage	Phase	NCI number
Pembrolizumab + chemotherapy	PD-1	Neoadjuvant	Ib	NCT02622074
Pembrolizumab + eribulin	PD-1	Metastatic	Ib/II	NCT02513472
Pembrolizumab + cyclophosphamide	PD-1	Metastatic	II	NCT02768701
Pembrolizumab + niraparib	PD-1, PARP	Metastatic	I/II	NCT02657889
Pembrolizumab + gemcitabine/ carboplatin	PD-1	Metastatic	II	NCT02755272
Atezolizumab + nab-paclitaxel	PD-L1	Metastatic	III	NCT02425891
Veliparib + atezolizumab	PARP, PD-L1	III-IV	II	NCT02849496
Pembrolizumab + chemotherapy	PD-1	IV	II	NCT02734290
MEDI4736 + nab-paclitaxel	PD-L1	Neoadjuvant	I/II	NCT02489448

correlated with greater pathologic complete response rates [29]. Mittendorf and colleagues reported overexpression of programmed death ligand 1 (PD-L1) in 20% of patients with TNBC, which correlated with higher numbers of TILs [56]. Overexpression of PD-L1 suggests that antibodies to PD-L1 may be efficacious in TNBC. In a phase I clinical trial with pembrolizumab, a humanized monoclonal antibody that blocks interaction of PD-L1 and PD-L2 with PD-1 receptors, overall response rate among metastatic TNBC patients was 18.5% with some durable responses. All patients on trial had tumors which stained positive for PD-L1 expression [57]. A phase I study of atezolizumab, a humanized monoclonal antibody which inhibits PD-L1 binding to PD-1 and B7, in combination with nab-paclitaxel demonstrated that the combination was tolerable with activity among metastatic TNBC patients [58].

Conclusion

Triple-negative breast cancer remains the most difficult to treat of the breast cancer subtypes due to a lack of targeted agents. Ongoing clinical trials focused particularly on targeted therapies, and immunotherapies offer the most promising future treatment alternatives. Refining treatment by subtype of TNBC is strategy that may also lead to progress in the treatment of TNBC. Among standard chemotherapy options, the use of platinum agents has impacted pCR rates in the neoadjuvant setting and response rates in the metastatic setting. Studies of platinum agents in the adjuvant and neoadjuvant setting are ongoing to determine if this option should become a standard of care for TNBC.

References

1. Bosch A, Eroles P, Zaragoza R, Vina JR, Lluch A. Triple-negative breast cancer: molecular features, pathogenesis, treatment and current lines of research. Cancer Treat Rev. 2010;36(3):206–15.
2. Foulkes WD, Smith IE, Reis-Filho JS. Triple-negative breast cancer. N Engl J Med. 2010;363(20):1938–48.
3. Millikan RC, Newman B, Tse CK, Moorman PG, Conway K, Dressler LG, et al. Epidemiology of basal-like breast cancer. Breast Cancer Res Treat. 2008;109(1):123–39.
4. Bauer KR, Brown M, Cress RD, Parise CA, Caggiano V. Descriptive analysis of estrogen receptor (ER)-negative, progesterone receptor (PR)-negative, and HER2-negative invasive breast cancer, the so-called triple-negative phenotype: a population-based study from the California cancer Registry. Cancer. 2007;109(9):1721–8.
5. Cui Y, Deming-Halverson SL, Shrubsole MJ, Beeghly-Fadiel A, Fair AM, Sanderson M, et al. Associations of hormone-related factors with breast cancer risk according to hormone receptor status among white and African American women. Clin Breast Cancer. 2014;14(6):417–25.
6. Ray M, Polite BN. Triple-negative breast cancers: a view from 10,000 feet. Cancer J. 2010;16(1):17–22.
7. Ambrosone CB, Zirpoli G, Ruszczyk M, Shankar J, Hong CC, McIlwain D, et al. Parity and breastfeeding among African-American women: differential effects on breast cancer risk by estrogen receptor status in the Women's Circle of Health Study. Cancer Causes Control: CCC. 2014;25(2):259–65.

8. Palmer JR, Viscidi E, Troester MA, Hong CC, Schedin P, Bethea TN, et al. Parity, lactation, and breast cancer subtypes in African American women: results from the AMBER Consortium. J Natl Cancer Inst. 2014;106(10):dju237.
9. Phipps AI, Li CI. Breastfeeding and triple-negative breast cancer: potential implications for racial/ethnic disparities. J Natl Cancer Inst. 2014;106(10):dju281.
10. Vona-Davis L, Rose DP, Hazard H, Howard-McNatt M, Adkins F, Partin J, et al. Triple-negative breast cancer and obesity in a rural Appalachian population. Cancer Epidemiol Biomark Prev. 2008;17(12):3319–24.
11. Kwan ML, Kushi LH, Weltzien E, Maring B, Kutner SE, Fulton RS, et al. Epidemiology of breast cancer subtypes in two prospective cohort studies of breast cancer survivors. Breast Cancer Res. 2009;11(3):R31.
12. Chen L, Cook LS, Tang MT, Porter PL, Hill DA, Wiggins CL, et al. Body mass index and risk of luminal, HER2-overexpressing, and triple negative breast cancer. Breast Cancer Res Treat. 2016;157(3):545–54.
13. Pierobon M, Frankenfeld CL. Obesity as a risk factor for triple-negative breast cancers: a systematic review and meta-analysis. Breast Cancer Res Treat. 2013;137(1):307–14.
14. Kawai M, Malone KE, Tang MT, Li CI. Height, body mass index (BMI), BMI change, and the risk of estrogen receptor-positive, HER2-positive, and triple-negative breast cancer among women ages 20 to 44 years. Cancer. 2014;120(10):1548–56.
15. Tun NM, Villani G, Ong K, Yoe L, Bo ZM. Risk of having BRCA1 mutation in high-risk women with triple-negative breast cancer: a meta-analysis. Clin Genet. 2014;85(1):43–8.
16. Fostira F, Tsitlaidou M, Papadimitriou C, Pertesi M, Timotheadou E, Stavropoulou AV, et al. Prevalence of BRCA1 mutations among 403 women with triple-negative breast cancer: implications for genetic screening selection criteria: a Hellenic Cooperative Oncology Group Study. Breast Cancer Res Treat. 2012;134(1):353–62.
17. Saura C, Saanchez-Olle G, Bossch N, et al. High prevalence of *BRCA1/2* germline mutation in female breast cancer patients with triple-negative phenotype (TNBC) and family history. JCO, 2010 ASCO Annual Meeting Abstracts. 2010;28(15):Abstract 1534.
18. Meyer P, Landgraf K, Hogel B, Eiermann W, Ataseven B. BRCA2 mutations and triple-negative breast cancer. PLoS One. 2012;7(5):e38361.
19. NCCN Guidelines Panel BC. Genetic/familial high-risk assessment: breast and ovarian 2016 [updated 2.2016].
20. Henderson IC, Berry DA, Demetri GD, Cirrincione CT, Goldstein LJ, Martino S, et al. Improved outcomes from adding sequential paclitaxel but not from escalating doxorubicin dose in an adjuvant chemotherapy regimen for patients with node-positive primary breast cancer. J Clin Oncol. 2003;21(6):976–83.
21. Mamounas EP, Bryant J, Lembersky B, Fehrenbacher L, Sedlacek SM, Fisher B, et al. Paclitaxel after doxorubicin plus cyclophosphamide as adjuvant chemotherapy for node-positive breast cancer: results from NSABP B-28. J Clin Oncol. 2005;23(16):3686–96.
22. Sparano JA, Wang M, Martino S, Jones V, Perez EA, Saphner T, et al. Weekly paclitaxel in the adjuvant treatment of breast cancer. N Engl J Med. 2008;358(16):1663–71.
23. Liedtke C, Mazouni C, Hess KR, Andre F, Tordai A, Mejia JA, et al. Response to neoadjuvant therapy and long-term survival in patients with triple-negative breast cancer. J Clin Oncol. 2008;26(8):1275–81.
24. Rouzier R, Perou CM, Symmans WF, Ibrahim N, Cristofanilli M, Anderson K, et al. Breast cancer molecular subtypes respond differently to preoperative chemotherapy. Clin Cancer Res. 2005;11(16):5678–85.
25. Wang S, Yang H, Tong F, Zhang J, Yang D, Liu H, et al. Response to neoadjuvant therapy and disease free survival in patients with triple-negative breast cancer. Gan To Kagaku Ryoho. 2009;36(2):255–8.
26. Carey LA, Dees EC, Sawyer L, Gatti L, Moore DT, Collichio F, et al. The triple negative paradox: primary tumor chemosensitivity of breast cancer subtypes. Clin Cancer Res. 2007;13(8):2329–34.
27. Perez EA, Moreno-Aspitia A, Aubrey Thompson E, Andorfer CA. Adjuvant therapy of triple negative breast cancer. Breast Cancer Res Treat. 2010;120(2):285–91.

28. Sikov WM, Berry DA, Perou CM, Singh B, Cirrincione CT, Tolaney SM, et al. Impact of the addition of carboplatin and/or bevacizumab to neoadjuvant once-per-week paclitaxel followed by dose-dense doxorubicin and cyclophosphamide on pathologic complete response rates in stage II to III triple-negative breast cancer: CALGB 40603 (Alliance). J Clin Oncol. 2015;33(1):13–21.
29. von Minckwitz G LS, Schneeweiss A, et al. Early survival analysis of the randomized phase II trial investigating the addition of carboplatin to neoadjuvant therapy for triple-negative and HER2-positive early breast cancer (GeparSixto). 2015 San Antonio Breast Cancer Symposium; December 9, 2015 2015.
30. Collignon J, Lousberg L, Schroeder H, Jerusalem G. Triple-negative breast cancer: treatment challenges and solutions. Breast Cancer. 2016;8:93–107.
31. Isakoff SJ, Mayer EL, He L, Traina TA, Carey LA, Krag KJ, et al. TBCRC009: a multicenter phase II clinical trial of platinum monotherapy with biomarker assessment in metastatic triple-negative breast cancer. J Clin Oncol. 2015;33(17):1902–9.
32. Gerratana L, Fanotto V, Pelizzari G, Agostinetto E, Puglisi F. Do platinum salts fit all triple negative breast cancers? Cancer Treat Rev. 2016;48:34–41.
33. Zeichner SB, Terawaki H, Gogineni K. A review of systemic treatment in metastatic triple-negative breast cancer. Breast Cancer: Basic Clin Res. 2016;10:25–36.
34. Anders CK, Winer EP, Ford JM, Dent R, Silver DP, Sledge GW, et al. Poly(ADP-ribose) polymerase inhibition: "targeted" therapy for triple-negative breast cancer. Clin Cancer Res. 2010;16(19):4702–10.
35. Fong PC, Boss DS, Yap TA, Tutt A, Wu P, Mergui-Roelvink M, et al. Inhibition of poly(ADP-ribose) polymerase in tumors from BRCA mutation carriers. N Engl J Med. 2009;361(2):123–34.
36. O'Shaughnessy J, Osborne C, Pippen JE, Yoffe M, Patt D, Rocha C, et al. Iniparib plus chemotherapy in metastatic triple-negative breast cancer. N Engl J Med. 2011;364(3):205–14.
37. O'Shaughnessy J, Schwartzberg S, Danso M, Rugo H, Miller K, Yardley D. A randomized phase III study of iniparib (BSI-201) in combination with gemcitabine/carboplatin (G/C) in metastatic triple-negative breast cancer (TNBC). J Clin Oncol. 2011;29 (suppl; abstr 1007).
38. Liu XSY, Maag DX, et al. Iniparib nonselectively modifies cysteine-containing proteins in tumor cells and is not a bona fide PARP inhibitor. Clin Cancer Res. 2012;18:10–23.
39. Patel AG, De Lorenzo S, Flatten K, Poirier G, Kaufmann SH. Failure of iniparib to inhibit poly(ADP-ribose) polymerase in vitro. Clin Cancer Res. 2012;18(6):1655–62.
40. Rugo HS, Olopade OI, DeMichele A, Yau C, Van 't veer LJ, Buxton MB, et al. Adaptive randomization of Veliparib-carboplatin treatment in breast cancer. N Engl J Med. 2016;375(1):23–34.
41. Wulfkuhle JD YC, Wolf DM, et al. Prediction of complete pathologic response to veliparib/carboplatin plus standard neoadjuvant therapy in HER2 negative breast cancer: exploratory protein pathway marker results from the I-SPY 2 trial. 2015 San Antonio Breast Cancer Symposium; December 10, 2015; San Antonio, TX2015.
42. Massihnia D, Galvano A, Fanale D, Perez A, Castiglia M, Incorvaia L, et al. Triple negative breast cancer: shedding light onto the role of pi3k/akt/mtor pathway. Oncotarget. 2016;
43. Tripathy D, Chien AJ, Hylton N, et al.. Adaptively randomized trial of neoadjuvant chemotherapy with or without the Akt inhibitor MK-2206. ASCO Annual Meeting; May 30, 2015; Chicago, IL2015.
44. Ibrahim YH, Garcia-Garcia C, Serra V, He L, Torres-Lockhart K, Prat A, et al. PI3K inhibition impairs BRCA1/2 expression and sensitizes BRCA-proficient triple-negative breast cancer to PARP inhibition. Cancer Discov. 2012;2(11):1036–47.
45. Wulfkuhle JD YC, Wolf DM, et al.. Protein activation mapping and exploratory predictive markers for pCR in triple-negative breast cancer patients treated with neratinib in the I-SPY2 trial. ASCO Annual Meeting; May 30, 2015; Chicago, IL.
46. Goldenberg DM, Cardillo TM, Govindan SV, Rossi EA, Sharkey RM. Trop-2 is a novel target for solid cancer therapy with sacituzumab govitecan (IMMU-132), an antibody-drug conjugate (ADC). Oncotarget. 2015;6(26):22496–512.
47. Lin H, Huang JF, Qiu JR, Zhang HL, Tang XJ, Li H, et al. Significantly upregulated TACSTD2 and cyclin D1 correlate with poor prognosis of invasive ductal breast cancer. Exp Mol Pathol. 2013;94(1):73–8.

48. Wu M, Liu L, Chan C. Identification of novel targets for breast cancer by exploring gene switches on a genome scale. BMC Genomics. 2011;12:547.
49. Bardia A DJ, Mayer IA, et al.. Safety and efficacy of anti-Trop-2 antibody drug conjugate, sacituzumab govitecan in heavily pretreated patients with TNBC. San Antonio Breast Cancer; December 10, 2015; San Antonio, TX2015.
50. Yardley DA, Weaver R, Melisko ME, Saleh MN, Arena FP, Forero A, et al. EMERGE: a randomized phase II study of the antibody-drug conjugate Glembatumumab Vedotin in advanced glycoprotein NMB-expressing breast cancer. J Clin Oncol. 2015;33(14):1609–19.
51. Lehmann BD, Bauer JA, Chen X, Sanders ME, Chakravarthy AB, Shyr Y, et al. Identification of human triple-negative breast cancer subtypes and preclinical models for selection of targeted therapies. J Clin Invest. 2011;121(7):2750–67.
52. Lehmann BD, Jovanovic B, Chen X, Estrada MV, Johnson KN, Shyr Y, et al. Refinement of triple-negative breast cancer molecular subtypes: implications for neoadjuvant chemotherapy selection. PLoS One. 2016;11(6):e0157368.
53. Kalimutho M, Parsons K, Mittal D, Lopez JA, Srihari S, Khanna KK. Targeted therapies for triple-negative breast cancer: combating a stubborn disease. Trends Pharmacol Sci. 2015;36(12):822–46.
54. Gucalp A, Tolaney S, Isakoff SJ, Ingle JN, Liu MC, Carey LA, et al. Phase II trial of bicalutamide in patients with androgen receptor-positive, estrogen receptor-negative metastatic breast cancer. Clin Cancer Res. 2013;19(19):5505–12.
55. Traina TA, Miller, K., Yardley, D., et al. Results from a phase 2 study of enzalutamide, an androgen receptor inhibitor, in advanced AR+ triple-negative breast cancer. ASCO Annual Meeting; June 1, 20152015.
56. Mittendorf EA, Philips AV, Meric-Bernstam F, Qiao N, Wu Y, Harrington S, et al. PD-L1 expression in triple-negative breast cancer. Cancer Immunol Res. 2014;2(4):361–70.
57. Nanda R CL, Dees EC, Berger R, Gupta S, Geva R, Pusztai L, Dolled-Filhart M, Emancipator K, Gonzalez EJ, Houp J, Pathiraja K, Karantza V, Iannone R, Gause CK, Cheng JD, Buisseret L. A phase Ib study of pembrolizumab (MK-3475) in patients with advanced triple-negative breast cancer. 2014 San Antonio Breast Cancer Symposium; December 10, 2014; San Antonio, TX2014.
58. Adams S, Diamond J., Hamilton E, et al. Safety and clinical activity of atezolizumab in combination with nab-paclitaxel in patients with metastatic triple-negative breast cancer. San Antonio Breast Cancer Symposium; December 11, 2015; San Antonio, TX2015.

New Treatments for Metastatic Breast Cancer

12

Ana Christina Garrido-Castro and Beth Overmoyer

Introduction

As the mechanisms that mediate resistance to standard endocrine or HER2-directed therapies are elucidated, novel targets have emerged for the treatment of metastatic breast cancer (MBC). Blockade of oncogenic signaling pathways, cell-cycle regulatory checkpoints, or epigenetic modulators has become strategies of interest, expecting to overcome or delay the appearance of resistance to standard regimens [1–5]. The investigation of these novel targeted therapies pertains to all subtypes of breast cancer. This changes the focus of classification away from traditional targets, e.g., hormonal and HER2 receptor, to a more global categorization of therapies that encompass the traditional targets. Several compounds are emerging after revealing promising preliminary antitumoral activity in phase I trials (Table 12.1). In this section, we seek to review the most recent efforts in later-stage drug development for the treatment of MBC, focusing on novel molecular targets.

A.C. Garrido-Castro, MD • B. Overmoyer, MD, FACP (✉)
Department of Medical Oncology, Harvard Medical School, Dana-Farber Cancer Institute, Susan F. Smith Center for Women's Cancer, 450 Brookline Ave, Boston, MA 02215, USA
e-mail: Ana_Garrido-Castro@dfci.harvard.edu; bovermoyer@partners.org

M. Howard-McNatt (ed.), *Changing Paradigms in the Management of Breast Cancer*, DOI 10.1007/978-3-319-60336-0_12

Table 12.1 Ongoing phase I clinical trials with novel drugs in advanced breast cancer

	Hormone receptor-positive/HER2-negative		HER2-positive		Triple-negative	
CDK inhibitors	Palbociclib with bazedoxifene in HR-positive breast cancer	NCT02448771	CDK4/CDK6 inhibitor, ribociclib (LEE011), in combination with trastuzumab or T-DM1 for HER2-positive advanced/MBC	NCT02657343	Palbociclib with bicalutamide for the treatment of androgen receptor-positive MBC	NCT02605486
	Palbociclib with bicalutamide for the treatment of androgen receptor-positive MBC	NCT02605486	PD-0332991 in combination with T-DM1 in the treatment of patients with advanced HER2-positive BC	NCT01976169	Sapacitabine and seliciclib in patients with advanced solid tumors	NCT00999401
	Sapacitabine and seliciclib in patients with advanced solid tumors	NCT00999401			Dinaciclib with pembrolizumab in patients with advanced BC and assessment of MYC oncogene overexpression	NCT01676753
PI3K/mTOR inhibitors	MLN0128 with exemestane or fulvestrant in postmenopausal women with ER/PR+ MBC	NCT02049957	Everolimus, letrozole, and trastuzumab in HR- and HER2-positive patients	NCT02152943	Eribulin and everolimus in patients with triple-negative MBC	NCT02120469
	Tamoxifen plus goserelin with alpelisib (BYL719) or buparlisib (BKM120) in premenopausal patients with HR-positive/HER2-negative, locally advanced, or MBC	NCT02058381	BYL719 and T-DM1 in HER2-positive MBC with progression on prior trastuzumab- and taxane-based therapy	NCT02038010	Dose escalation of MK-2206 with weekly paclitaxel in patients with locally advanced or metastatic solid tumors with an expansion in advanced BC	NCT01263145
	BYL719 and nab-paclitaxel in locally recurrent or metastatic HER2-negative breast cancer	NCT02379247	Copanlisib in combination with trastuzumab in HER2-positive breast cancer	NCT02705859	BYL719 and nab-paclitaxel in locally recurrent or metastatic HER2-negative breast cancer	NCT02379247

	AZD2014 plus fulvestrant in patients with estrogen receptor-positive MBC	NCT01597388	LJM716, BYL719, and trastuzumab in patients with HER2+ MBC	NCT02167854	AZD2014 with selumetinib in patients with advanced cancers	NCT02583542
	GDC-0032 with either docetaxel or paclitaxel in patients with HER2-negative, locally advanced, or metastatic breast cancer or NSCLC	NCT01862081	Taselisib (GDC-0032) in combination with anti-HER2 therapies in participants with advanced HER2+ breast cancer	NCT02390427	GDC-0032 with either docetaxel or paclitaxel in patients with HER2-negative, locally advanced, or MBC or NSCLC	NCT01862081
	Ascending doses of AZD5363 under adaptable dosing schedules in patients with advanced solid malignancies	NCT01226316	Ascending doses of AZD5363 under adaptable dosing schedules in patients with advanced solid malignancies	NCT01226316	PQR309 and eribulin in metastatic HER2-negative and triple-negative breast cancer	NCT02723877
	AZD5363 combined with paclitaxel in breast cancer patients	NCT01625286	Lapatinib, everolimus, and capecitabine for HER2-positive MBC with CNS progression after trastuzumab	NCT01783756	AZD5363 combined with paclitaxel in breast cancer patients	NCT01625286
	MK2206 with anastrozole, fulvestrant, or anastrozole and fulvestrant in postmenopausal women with MBC	NCT01344031			LY2780301 in combination with weekly paclitaxel in HER2-negative MBC	NCT01980277
	Dose escalation of MK-2206 with weekly paclitaxel in patients with locally advanced or metastatic solid tumors with an expansion in advanced breast cancer	NCT01263145				
	PQR309 and eribulin in metastatic HER2-negative and triple-negative breast cancer	NCT02723877				
	LY2780301 in combination with weekly paclitaxel in HER2-negative MBC	NCT01980277				

(continued)

Table 12.1 (continued)

	Hormone receptor-positive/HER2-negative		HER2-positive	Triple-negative
Combined CDK and PI3K/mTOR inhibition	LEE011 with everolimus and exemestane in HR-positive HER2-negative advanced breast cancer	NCT01857193		
	Ribociclib with everolimus + exemestane in HR+ HER2− locally advanced/MBC post progression on CDK4/CDK6 inhibitor	NCT02732119		
	LEE011 with fulvestrant and BYL719 or BKM120 in advanced breast cancer	NCT02088684		
	LEE011 and BYL719 with letrozole in adult patients with advanced ER+ breast cancer	NCT01872260		
	LEE011 with buparlisib and letrozole for HR+, HER2-negative postmenopausal women with locally advanced or MBC	NCT02154776		
	Palbociclib with everolimus and exemestane in ER-positive HER2-negative MBC	NCT02871791		
	AZD2014 and palbociclib on a background of hormonal therapy in patients with locally advanced/metastatic ER-positive breast cancer	NCT02599714		
	GDC-0077 as a single agent and in combination with endocrine and targeted therapies in locally advanced or metastatic PIK3CA-mutant HR-positive breast cancer	NCT03006172		
	Gedatolisib with palbociclib and either letrozole or fulvestrant in metastatic or locally advanced/recurrent breast cancer	NCT02684032		

Combined IGFR and mTOR inhibition	BI 836845 and everolimus in combination with exemestane in women with HR+/ HER2− advanced breast cancer	NCT02123823				
FGFR inhibitors	AZD4547 with either anastrozole or letrozole in ER+ patients who have progressed on treatment with anastrozole or letrozole	NCT01791985			Dose-escalation study of INCB054828 in subjects with advanced malignancies	NCT02393248
	Dose-escalation study of INCB054828 in subjects with advanced malignancies	NCT02393248				
JAK inhibitors	Ruxolitinib in combination with weekly paclitaxel in HER2-negative MBC	NCT02041429	Ruxolitinib in combination with trastuzumab in HER2-positive MBC	NCT02066532	Ruxolitinib in combination with weekly paclitaxel in HER2-negative MBC	NCT02041429
Kinase receptor inhibitors			Trastuzumab emtansine (T-DM1) with neratinib in HER2-positive MBC	NCT02236000	Galunisertib, LY2157299 (TGFβR1 inhibitor), with paclitaxel in patients with androgen receptor-negative, triple-negative MBC	NCT02672475
			KD019 (tesevatinib) and trastuzumab in subjects with HER2-positive MBC	NCT02154529		

(continued)

Table 12.1 (continued)

	Hormone receptor-positive/HER2-negative		HER2-positive		Triple-negative	
Immune therapy	Anti-PD-L1, MEDI4736, with tremelimumab in subjects with advanced solid tumors	NCT01975831	Durvalumab in patients with HER2-positive MBC receiving trastuzumab	NCT02649686	Pembrolizumab plus chemotherapy in triple-negative MBC	NCT02734290
	Mesothelin-specific chimeric antigen receptor-positive T cells in patients with mesothelin-expressing MBC	NCT02792114	Anti-PD-1 monoclonal antibody (MK-3475) in advanced, trastuzumab-resistant, HER2-positive breast cancer	NCT02129556	Eribulin with pembrolizumab in subjects with triple-negative MBC	NCT02513472
	Nivolumab with nab-paclitaxel plus or minus gemcitabine in pancreatic cancer, nab-paclitaxel/carboplatin in stage IIIB/IV NSCLC or nab-paclitaxel in recurrent MBC	NCT02309177	Pembrolizumab and monoclonal antibody therapy (T-DM1 or trastuzumab) in patients with advanced cancer	NCT02318901	Pembrolizumab with INCB039110 (JAK inhibitor) and/or pembrolizumab with INCB050465 (PI3K-delta inhibitor) in advanced solid tumors	NCT02646748
	Entinostat, nivolumab, and ipilimumab in patients with solid tumors that are metastatic or cannot be removed by surgery or HER2-negative, locally advanced, or MBC	NCT02453620	Atezolizumab with trastuzumab emtansine or with trastuzumab and pertuzumab in HER2-positive breast cancer	NCT02605915	Entinostat, nivolumab, and ipilimumab in patients with solid tumors that are metastatic or cannot be removed by surgery or HER2-negative, locally advanced, or MBC	NCT02453620
			Adenoviral transduced autologous dendritic cell vaccine expressing HER2/Neu ECTM in adults with tumors with 1–3+ HER2/Neu expression	NCT01730118	Varlilumab (CDX-1127, anti-CD27 agonist) with atezolizumab (MPDL3280A, anti-PD-L1) in patients with advanced cancer	NCT02543645
			Chimeric antigen receptor-modified T cells for HER2-positive recurrent and MBC	NCT02547961	Avelumab with other immunotherapies in advanced malignancies (avelumab plus PF-05082566, anti-4-1BB antibody, in triple-negative cohort)	NCT02554812
					Nivolumab with nab-paclitaxel plus or minus gemcitabine in pancreatic cancer, nab-paclitaxel/carboplatin in stage IIIB/IV NSCLC, or nab-paclitaxel in recurrent MBC	NCT02309177
					Durvalumab with paclitaxel in patients with triple-negative PD-L1 positive MBC	NCT02628132

PARP inhibitors	Veliparib and carboplatin in patients with HER2-negative MBC	NCT01251874			Veliparib and carboplatin in patients with HER2-negative MBC	NCT01251874
Combined immune therapy and PARP inhibition					Durvalumab with olaparib in advanced solid tumors, including TNBC	NCT02484404
					Niraparib with pembrolizumab in patients with triple-negative breast cancer or ovarian cancer	NCT02657889
HDAC inhibitors	ACY-1215 (ricolinostat) with nab-paclitaxel in unresectable or MBC	NCT02632071	ACY-1215 (ricolinostat) with nab-paclitaxel in unresectable or MBC	NCT02632071	ACY-1215 (ricolinostat) with nab-paclitaxel in unresectable or MBC	NCT02632071
	Panobinostat (LBH589) and letrozole in patients with MBC	NCT01105312	Entinostat, lapatinib, and trastuzumab in patients with locally recurrent or distant relapsed MBC previously treated with trastuzumab only	NCT01434303	Panobinostat (LBH589) and letrozole in patients with MBC	NCT01105312
	Ixabepilone and vorinostat in MBC	NCT01084057	Ixabepilone and vorinostat in MBC	NCT01084057	Ixabepilone and vorinostat in MBC	NCT01084057
					Romidepsin plus cisplatin in locally recurrent or metastatic triple-negative breast cancer	NCT02393794
Antibody-drug conjugates (ADC)	SGN-LIV1A in breast cancer patients	NCT01969643	SGN-LIV1A in breast cancer patients	NCT01969643	SGN-LIV1A in breast cancer patients	NCT01969643
	U3-1402 in patients with HER3-positive MBC	NCT02980341	U3-1402 in patients with HER3-positive MBC	NCT02980341	U3-1402 in patients with HER3-positive MBC	NCT02980341
	IMMU-132 (hRS7-SN38) in patients with epithelial cancers	NCT01631552	IMMU-132 (hRS7-SN38) in patients with epithelial cancers	NCT01631552	IMMU-132 (hRS7-SN38) in patients with epithelial cancers	NCT01631552
			ARX788 as a single agent in subjects with advanced cancers with HER2 expression	NCT02512237		
			First-in-human study of DS-8201A, in subjects with advanced solid malignant tumors	NCT02564900		

(continued)

Table 12.1 (continued)

	Hormone receptor-positive/HER2-negative		HER2-positive		Triple-negative	
HSP inhibitors			Ganetespib with paclitaxel, trastuzumab, and pertuzumab in HER2+ MBC	NCT02060253		
Bromodomain inhibitors	GSK525762 in subjects with NUT midline carcinoma (NMC) and other cancers	NCT01587703			GSK525762 in subjects with NUT midline carcinoma (NMC) and other cancers	NCT01587703
					MK-8628, a small molecule inhibitor of the bromodomain and extra-terminal (BET) proteins, in subjects with selected advanced solid tumors	NCT02698176

Targeting Checkpoints in Breast Cancer: Cell-Cycle and Immune Regulation

Cell-Cycle Regulation: The Role of CDK and Cyclins in Breast Cancer

The transition into each phase of the cell cycle (G1, S, G2, and mitosis) is controlled by checkpoints wherein defects in DNA synthesis are detected [6]. Activation of these checkpoints induces cell-cycle arrest and enables DNA repair. A subset of three interphase cyclin-dependent kinases (CDK2, CDK4, and CDK6), a mitotic CDK (CDK1), and ten cyclins (classified in four groups: A-, B-, D-, and E-type cyclins) form CDK-cyclin complexes that regulate these checkpoints [7], as depicted in Fig. 12.1. Mitogenic stimuli result in expression of D-type cyclins which associate with CDK4 and CDK6, producing hyperphosphorylation and inactivation of the retinoblastoma tumor suppressor protein (Rb) thus allowing transition from G1 to S phase. CDK2-cyclin E complexes further phosphorylate and completely inactivate Rb, resulting in transcription and synthesis of numerous proteins that initiate S phase [8]. Cancer cells may overcome the restriction point in G1 phase through constitutive activation of cyclin D-CDK4/CDK6 or loss of pRb and other inhibitory proteins [9, 10].

Crosstalk between several oncogenic signaling pathways and cell-cycle machinery has become patent in breast cancer (Fig. 12.1). Cyclin D1 can directly bind to ERα, even in the absence of estradiol, and induce ER-mediated transcription [11]. Cyclin D1 amplification, CDK4 gain, and a greater frequency of alterations of the Rb pathway have been reported in luminal A, luminal B, and HER2-enriched tumors [12]. In contrast to basal subtypes, ER-positive cancer cell lines have been proven the most sensitive to CDK4/CDK6 inhibitors [13]. CDK4/CDK6 inhibitors can also resensitize HER2-amplified tumors that have developed resistance to HER2-directed therapies by reducing TSC2 phosphorylation and attenuating mTOR signaling [5]. Altogether, this evidence supports the rationale for the development of CDK4/CDK6 inhibitors in ER-positive and HER2-positive breast cancer, in combination with endocrine and other targeted therapies.

The current landscape of the treatment of ER-positive breast cancer has rapidly changed with the development of three selective CDK4/CDK6 inhibitors, palbociclib (PD0332991), ribociclib (LEE011), and abemaciclib (LY2835219), each with distinct pharmacokinetic and safety profiles. Abemaciclib has more potent inhibitory activity against CDK4, compared to palbociclib and ribociclib [14], and can also penetrate the central nervous system (CNS) [15]. A greater incidence of fatigue and gastrointestinal disorders has been reported with abemaciclib, compared to higher-grade 3–4 neutropenia observed with the other CDK4/CDK6 inhibitors [16–18]. In terms of efficacy (Table 12.2), palbociclib received US Food and Drug Administration (FDA) accelerated approval in combination with letrozole based on a 10-month progression-free survival (PFS) improvement in postmenopausal women who had no prior therapy for advanced ER-positive disease [19, 20]. Palbociclib was also approved in combination with fulvestrant following progression on prior endocrine therapy, based on data reported from the PALOMA-3 trial

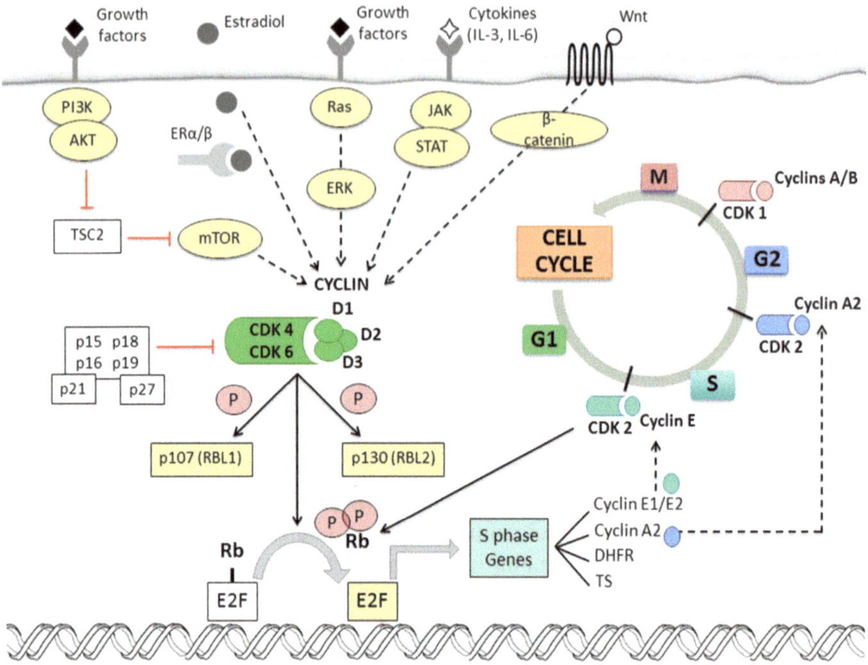

Fig. 12.1 Crosstalk between cell-cycle machinery and oncogenic signaling pathways (Modified with permission from Garrido-Castro A.C., Goel S. Curr Breast Cancer Rep (2017)). The transition into each phase of the cell cycle (*G1*, *S*, *G2*, and mitosis) is tightly controlled by checkpoints that are regulated by CDK-cyclin complexes. Mitogenic stimuli activate intracellular signaling pathways (i.e., *PI3K/AKT/mTOR*, *Ras/Raf/MAPK*, *JAK/STAT*, etc.) that induce the expression of D-type cyclins (*D1*, *D2*, and *D3*). Cyclin D preferentially associates with CDK4 and CDK6, producing hyperphosphorylation and inactivation of retinoblastoma (*Rb*) by uncoupling it from E2F transcription factors, thus allowing cell-cycle transition from G1 to S phase. In addition, these complexes partially inactivate the inhibitory pocket proteins RBL1 (also known as p107) and RBL2 (also known as p130), enabling the expression of E-type cyclins. CDK2-cyclin E complexes further phosphorylate and completely inactivate these pocket proteins and Rb. This results in transcription and synthesis of numerous proteins that initiate S phase, such as dihydrofolate reductase (*DHFR*) and thymidylate synthase (*TS*). A-type cyclins drive the transition from S phase to G2 during later stages of DNA replication and finally activate CDK1 to induce mitosis. After the rupture of the nuclear membrane, degradation of A-type cyclins leads to binding of CDK1 to cyclin B, responsible for entry into mitosis. CDK activation is primarily controlled by binding to cyclins, which show a cyclical pattern of synthesis and degradation. In addition to decreasing levels of D-type cyclins as cells progress through S phase, endogenous inhibition of CDK4/CDK6 is also enabled by two families of CDK inhibitors: the INK4 family (p16INK4A, p15INK4B, p18INK4C, and p19INK4D) and the Cip/Kip family (p21, p27, and p57). Estrogen steroids, such as 17-β-estradiol, promote cell-cycle progression by increasing CCND1 transcription, assembly of active cyclin D1-CDK4 complexes, and, ultimately, pRb phosphorylation. Cyclin D1 can also directly bind to ERα and induce ER-mediated transcription, even in the absence of estradiol

[21, 22]. Recently, a randomized placebo-controlled phase III study, MONALEESA-2, met its primary endpoint by demonstrating a significant increase in PFS in patients treated with ribociclib and letrozole in the first-line metastatic setting [23]; at the time of writing, this combination awaits regulatory approval. Abemaciclib was granted FDA Breakthrough Therapy designation after revealing promising antitumoral activity in phase I/II studies, despite inclusion of heavily pretreated patients [18, 24]. Randomized phase III trials of abemaciclib in combination with hormonal therapies in the early-line metastatic setting are ongoing (NCT02107703, NCT02246621).

In HER2-positive disease, CDK4/CDK6 inhibitors are currently being explored in phase I/II trials combined with trastuzumab or the antibody-drug conjugate, trastuzumab emtansine (T-DM1), with or without endocrine therapy (NCT02657343, NCT02448420, NCT01976169, NCT02675231). Despite the absence of preclinical data favoring CDK4/CDK6 inhibition in triple-negative breast cancer (TNBC), other CDK targets are under investigation in this subtype. Dinaciclib, a potent inhibitor of CDK1, CDK2, CDK5, and CDK9, has demonstrated encouraging in vitro and in vivo activity [25, 26]. In addition, dinaciclib sensitizes TNBC cell lines to PARP inhibition [27], which encouraged the ongoing phase I trial in combination with veliparib (NCT01434316).

Immune Checkpoint Blockade

The interaction between immunity and cancer has been subject of great interest over the past decades. However, not until recently have immunotherapeutic strategies demonstrated an improvement in patient outcomes in breast cancer. Neoantigens, i.e., peptides arising from cancer specific mutations, are processed by dendritic cells and presented on major histocompatibility class I (MHC-I) and class II (MHC-II) molecules to T cells [28]. The activation of effector T-cell responses against neoantigens requires the establishment of an immunological synapse in which two signals must be present: (1) the interaction between the antigen-MHC complex and the T-cell receptor (TCR) and (2) the presence of the co-stimulatory molecule, CD28, which binds to its ligands B7-1 (also known as CD80) and B7-2 (CD86) that are expressed by antigen-presenting cells (APC), such as dendritic cells [29]. Both interactions will then stimulate TCR signaling through PI3K-AKT, Ras-Raf-MAPK, and NF-κB pathways, causing secretion of cytokines and promoting proliferation of activated T cells which infiltrate into tumor beds, recognize, and kill cancer cells. However, binding of T-cell inhibitory checkpoint molecules, PD-1 and CTLA-4, to their respective ligands, PD-L1/PD-L2 and CD80/CD86, induces the recruitment of phosphatases that block TCR signaling [28]. Inhibition of these checkpoints has become an attractive strategy, especially for tumors with elevated lymphocytic infiltration.

Traditionally, breast cancer has not been considered highly immunogenic, in part due to the lower prevalence of somatic mutations and less likelihood of formation of neoantigens compared to other tumors, such as melanoma, lung, or urothelial carcinoma [30]. Nevertheless, the presence of tumor-infiltrating lymphocytes (TILs) is prognostic in early-stage triple-negative or HER2-amplified breast cancer [31].

Table 12.2 Results of phase II/III clinical trials with CDK4/CDK6 inhibitors in advanced breast cancer

	CDK inhibitors				
	Palbociclib			Ribociclib	Abemaciclib
Clinical trial	PALOMA-1	PALOMA-2	PALOMA-3	MONALEESA-2	MONARCH-1
Trial design	Phase II open-label	Phase III double-blind	Phase III double-blind	Phase III double-blind	Phase II single-arm
Study arms	Palbociclib + letrozole vs. letrozole	Palbociclib + letrozole vs. placebo + letrozole	Palbociclib + fulvestrant vs. placebo + fulvestrant (+/− goserelin)	Ribociclib + letrozole vs. placebo + letrozole	Abemaciclib
Study drug dose	125 mg QD 3 w on/1 w off	125 mg QD 3 w on/1 w off	125 mg QD 3 w on/1 w off	600 mg QD 3w on/1w off	200 mg BID continuously
Characteristics					
Menopausal status	Postmenopausal	Postmenopausal	All	Postmenopausal	All
Prior ET allowed for advanced disease	No	No	Yes[a]	No	Yes
Total pts, n	165	666	521	668	132
Efficacy					
Median PFS (experimental arm vs. control arm), mo	20.2 vs. 10.2	24.8 vs. 14.5	9.5 vs. 4.6	NR vs. 14.7	6.0
HR PFS (95% CI)	0.49 (0.32–0.75)	0.58 (0.46–0.72)	0.46 (0.36–0.59)	0.56 (0.43–0.72)	NA
Median OS (experimental arm vs. control arm), mo	37.5 vs. 33.3	NA	NA	NA	17.7
HR OS (95% CI)	0.81 (0.49–1.35)	NA	NA	NA	NA
ORR (ITT), %	43 vs. 33	42 vs. 35	19 vs. 9	41 vs. 28	20

	CDK inhibitors				
	Palbociclib			Ribociclib	Abemaciclib
CBR (ITT), %	81 vs. 58	85 vs. 70	67 vs. 40	80 vs. 73	42.4
Safety					
Grade 3–4 neutropenia, %	54 vs. 1	67 vs. 1	65 vs. 1	59 vs. 1	27
Grade 3–4 diarrhea, %	4 vs. 0	1 vs. 1	0 vs. 1	1 vs. 1	20
Grade 3–4 elevated liver enzymes (ALT; AST), %	0 vs. 0; 1 vs. 0	NA	2 vs. 0; 3 vs. 2	9 vs. 1; 6 vs. 1	NA

Percentages are reported, respectively, per study arms of treatment

ET endocrine therapy, *w* weeks, *mo* months, *pts* patients, *n* number, *NA* not available/not applicable, *NR* not reached, *PFS* progression-free survival, *OS* overall survival, *HR* hazard ratio, *ORR* overall response rate, *CBR* clinical benefit rate, *ITT* intention-to-treat, *ALT* alanine transaminase, *AST* aspartate transaminase

[a]Patients who received no prior lines of therapy in the context of metastatic disease: 24% vs. 26%

Results from several trials evaluating immune checkpoint inhibitors in the metastatic setting have been reported (Table 12.3) [32–36]. However, comparisons are limited due to broad variations in the inclusion criteria of each study, including differences in tumor subtype, prior number of therapies allowed, preselection based on PD-L1 positivity, and assays used to quantify PD-L1 expression. Common adverse events that have been reported with these agents include arthralgia, fatigue, nausea, diarrhea, and pyrexia. The occurrence of specific immune-related toxicities, such as endocrinopathies, pneumonitis, or hepatitis, is rare and has been attributed to the release of the breaks on autoimmunity. Single-agent checkpoint inhibitors, pembrolizumab and atezolizumab, have achieved overall response rates (ORR) of approximately 19% in heavily pretreated patients with PD-L1-positive TNBC [32, 36]. Conversely, in the JAVELIN trial, ORR in unselected TNBC patients treated with the PD-L1 antibody avelumab was 8.6% and ranged from 6.1% in patients with ≥1% of PD-L1-positive tumor cells to 44.4% in those with ≥10% of PD-L1-positive cells [35], underscoring the need for standardization of assays in the search for predictive biomarkers of response.

Limited activity has been observed in the setting of HER2-positive and ER-positive disease [34, 35]. Although treatment with single-agent pembrolizumab has achieved modest response rates in patients with ER-positive PD-L1-positive tumors, strikingly higher response rates (67–89%) seen with atezolizumab combined with *nab*-paclitaxel, as first-line therapy for patients with metastatic TNBC [33], have encouraged larger trials of immune checkpoint inhibitors combined with chemotherapy in both hormone receptor-positive and hormone receptor-negative breast cancer (NCT02425891, NCT02819518, NCT02628132, NCT02755272, NCT02648477, NCT02513472). Combinations with agonists of stimulatory checkpoints (OX40, 4-1BB) or antibodies that block other inhibitory checkpoints (CTLA-4, LAG-3, TIM-3) are also emerging.

Oncogenic Signaling Pathways

Phosphatidylinositol-3 Kinase/AKT/Mammalian Target of Rapamycin Pathway

The family of PI3 kinases is divided into three classes, of which class IA has been the most clearly implicated in human cancer [37]. Class IA PI3K is comprised of a p110 catalytic subunit (with three isoforms, p110α, p110β, and p110δ, encoded by *PIK3CA*, *PIK3CB*, and *PIK3CD*) and a p85 regulatory subunit that is responsible for inhibition of p110 in the absence of activating signals. Ligand binding results in the recruitment of class I PI3Ks to the plasma membrane and liberation of p110, initiating intracellular cascades that lead to cell growth and survival [38]. Genetic alterations that promote activation of the PI3K pathway (*PIK3CA*, *PIK3R1*, *AKT1*, *PTEN*) are present at a high frequency in breast cancer, particularly in luminal tumors [12]. Upregulation of the PI3K pathway is a known mechanism of resistance to endocrine treatment [39, 40], and preclinical studies have demonstrated that blocking PI3K and/or downstream effectors, AKT and mTOR, can restore sensitivity to endocrine therapy [41].

Table 12.3 Results of immunotherapy clinical trials in advanced breast cancer

	Pembrolizumab in PD-L1+ tumors: TNBC cohort (KEYNOTE-012)	Pembrolizumab in PD-L1+ ER+/HER2− breast cancer (KEYNOTE-028)	Atezolizumab in tumors unselected for PD-L1: TNBC cohort	Atezolizumab + *nab*-paclitaxel in tumors unselected for PD-L1: TNBC cohort	Avelumab in locally advanced or metastatic breast cancer: unselected for PD-L1 or HR/HER2 status (JAVELIN)			
Mechanism of action	Humanized IgG4 anti-PD-1	Humanized IgG4 Anti-PD-1	Humanized IgG1 anti-PD-L1	Humanized IgG1 anti-PD-L1	Fully human IgG1 anti-PD-L1			
Dose and schedule	10 mg/kg (Q2W)	10 mg/kg (Q2W)	15 mg/kg or 20 mg/kg or 1,200 mg flat dose (Q3W)	Atezolizumab: 800 mg (Q2W); Nab-paclitaxel: 125 mg/kg on days 1,8,15 (Q4W)	10 mg/kg (Q2W)			
Breast cancer subtype	Triple-negative	ER-positive, HER2-negative	Triple-negative	Triple-negative	All	TNBC cohort	HER2-positive cohort	HR-positive, HER2-negative cohort
PD-L1 positivity definition	≥1% TC or any staining in stroma	≥1% TC or any staining in stroma	≥5% IC	≥1% IC; ≥1% TC	≥1% TC; ≥10% IC	≥1% TC; ≥10% IC	≥1% TC; ≥10% IC	≥1% TC; ≥10% IC
PD-L1 inclusion criteria	Positive	Positive	All-comers[a]	All-comers	All-comers			
No. PD-L1+ pts/no. PD-L1 evaluable cases (%)	65/111 (58.6)	48/248 (19.4)	37/54 (68.5)	9/24 (37.5); 3/24 (12.5)	85/136 (62.5); 12/136 (8.8)	33/48 (68.8); 9/48 (18.8)	15/21 (71.4); 1/21 (4.8)	31/56 (55.4); 2/56 (3.6)
No. pts enrolled	32	25	54	32	168	58	26	72
No. pts included in efficacy analysis	27	25	21[a]	24	168	58	26	72
No. prior therapies for metastatic disease, median (range)	2 (0–9)	NA	NA	5 (1–10)	3 (0–10)	NA	NA	NA

(continued)

Table 12.3 (continued)

	Pembrolizumab in PD-L1+ tumors: TNBC cohort (KEYNOTE-012)	Pembrolizumab in PD-L1+ ER+/HER2− breast cancer (KEYNOTE-028)	Atezolizumab in tumors unselected for PD-L1: TNBC cohort	Atezolizumab + *nab*-paclitaxel in tumors unselected for PD-L1: TNBC cohort	Avelumab in locally advanced or metastatic breast cancer: unselected for PD-L1 or HR/HER2 status (JAVELIN)			
No. pts with ≥3 prior therapies for metastatic disease (%)	15 (46.9)	20 (80.0)	NA[b]	1 (4.2)	88 (52.4)	13 (22.4)	NA	NA
ORR, %	18.5	12.0[c]	19.0	70.8[d]	4.8	8.6	3.8	2.8
ORR in PD-L1+ cohort, %	18.5	12.0[c]	19.0	77.8	3.5; 33.3	6.1; 44.4	NA	NA
CBR, %	25.9	20.0[c]	NA	NA	28.0	31.0	NA	NA
Median DOR, wks (range)	NR (15.0 to 47.3+)	NR (8.7+ to 44.3+)	NR (18 to 56+)	NA	28.7 (6.1-NR)	NA	NA	NA
Median PFS, mo (95% CI)	1.9 (1.7–5.5)	NA	NA	NA	NA	NA	NA	NA
PFS rate at 6 mo, %	24.4	NA	27	NA	NA	NA	NA	NA
Median OS, mo (95% CI)	11.2 (5.3-NR)	NA	NA	NA	NA	NA	NA	NA

According to PD-L1 positivity in IC

TNBC triple-negative breast cancer, *ER* estrogen receptor, *HR* hormone receptor, *no* number, *pts* patients, *TC* tumor cells, *IC* immune cells, *ORR* overall response rate, *CBR* clinical benefit rate (defined as patients with complete response, partial response or stable disease for ≥24 wks), *wks* weeks, *mo* months, *DOR* duration of response, *NR* not reached, *NA* not available, *PFS* progression-free survival, *OS* overall survival

[a]All evaluable patients were PD-L1 positive. Data for PD-L1 negative tumors: NA

[b]No. pts with ≥4 lines of prior therapy for advanced disease: 48 (88.9%)

[c]If pts. with at least one scan post-baseline are considered, ORR was 14% and CBR was 23%

[d]Confirmed ORR, defined as at least two consecutive assessments of complete or partial response: 41.7 (22.1–63.4)

Everolimus, an mTOR inhibitor, is the only agent targeting this pathway that is currently approved by the FDA, in combination with exemestane, after progression on a nonsteroidal aromatase inhibitor (NSAI). Although there was a 4.6-month increase in PFS, compared to exemestane alone (7.8 versus 3.2 months, respectively) [42, 43], no OS benefit was noted, and approximately 40% of patients experienced grade 3–4 adverse events [44]. More recently, several pan-PI3K or p110α-specific inhibitors have emerged, the latter in hopes of sparing undesired toxicity due to blockade of other p110 isoforms.

Buparlisib (BKM120), an oral pan-PI3K inhibitor that targets all class I isoforms [45], was determined to be safe and efficacious in combination with letrozole or fulvestrant, in early dose-escalation studies in endocrine-resistant metastatic disease, reaching a clinical benefit rate (CBR) of 31–59% [46, 47]. Further evaluation of buparlisib in phase III randomized placebo-controlled trials revealed a statistically significant, though modest, 2-month increase in PFS when administered with fulvestrant after progression on AI (BELLE-2) [48] or after dual AI-mTOR inhibition (BELLE-3) [49] (Table 12.4). Of note, subgroup analyses according to mutational status have shown greater improvements in PFS in patients with *PIK3CA*-mutant tumors. Overall, the most common AE were hypertransaminasemia, hyperglycemia, fatigue, nausea, diarrhea, and rash. Buparlisib's ability to cross the blood-brain barrier also provoked mood disorders, such as anxiety or depression, in approximately 20% of patients.

Selective PI3K inhibitors have emerged, specifically targeting p110α or mutant *PIK3CA* isoforms. Taselisib (GDC-0032) is a β-sparing PI3K inhibitor that is almost 200× more potent than buparlisib against p110α [50]. Preliminary results from a phase II single-arm study evaluating taselisib and fulvestrant in 60 postmenopausal women, who failed to respond to at least one prior endocrine therapy in the adjuvant or metastatic setting, are illustrated in Table 12.4 [51]. Despite a lower occurrence of grade 3–4 toxicities, a broad span of AE was still noted. *PIK3CA* mutations were present in 20 of 45 evaluable cases (44.4%) and were associated with heightened clinical activity compared to those with wild-type tumors (ORR, 38.5% vs. 10.5%; CBR, 38.5% vs. 15.8%, respectively). Taselisib is currently being tested in a phase III randomized trial (SANDPIPER, NCT02340221) in combination with fulvestrant after progression on AI; enrollment will be enriched for *PIK3CA*-mutant tumors.

Alpelisib (BYL719) is a selective p110α inhibitor in advanced stages of development in ER-positive breast cancer. In earlier phase I trials, alpelisib demonstrated a more favorable toxicity profile compared to pan-PI3K inhibitors, both as a single agent and in combination with letrozole or fulvestrant [52–54]. SOLAR-1 is an ongoing phase III trial assessing the efficacy of alpelisib and fulvestrant after AI therapy (NCT02437318).

Inhibition of PI3K/AKT/mTOR is a strategy not only of interest in ER-positive disease. Constitutive activation of the PI3K pathway, through *PIK3CA* mutation or loss of PTEN function, can mediate resistance to trastuzumab [55, 56]. Preclinical studies demonstrated synergy between trastuzumab and PI3K/mTOR inhibitors; however, to date, this has not translated into clinically meaningful benefit [57, 58]. In the phase III BOLERO-3 study, patients with HER2-positive, trastuzumab-resistant disease were randomized to receive weekly trastuzumab and vinorelbine with

Table 12.4 Results of phase II/III clinical trials with PI3K inhibitors in advanced breast cancer

	PI3K inhibitors			
	Buparlisib			Taselisib
Clinical trial	BELLE-2	BELLE-3	BELLE-4	PMT4979g
Trial design	Phase III double-blind	Phase III double-blind	Phase II double-blind	Phase II single-arm
Study arms	Buparlisib + fulvestrant vs. placebo + fulvestrant	Buparlisib + fulvestrant vs. placebo + fulvestrant	Buparlisib + paclitaxel vs. placebo + paclitaxel	Taselisib + fulvestrant
Study drug dose	100 mg QD continuously	100 mg QD continuously	100 mg QD continuously	6 mg QD continuously
Characteristics				
Menopausal status	Postmenopausal	Postmenopausal	All	Postmenopausal
Prior ET allowed for advanced disease	Yes	Yes (after progression on AI + mTOR inhibitor)	Yes	Yes
Total pts, n	1,147	432	416[a]	60
Any prior ET[b], %	100	100	44 vs. 50	100
PIK3CA mut status[c], %	30 vs. 38	39[d]	26	44
Efficacy				
Median PFS (experimental arm vs. control arm), mo	6.9 vs. 5.0	3.9 vs. 1.8	8.0 vs. 9.2	NA
HR PFS (95% CI)	0.78 (0.67–0.89)	0.67 (0.53–0.84)	1.18 (0.82–1.68)	NA
ORR (ITT), %	12 vs. 8	8 vs. 2	23 vs. 27	17
CBR (ITT), %	44 vs. 42	25 vs. 15	26 vs. 33	25
Safety				
Grade 3–4 diarrhea, %	4 vs. 1	3 vs. 1	5 vs. 3	12
Grade 3–4 elevated liver enzymes (ALT; AST), %	26 vs. 1; 18 vs. 3	22 vs. 3; 18 vs. 3	7 vs. <1; NA	NA
Grade 3–4 hyperglycemia, %	15 vs. <1	12 vs. 0	9 vs. <1	7
Grade 3–4 rash, %	8 vs. 0	2 vs. 0	8 vs. 1	5

Percentages are reported, respectively, per study arms of treatment

ET endocrine therapy, *AI* aromatase inhibitor, *mo* months, *pts* patients, *n* number, *NA* not available/not applicable, *PFS* progression-free survival, *HR* hazard ratio, *ORR* overall response rate, *CBR* clinical benefit rate, *ITT* intention-to-treat, *ALT* alanine transaminase, *AST* aspartate transaminase

[a]At the time of the interim PFS analysis, 338 pts. had been randomized to treatment

[b]Including (neo)adjuvant setting

[c]When evaluable in baseline cfDNA (except BELLE-4 that reported PIK3CA status analyzed in tumor tissue)

[d]PIK3CA mutational status in the overall population (data not reported per arm of treatment)

everolimus or placebo. Everolimus extended median PFS from 5.78 to 7.0 months (HR 0.70), albeit with substantial toxicity [59]. Moreover, the addition of everolimus to trastuzumab and paclitaxel, as first-line treatment for HER2-positive advanced breast cancer, failed to improve PFS in BOLERO-1 [60]. Combinations of the novel selective PI3K inhibitors, taselisib and alpelisib, with HER2-directed therapies T-DM1 and pertuzumab are currently ongoing (NCT02390427, NCT02038010).

Although *PIK3CA* mutations are more prevalent in luminal disease, loss of *PTEN* and *INPP4B*, which sensitizes cell lines to PI3K inhibition [61], is more common in basal-like tumors [12]. Chemotherapy added to PI3K inhibition is under evaluation in TNBC. Drugs that provide dual PI3K/mTOR blockade (gedatolisib, PQR309), as well as inhibitors of AKT (AZD5363, MK-2206, GDC-0068) and mTOR (TAK-228 or MLN0128, AZD2014), are also being explored in combination with standard regimens across breast cancer subtypes.

Insulin-Like Growth Factor Receptor (IGF-1R) and Fibroblast Growth Factor Receptor (FGFR) Pathways

Increased activation of the tyrosine kinase receptor, IGF-1R, has been associated with cancer cell proliferation and migration [62] and can mediate resistance to endocrine and HER2-directed therapy due to the crosstalk between IGF-1R and the PI3K/MAPK pathways [63, 64]. Despite promising preclinical data, several IGF-1R-specific antibodies (figitumumab, cixutumumab, ganitumab) have failed to demonstrate benefit in combination with endocrine therapy in phase II clinical trials [65–67]. Nonetheless, IGF-1R signaling through AKT may play an important role in the onset of resistance to mTOR inhibitors [68], and combined blockade of IGF-1R and mTOR could improve clinical outcomes. A randomized phase II trial is assessing the efficacy of BI 836845, an IGF ligand-neutralizing antibody, with exemestane and everolimus [69].

Amplification of *FGFR* genes, present in approximately 10% of breast cancers [70], is associated with poor prognosis [71, 72] and promotes resistance to endocrine therapy through persistent MAPK activation [71]. In addition, FGF2 ligand mediates growth of basal-like breast cancer, and TNBC cell lines have demonstrated sensitivity to FGFR inhibitors in the presence of FGF2 [73]. Selective (i.e., BGJ398, JNJ-42756493, INCB054828) and nonselective (i.e., lucitanib, nintedanib, dovitinib, AZD4547) FGFR inhibitors have been tested in phase I/II trials in solid tumors, but limited evidence of clinical activity has been reported to date in breast cancer cohorts treated with selective single-agent inhibition [74–76]; combinations with immune or chemotherapy are ongoing (NCT02393248).

Cytokine-Mediated JAK/STAT Pathway

Janus kinase 2 (JAK2), a non-receptor tyrosine kinase that binds to the cytoplasmic tail of transmembrane cytokine receptors, activates STAT transcription factors that stimulate the expression of various cell-cycle regulators, including cyclins D1, D2, and E (Fig. 12.1) [77]. The IL6/JAK2/STAT3 pathway plays an important role in the proliferation and metastatic spread of CD44+/CD24+ stem cell-like breast cancer cells, a predominant population in inflammatory breast cancer [78]. Furthermore, activation of JAK2/STAT5 has been implicated in resistance to PI3K/mTOR inhibition in TNBC cell lines [79]. Ruxolitinib is an oral inhibitor of JAK1 and JAK2 that has shown promising antitumoral activity combined with paclitaxel in metastatic HER2-negative breast cancer (ORR, 21%; CBR, 84%) [80]. Ruxolitinib is currently being tested with other standard regimens (capecitabine, NCT02120417; trastuzumab, NCT02066532; exemestane, NCT01594216) in all subtypes of MBC.

Broad-Spectrum Tyrosine Kinase Inhibitors and Anti-angiogenesis

Despite initial FDA approval of bevacizumab (a humanized monoclonal antibody against vascular endothelial growth factor, VEGF) in combination with chemotherapy based on PFS improvement as first-line treatment for HER2-negative advanced breast cancer [81–84], the lack of OS benefit led to withdrawal of its indication in breast cancer in the USA. Emphasis has now been directed to broad-spectrum tyrosine kinase inhibitors (TKI) that target several families of growth factor receptors, including VEGF receptor (VEGFR) and platelet-derived growth factor receptor (PDGFR). Cabozantinib, an oral TKI with activity against VEGFR2, MET, and AXL, elicited an ORR of 13.6% and CBR of 46.7%, in ER-positive disease [85]. Lucitanib (E3810), a multi-TKI directed to FGFR1, VEGFR1-3, and macrophage colony-stimulating factor-1 receptor (CSF1R), achieved a PFS greater than 9 months and six confirmed partial responses in 12 patients with FGF-aberrant breast cancer [86]. Other VEGFR, PDGFR, and c-Kit inhibitors, such as sunitinib, sorafenib, or axitinib, have failed to improve survival in breast cancer [87–89]. It seems clear that some, but not all, patients may benefit from anti-angiogenic therapies, highlighting the need to identify biomarkers that could guide patient selection.

Antibody-Drug Conjugates

Antibody-drug conjugates (ADC) are a novel class of drugs linking an antibody (selective for a cancer cell surface antigen) to a highly cytotoxic agent, in order to optimize the delivery of chemotherapy to the tumor, improve efficacy, and minimize off-target systemic toxicity [90]. T-DM1 is the only ADC currently approved for the treatment of breast cancer, although there are several new compounds emerging. Sacituzumab govitecan, or IMMU-132, is an ADC targeting Trop-2 present on TNBC that delivers SN-38 (active metabolite of irinotecan). In a phase II trial involving heavily pretreated patients, ORR and CBR at 6 months were 29% and 45.5%, respectively, and median PFS and OS were 5.6 and 14.3 months, respectively [91]. The most frequent grade 3–4 AE were neutropenia, anemia, and mild GI toxicity. Based on these results, IMMU-132 was granted FDA Breakthrough

Therapy designation in 2016 for patients with pretreated metastatic TNBC and will be compared to treatment of physician's choice in a randomized phase III trial (NCT02574455). DS-8201a, an anti-HER2 ADC that delivers a new topoisomerase I inhibitor, showed promising efficacy in T-DM1-resistant and low HER2-expressing PDX models [92] and has now entered clinical development (NCT02564900).

Regulation of DNA Synthesis, Transcription, and Repair

Epigenetic Modulation

Upregulation of histone deacetylases (HDAC) alters the balance between histone acetylation and deacetylation, leading to epigenetic repression of tumor suppressor genes, and ultimately oncogenesis [93]. In preclinical models, the addition of HDAC inhibitors to antiestrogens enhances the antiproliferative effect of either agent alone [94] and reverses tamoxifen- and AI-induced resistance [3, 95].

Entinostat, a highly specific class I HDAC inhibitor, was granted FDA Breakthrough Therapy designation in 2013 based on the results of ENCORE-301, a phase II trial for postmenopausal women treated with exemestane in combination with either entinostat or placebo, after progressing on NSAI [96]. Entinostat extended both PFS and OS when added to exemestane, with absolute improvements of 2.0 and 8.3 months, respectively. E2112 is an ongoing randomized phase III trial seeking to confirm these results in a larger population (NCT02115282). HDAC inhibitors upregulate PD-L1 expression and synergize with PD-1 blockade in murine melanoma models [97]. This has provided the rationale for multiple combinations of entinostat with immunotherapies across all MBC subtypes, including TNBC and HER2-negative disease (NCT02708680, NCT02453620).

PARP Inhibitors and DNA Repair

Poly(ADP-ribose) polymerase-1 (PARP1) is a critical enzyme involved in base excision repair of DNA [98]. Loss of PARP1 function increases the number of DNA breaks that require homologous recombination repair (HRR). Defects in HRR genes (e.g., *BRCA1*/*BRCA2*) lead to failure to efficiently repair DNA double-stranded breaks (DSB), thus promoting the use of alternative DNA repair processes which can induce DNA mutagenesis. Basal-like breast cancers are associated with *BRCA1* phenotype, and BRCA-related tumors are more likely to exhibit ER negativity [99], making PARP inhibition a strategy of great interest in *BRCA*-mutant breast cancer, particularly in TNBC.

Olaparib, veliparib, niraparib, and talazoparib have shown single-agent antitumoral activity in *BRCA*-associated MBC [100–103]. In a phase II study in 54 patients with germline *BRCA1*/*BRCA2* mutations, olaparib achieved a 41% ORR, and responses were seen in both hormone receptor-positive/HER2-negative and TNBC disease [103]. Several phase III trials are now comparing these agents with physician's choice of chemotherapy in *BRCA*-carriers (OlympiaD, NCT02000622; BRAVO, NCT01905592; EMBRACA, NCT01945775). Loss of PARP induces tumor sensitization to DNA cross-linking agents, explaining the synergy observed in preclinical models treated with PARP inhibitors and drugs such as cisplatin, carboplatin, cyclophosphamide, or temozolomide [104]. These combinations have shown promising preliminary activity in patients with BRCA-mutant and non-BRCA-associated tumors [105–107]. Furthermore, reports that BRCA-deficient TNBC harbors a higher mutational load, number of neoantigens, and increased immune cell activation [108] have encouraged ongoing phase I assessment of anti-PD-1/anti-L1 blockade with PARP inhibition (NCT02484404, NCT02657889).

Heat Shock Protein (Hsp) 90

Heat shock proteins are molecular chaperones that modulate the folding and transport across cell membranes of many cellular proteins [109]. Hsp90 is highly expressed in mammalian cells, and its overexpression has been implicated in the oncogenesis of ductal breast carcinomas [110]. The Hsp90 inhibitor tanespimycin demonstrated an ORR of 22% and 6-month median PFS when added to trastuzumab, after progression on prior trastuzumab-based regimens in HER2-positive MBC [111]. Although ganetespib showed limited efficacy as a single agent across all subtypes of MBC, activity was highest in the HER2-positive cohort [112]. Ganetespib is currently being explored in combination with trastuzumab, pertuzumab, and paclitaxel (NCT02060253) and also with fulvestrant (NCT01560416).

Central Nervous System Disease

The incidence of CNS metastases is increasing in patients with breast cancer, partly due to improvement in survival with systemic therapies that manage to control extracranial disease. To date, there are no FDA-approved systemic therapies for the treatment of breast cancer brain metastases. Cytotoxic agents, such as capecitabine, temozolomide, or cisplatin, have been assessed in small prospective trials, demonstrating modest CNS response and PFS rates of less than 3 months [113]. Etirinotecan pegol (NKTR-102) is a topoisomerase I inhibitor, and although NKTR-102 did not significantly improve OS when compared to physician's choice of treatment, the subgroup of patients with brain metastasis benefited from the experimental drug (HR 0.51). A phase III trial limited to patients with stable brain metastases is now ongoing (NCT02915744).

Several novel targeting agents have also shown specific activity in patients with CNS metastases. Given that concentrations of abemaciclib in cerebrospinal fluid reach those of unbound drug in plasma [18], evaluation of abemaciclib in patients with brain metastases secondary to hormone receptor-positive breast cancer is ongoing (NCT02308020). Various agents have demonstrated activity in

HER2-positive CNS metastases; however limited data exist comparing novel treatments to standard of care regimens. Neratinib, a potent oral TKI of ErbB1, HER2, and ErbB4, was evaluated in monotherapy in a single-arm phase II trial in patients whose CNS disease had progressed after any CNS-directed therapy [114]. Objective CNS response rate was 8% in this heavily pretreated population, not differing significantly from those seen with lapatinib [115]. A phase II trial with neratinib and capecitabine for the treatment of HER2-positive brain metastases is ongoing (NCT01494662). Recently, results were reported from a phase I study of tucatinib (ONT-380), a novel HER2-selective TKI with CNS penetration, in combination with T-DM1 [116]. In patients with previously treated or untreated asymptomatic CNS lesions, median PFS was 6.5 months; of 12 patients with measurable CNS disease, two complete and two partial responses were observed, and three others achieved stable CNS disease >6 months. The effect of tucatinib in patients with brain metastases is being investigated in a phase II study in combination with capecitabine and trastuzumab in patients who have received prior treatment with a taxane, trastuzumab, pertuzumab, and T-DM1 (NCT02614794).

Leptomeningeal metastases confer a poor prognosis across all breast cancer subtypes, and there are very few prospective trials in this population to guide treatment decisions [113]. Case reports of activity with intrathecal trastuzumab have led to the design of two studies in HER2-positive leptomeningeal disease (NCT01325207, NCT01373710) and a phase I trial of intrathecal trastuzumab plus pertuzumab in patients with untreated asymptomatic or low symptomatic brain metastases (NCT02598427).

Conclusions

The landscape of treatment of MBC has evolved rapidly over the past years and continues to progress as additional mechanisms of resistance to current therapies are discovered. Promising PFS and response rates are being reported from large phase III trials with CDK4/CDK6, PI3K, and PARP inhibitors, though we eagerly await OS analyses to determine the long-term impact of these new agents. As the selection of treatments for MBC grows, physicians face the important challenge of identifying patients who are most likely to respond while sparing undesired toxicities to those who may not benefit from these therapies. Beyond the sensitivity of HRR-deficient tumors to PARP inhibition, the search for biomarkers of response to novel drugs, such as CDK4/CDK6 or PI3K inhibitors, has not yet yielded clinically meaningful results. Exploratory analyses of studies of palbociclib showed that neither Ki67 staining, Rb localization, p16 nuclear expression, nor *CCND1* amplification was predictive for PFS or ORR [19, 117, 118]. Mutations in the ER gene (*ESR1*) conferred worse prognosis but were not predictive of response in PALOMA-3; both *ESR1*-mutant and wild-type populations significantly benefited from palbociclib (HR for PFS: 0.43 and 0.49, respectively) [119]. Assessment of the efficacy of PI3K inhibitors according to *PIK3CA* status has also revealed conflicting data. Patients with *PIK3CA* mutations detected in archival tumor samples in BELLE-2 did not benefit from the addition of buparlisib to fulvestrant; however, when analyzed in circulating free DNA (cfDNA), a significant improvement in PFS was noted [48]. Conversely, while buparlisib increased PFS in all patients in BELLE-3 with *PIK3CA*-mutant tumors, either in primary tumor or cfDNA samples, significant benefit was also seen in the cfDNA wild-type group [49]. The correlation between detection methods remains unclear, and the acquisition of new tumor biopsies, rather than archival specimens, seems essential for the correct assessment of marker status, particularly in pretreated patients.

In the era of next-generation sequencing, knowledge of the genomic drivers of breast cancer and resistance to treatment is expanding. Molecular profiling is now being routinely performed, providing physicians with extensive data regarding mutations, copy number variations, etc. However, the clinical implications of most of these alterations are still unknown. Comprehensive analyses of large patient cohorts with detailed clinical and genomic data are needed to clarify their importance and potential applicability to therapeutic decisions. Despite the advances that have been made over the past decade, greater efforts need to be made to understand the biology and aggressive nature of subtypes of MBC in order to develop more potent and effective drugs that can significantly impact patient outcomes.

References

1. Schiff R, Massarweh S, Shou J, Osborne CK. Breast cancer endocrine resistance: how growth factor signaling and estrogen receptor coregulators modulate response. Clin Cancer Res. 2003;9(1 Pt 2):447S–54S.
2. Alves CL, Elias D, Lyng MB, Bak M, Kirkegaard T, Lykkesfeldt AE, et al. High CDK6 protects cells from fulvestrant-mediated apoptosis and is a predictor of resistance to fulvestrant in estrogen receptor-positive metastatic breast cancer. Clin Cancer Res. 2016;22:5514–26.
3. Raha P, Thomas S, Thurn KT, Park J, Munster PN. Combined histone deacetylase inhibition and tamoxifen induces apoptosis in tamoxifen-resistant breast cancer models, by reversing Bcl-2 overexpression. Breast Cancer Res. 2015;17:26.
4. Garcia-Garcia C, Ibrahim YH, Serra V, Calvo MT, Guzman M, Grueso J, et al. Dual mTORC1/2 and HER2 blockade results in antitumor activity in preclinical models of breast cancer resistant to anti-HER2 therapy. Clin Cancer Res. 2012;18(9):2603–12.
5. Goel S, Wang Q, Watt AC, Tolaney SM, Dillon DA, Li W, et al. Overcoming therapeutic resistance in HER2-positive breast cancers with CDK4/6 inhibitors. Cancer Cell. 2016;29(3):255–69.
6. Alberts B. Molecular biology of the cell, vol. xxxiv. 4th ed. New York: Garland Science; 2002. 1548 p. p
7. Malumbres M, Barbacid M. Cell cycle, CDKs and cancer: a changing paradigm. Nat Rev Cancer. 2009;9(3):153–66.
8. Schwartz GK, Shah MA. Targeting the cell cycle: a new approach to cancer therapy. J Clin Oncol. 2005;23(36):9408–21.
9. Spring L, Bardia A, Modi S. Targeting the cyclin D-cyclin-dependent kinase (CDK) 4/6-retinoblastoma pathway with selective CDK 4/6 inhibitors in hormone receptor-positive breast cancer: rationale, current status, and future directions. Discov Med. 2016;21(113):65–74.
10. Finn RS, Aleshin A, Slamon DJ. Targeting the cyclin-dependent kinases (CDK) 4/6 in estrogen receptor-positive breast cancers. Breast Cancer Res. 2016;18(1):17.

11. Zwijsen RM, Wientjens E, Klompmaker R, van der Sman J, Bernards R, Michalides RJ. CDK-independent activation of estrogen receptor by cyclin D1. Cell. 1997;88(3):405–15.
12. Cancer Genome Atlas N. Comprehensive molecular portraits of human breast tumours. Nature. 2012;490(7418):61–70.
13. Finn RS, Dering J, Conklin D, Kalous O, Cohen DJ, Desai AJ, et al. PD 0332991, a selective cyclin D kinase 4/6 inhibitor, preferentially inhibits proliferation of luminal estrogen receptor-positive human breast cancer cell lines in vitro. Breast Cancer Res BCR. 2009;11(5):R77.
14. O'Leary B, Finn RS, Turner NC. Treating cancer with selective CDK4/6 inhibitors. Nat Rev Clin Oncol. 2016;13(7):417–30.
15. Raub TJ, Wishart GN, Kulanthaivel P, Staton BA, Ajamie RT, Sawada GA, et al. Brain exposure of two selective dual CDK4 and CDK6 inhibitors and the antitumor activity of CDK4 and CDK6 inhibition in combination with temozolomide in an intracranial glioblastoma xenograft. Drug Metab Dispos. 2015;43(9):1360–71.
16. Flaherty KT, Lorusso PM, Demichele A, Abramson VG, Courtney R, Randolph SS, et al. Phase I, dose-escalation trial of the oral cyclin-dependent kinase 4/6 inhibitor PD 0332991, administered using a 21-day schedule in patients with advanced cancer. Clin Cancer Res. 2012;18(2):568–76.
17. Infante JR, Shapiro GI, Witteven O, Gerecitano JF, Ribrag V, Chugh R, et al., editors. A phase I study of the single-agent CDK4/6 inhibitor LEE011 in patients with advanced solid tumors and lymphomas. 2014 American Society of Clinical Oncology (ASCO) Annual Meeting; May 30–June 3, 2014; Chicago, IL (USA): J Clin Oncol. 2014; 32:5s, (suppl; abstr 2528^).
18. Patnaik A, Rosen LS, Tolaney SM, Tolcher AW, Goldman JW, Gandhi L, et al. Efficacy and safety of abemaciclib, an inhibitor of CDK4 and CDK6, for patients with breast cancer, non-small cell lung cancer, and other solid tumors. Cancer Discov. 2016;6(7):740–53.
19. Finn RS, Crown JP, Lang I, Boer K, Bondarenko IM, Kulyk SO, et al. The cyclin-dependent kinase 4/6 inhibitor palbociclib in combination with letrozole versus letrozole alone as first-line treatment of oestrogen receptor-positive, HER2-negative, advanced breast cancer (PALOMA-1/TRIO-18): a randomised phase 2 study. Lancet Oncol. 2015;16(1):25–35.
20. Finn RS, Martin M, Rugo HS, Jones S, Im S-A, Gelmon KA, et al., editors. PALOMA-2: primary results from a phase 3 trial of palbociclib plus letrozole compared with placebo plus letrozole in postmenopausal women with ER+/HER2- advanced breast cancer. 2016 American Society of Clinical Oncology (ASCO) Annual Meeting; June 3–7, 2016; Chicago, IL (USA): J Clin Oncol. 2016; 34 (suppl; abstr 507).
21. Turner NC, Ro J, Andre F, Loi S, Verma S, Iwata H, et al. Palbociclib in hormone-receptor-positive advanced breast cancer. N Engl J Med. 2015;373(3):209–19.
22. Cristofanilli M, Turner NC, Bondarenko I, Ro J, Im S-A, Masuda N, et al. Fulvestrant plus palbociclib versus fulvestrant plus placebo for treatment of hormone-receptor-positive, HER2-negative metastatic breast cancer that progressed on previous endocrine therapy (PALOMA-3): final analysis of the multicentre, double-blind, phase 3 randomised controlled trial. Lancet Oncol. 2016;17(4):425–39.
23. Hortobagyi GN, Stemmer SM, Burris HA, Yap YS, Sonke GS, Paluch-Shimon S, et al. Ribociclib as first-line therapy for HR-positive, advanced breast cancer. N Engl J Med. 2016;375(18):1738–48.
24. Dickler M, Tolaney SM, Rugo HS, Cortes J, Dieras V, Patt DA, et al., editors. MONARCH-1: results from a phase 2 study of abemaciclib, a CDK4 and CDK6 inhibitor, as monotherapy, in patients with HR+/HER2- breast cancer, after chemotherapy for metastatic disease. 2016 American Society of Clinical Oncology (ASCO) Annual Meeting; June 3–7, 2016; Chicago, IL (USA): J Clin Oncol. 2016; 34 (suppl; abstr 510).
25. Rajput S, Khera N, Guo Z, Hoog J, Li S, Ma CX. Inhibition of cyclin dependent kinase 9 by dinaciclib suppresses cyclin B1 expression and tumor growth in triple negative breast cancer. Oncotarget. 2016;7(35):56864–75.
26. Horiuchi D, Kusdra L, Huskey NE, Chandriani S, Lenburg ME, Gonzalez-Angulo AM, et al. MYC pathway activation in triple-negative breast cancer is synthetic lethal with CDK inhibition. J Exp Med. 2012;209(4):679–96.

27. Johnson SF, Johnson N, Chi D, Primack B, D'Andrea AD, Lim E, et al. Abstract 1788: the CDK inhibitor dinaciclib sensitizes triple-negative breast cancer cells to PARP inhibition. Cancer Res. 2013;73(8 Suppl):1788.
28. Chen DS, Mellman I. Oncology meets immunology: the cancer-immunity cycle. Immunity. 2013;39(1):1–10.
29. Acuto O, Michel F. CD28-mediated co-stimulation: a quantitative support for TCR signalling. Nat Rev Immunol. 2003;3(12):939–51.
30. Alexandrov LB, Nik-Zainal S, Wedge DC, Aparicio SA, Behjati S, Biankin AV, et al. Signatures of mutational processes in human cancer. Nature. 2013;500(7463):415–21.
31. Savas P, Salgado R, Denkert C, Sotiriou C, Darcy PK, Smyth MJ, et al. Clinical relevance of host immunity in breast cancer: from TILs to the clinic. Nat Rev Clin Oncol. 2016;13(4):228–41.
32. Nanda R, Chow LQM, Dees EC, Berger R, Gupta S, Geva R, et al. Pembrolizumab in patients with advanced triple-negative breast cancer: phase Ib KEYNOTE-012 study. J Clin Oncol. 2016;34(21):2460–7.
33. Emens L, Adams S, Loi S, Schmid P, Schneeweiss A, Rugo H, et al. Abstract OT1-01-06: a phase III randomized trial of atezolizumab in combination with nab-paclitaxel as first line therapy for patients with metastatic triple-negative breast cancer (mTNBC). Cancer Res. 2016;76(4 Suppl):OT1-01-6-OT1--6.
34. Rugo H, Delord J-P, Im S-A, Ott P, Piha-Paul S, Bedard P, et al. Abstract S5-07: preliminary efficacy and safety of pembrolizumab (MK-3475) in patients with PD-L1–positive, estrogen receptor-positive (ER+)/HER2-negative advanced breast cancer enrolled in KEYNOTE-028. Cancer Res. 2016;76(4 Suppl):S5-07-S5.
35. Dirix L, Takacs I, Nikolinakos P, Jerusalem G, Arkenau H-T, Hamilton E, et al. Abstract S1-04: avelumab (MSB0010718C), an anti-PD-L1 antibody, in patients with locally advanced or metastatic breast cancer: a phase Ib JAVELIN solid tumor trial. Cancer Res. 2016;76(4 Suppl):S1-04-S1.
36. Emens LA, Braiteh FS, Cassier P, DeLord J-P, Eder JP, Shen X, et al. Abstract PD1-6: inhibition of PD-L1 by MPDL3280A leads to clinical activity in patients with metastatic triple-negative breast cancer. Cancer Res. 2015;75(9 Suppl):PD1-6.
37. Courtney KD, Corcoran RB, Engelman JA. The PI3K pathway as drug target in human cancer. J Clin Oncol. 2010;28(6):1075–83.
38. Thorpe LM, Yuzugullu H, Zhao JJ. PI3K in cancer: divergent roles of isoforms, modes of activation and therapeutic targeting. Nat Rev Cancer. 2015;15(1):7–24.
39. Hoeflich KP, Guan J, Edgar KA, O'Brien C, Savage H, Wilson TR, et al. The PI3K inhibitor taselisib overcomes letrozole resistance in a breast cancer model expressing aromatase. Genes Cancer. 2016;7(3–4):73–85.
40. Miller TW, Balko JM, Arteaga CL. Phosphatidylinositol 3-kinase and antiestrogen resistance in breast cancer. J Clin Oncol. 2011;29(33):4452–61.
41. Boulay A, Rudloff J, Ye J, Zumstein-Mecker S, O'Reilly T, Evans DB, et al. Dual inhibition of mTOR and estrogen receptor signaling in vitro induces cell death in models of breast cancer. Clin Cancer Res. 2005;11(14):5319–28.
42. Baselga J, Campone M, Piccart M, Burris HA 3rd, Rugo HS, Sahmoud T, et al. Everolimus in postmenopausal hormone-receptor-positive advanced breast cancer. N Engl J Med. 2012;366(6):520–9.
43. Yardley DA, Noguchi S, Pritchard KI, Burris HA 3rd, Baselga J, Gnant M, et al. Everolimus plus exemestane in postmenopausal patients with HR(+) breast cancer: BOLERO-2 final progression-free survival analysis. Adv Ther. 2013;30(10):870–84.
44. Piccart M, Hortobagyi GN, Campone M, Pritchard KI, Lebrun F, Ito Y, et al. Everolimus plus exemestane for hormone-receptor-positive, human epidermal growth factor receptor-2-negative advanced breast cancer: overall survival results from BOLERO-2dagger. Ann Oncol. 2014;25(12):2357–62.

45. Maira SM, Pecchi S, Huang A, Burger M, Knapp M, Sterker D, et al. Identification and characterization of NVP-BKM120, an orally available pan-class I PI3-kinase inhibitor. Mol Cancer Ther. 2012;11(2):317–28.
46. Mayer IA, Abramson VG, Isakoff SJ, Forero A, Balko JM, Kuba MG, et al. Stand up to cancer phase Ib study of pan-phosphoinositide-3-kinase inhibitor buparlisib with letrozole in estrogen receptor-positive/human epidermal growth factor receptor 2-negative metastatic breast cancer. J Clin Oncol. 2014;32(12):1202–9.
47. Ma CX, Luo J, Naughton M, Ademuyiwa F, Suresh R, Griffith M, et al. A phase I trial of BKM120 (buparlisib) in combination with fulvestrant in postmenopausal women with estrogen receptor-positive metastatic breast cancer. Clin Cancer Res. 2016;22(7):1583–91.
48. Baselga J, Im S-A, Iwata H, Clemons M, Ito Y, Awada A, et al., editors. PIK3CA status in circulating tumor DNA predicts efficacy of buparlisib plus fulvestrant in postmenopausal women with endocrine-resistant HR+/HER2- advanced breast cancer: first results from the randomized, phase III BELLE-2 trial. 38th Annual San Antonio Breast Cancer Symposium; Dec 8-12, 2015; San Antonio, TX (USA): Cancer Res. 2016;76(4 suppl):abstr S6–01.
49. Di Leo A, Seok Lee K, Ciruelos E, Lonning P, Janni W, O'Regan R, et al., editors. BELLE-3: a phase III study of buparlisib and fulvestrant in postmenopausal women with HR+, HER2-, AI-treated locally advanced or metastatic breast cancer, who progressed on or after mTOR inhibitor-based treatment. 39th Annual San Antonio Breast Cancer Symposium; Dec 6–10. San Antonio, TX (USA); 2016.
50. Ndubaku CO, Heffron TP, Staben ST, Baumgardner M, Blaquiere N, Bradley E, et al. Discovery of 2-{3-[2-(1-isopropyl-3-methyl-1H-1,2-4-triazol-5-yl)-5,6-dihydrobenzo[f]imidazo[1,2-d][1,4]oxazepin-9-yl]-1H-pyrazol-1-yl}-2-methylpropanamide (GDC-0032): a beta-sparing phosphoinositide 3-kinase inhibitor with high unbound exposure and robust in vivo antitumor activity. J Med Chem. 2013;56(11):4597–610.
51. Dickler M, Saura C, Richards D, Krop I, Cervantes A, Bedard PL, et al., editors. A phase II study of the PI3K inhibitor taselisib (GDC-0032) combined with fulvestrant (F) in patients (pts) with HER2-negative (HER2-), hormone receptor-positive (HR+) advanced breast cancer (BC). 2016 American Society of Clinical Oncology (ASCO) Annual Meeting; June 3–7, 2016; Chicago, IL (USA): J Clin Oncol. 2016;34(suppl; abstr 520).
52. Gonzalez-Angulo AM, Juric D, Argilés G, Schellens J, Burris H, Berlin J, et al., editors. Safety, pharmacokinetics, and preliminary activity of the α-specific PI3K inhibitor BYL719: results from the first-in-human study. 2013 American Society of Clinical Oncology (ASCO) Annual Meeting; May 31-June 4, 2013; Chicago, IL (USA): J Clin Oncol. 2013;31(suppl; abstr 2531).
53. Mayer IA, Abramson VG, Formisano L, Balko JM, Estrada MV, Sanders ME, et al. A phase Ib study of alpelisib (BYL719), a PI3Kalpha-specific inhibitor, with letrozole in ER+/HER2- metastatic breast cancer. Clin Cancer Res. 2017;23(1):26–34.
54. Janku F, Juric D, Cortes J, Rugo H, Burris HA, Schuler M, et al., editors. Phase I study of the PI3K alpha inhibitor BYL719 plus fulvestrant in patients with PIK3CA-altered and wild type ER+/HER2-locally advanced or metastatic breast cancer. 37th Annual San Antonio Breast Cancer Symposium; December 9-13, 2014; San Antonio, TX (USA): Cancer Res. 2015;75(9 suppl):abstr PD5–5.
55. Berns K, Horlings HM, Hennessy BT, Madiredjo M, Hijmans EM, Beelen K, et al. A functional genetic approach identifies the PI3K pathway as a major determinant of trastuzumab resistance in breast cancer. Cancer Cell. 2007;12(4):395–402.
56. Dave B, Migliaccio I, Gutierrez MC, Wu MF, Chamness GC, Wong H, et al. Loss of phosphatase and tensin homolog or phosphoinositol-3 kinase activation and response to trastuzumab or lapatinib in human epidermal growth factor receptor 2-overexpressing locally advanced breast cancers. J Clin Oncol. 2011;29(2):166–73.
57. Miller TW, Forbes JT, Shah C, Wyatt SK, Manning HC, Olivares MG, et al. Inhibition of mammalian target of rapamycin is required for optimal antitumor effect of HER2 inhibitors against HER2-overexpressing cancer cells. Clin Cancer Res. 2009;15(23):7266–76.

58. Yao E, Zhou W, Lee-Hoeflich ST, Truong T, Haverty PM, Eastham-Anderson J, et al. Suppression of HER2/HER3-mediated growth of breast cancer cells with combinations of GDC-0941 PI3K inhibitor, trastuzumab, and pertuzumab. Clin Cancer Res. 2009;15(12):4147–56.
59. Andre F, O'Regan R, Ozguroglu M, Toi M, Xu B, Jerusalem G, et al. Everolimus for women with trastuzumab-resistant, HER2-positive, advanced breast cancer (BOLERO-3): a randomised, double-blind, placebo-controlled phase 3 trial. Lancet Oncol. 2014;15(6):580–91.
60. Hurvitz SA, Andre F, Jiang Z, Shao Z, Mano MS, Neciosup SP, et al. Combination of everolimus with trastuzumab plus paclitaxel as first-line treatment for patients with HER2-positive advanced breast cancer (BOLERO-1): a phase 3, randomised, double-blind, multicentre trial. Lancet Oncol. 2015;16(7):816–29.
61. Fedele CG, Ooms LM, Ho M, Vieusseux J, O'Toole SA, Millar EK, et al. Inositol polyphosphate 4-phosphatase II regulates PI3K/Akt signaling and is lost in human basal-like breast cancers. Proc Natl Acad Sci U S A. 2010;107(51):22231–6.
62. Pollak MN, Schernhammer ES, Hankinson SE. Insulin-like growth factors and neoplasia. Nat Rev Cancer. 2004;4(7):505–18.
63. Zhang Y, Moerkens M, Ramaiahgari S, de Bont H, Price L, Meerman J, et al. Elevated insulin-like growth factor 1 receptor signaling induces antiestrogen resistance through the MAPK/ERK and PI3K/Akt signaling routes. Breast Cancer Res. 2011;13(3):R52.
64. Gallardo A, Lerma E, Escuin D, Tibau A, Munoz J, Ojeda B, et al. Increased signalling of EGFR and IGF1R, and deregulation of PTEN/PI3K/Akt pathway are related with trastuzumab resistance in HER2 breast carcinomas. Br J Cancer. 2012;106(8):1367–73.
65. Ryan P, Neven P, Blackwell K, Dirix L, Barrios C, Miller W, et al. P1-17-01: figitumumab plus exemestane versus exemestane as first-line treatment of postmenopausal hormone receptor-positive advanced breast cancer: a randomized, open-label phase II trial. Cancer Res. 2011;71(24 Suppl):P1-17-01-P1-17-01.
66. Gradishar WJ, Yardley DA, Layman R, Sparano JA, Chuang E, Northfelt DW, et al. Clinical and translational results of a phase II, randomized trial of an anti-IGF-1R (cixutumumab) in women with breast cancer that progressed on endocrine therapy. Clin Cancer Res. 2016;22(2):301–9.
67. Robertson JF, Ferrero JM, Bourgeois H, Kennecke H, de Boer RH, Jacot W, et al. Ganitumab with either exemestane or fulvestrant for postmenopausal women with advanced, hormone-receptor-positive breast cancer: a randomised, controlled, double-blind, phase 2 trial. Lancet Oncol. 2013;14(3):228–35.
68. O'Reilly KE, Rojo F, She QB, Solit D, Mills GB, Smith D, et al. mTOR inhibition induces upstream receptor tyrosine kinase signaling and activates Akt. Cancer Res. 2006;66(3):1500–8.
69. Cortes J, Martinez Janez N, Sablin M-P, Perez-Fidalgo JA, Neven P, Hedayati E, et al., editors. Phase 1b/2 trial of BI 836845, an insulin-like growth factor (IGF) ligand-neutralizing antibody, combined with exemestane (Ex) and everolimus (Ev) in hormone receptor-positive (HR+) locally advanced or metastatic breast cancer (BC): primary phase 1b results. 2016 American Society of Clinical Oncology (ASCO) Annual Meeting; June 3–7, 2016; Chicago, IL (USA): J Clin Oncol. 2016;34(suppl; abstr 530).
70. Courjal F, Cuny M, Simony-Lafontaine J, Louason G, Speiser P, Zeillinger R, et al. Mapping of DNA amplifications at 15 chromosomal localizations in 1875 breast tumors: definition of phenotypic groups. Cancer Res. 1997;57(19):4360–7.
71. Turner N, Pearson A, Sharpe R, Lambros M, Geyer F, Lopez-Garcia MA, et al. FGFR1 amplification drives endocrine therapy resistance and is a therapeutic target in breast cancer. Cancer Res. 2010;70(5):2085–94.
72. Elbauomy Elsheikh S, Green AR, Lambros MB, Turner NC, Grainge MJ, Powe D, et al. FGFR1 amplification in breast carcinomas: a chromogenic in situ hybridisation analysis. Breast Cancer Res. 2007;9(2):R23.
73. Sharpe R, Pearson A, Herrera-Abreu MT, Johnson D, Mackay A, Welti JC, et al. FGFR signaling promotes the growth of triple-negative and basal-like breast cancer cell lines both in vitro and in vivo. Clin Cancer Res. 2011;17(16):5275–86.

74. Andre F, Cortes J. Rationale for targeting fibroblast growth factor receptor signaling in breast cancer. Breast Cancer Res Treat. 2015;150(1):1–8.
75. Tabernero J, Bahleda R, Dienstmann R, Infante JR, Mita A, Italiano A, et al. Phase I dose-escalation study of JNJ-42756493, an oral pan-fibroblast growth factor receptor inhibitor, in patients with advanced solid tumors. J Clin Oncol. 2015;33(30):3401–8.
76. Nogova L, Sequist LV, Perez Garcia JM, Andre F, Delord JP, Hidalgo M, et al. Evaluation of BGJ398, a fibroblast growth factor receptor 1-3 kinase inhibitor, in patients with advanced solid tumors harboring genetic alterations in fibroblast growth factor receptors: results of a global phase I, dose-escalation and dose-expansion study. J Clin Oncol. 2017;35(2):157–65.
77. Desrivieres S, Kunz C, Barash I, Vafaizadeh V, Borghouts C, Groner B. The biological functions of the versatile transcription factors STAT3 and STAT5 and new strategies for their targeted inhibition. J Mammary Gland Biol Neoplasia. 2006;11(1):75–87.
78. Marotta LL, Almendro V, Marusyk A, Shipitsin M, Schemme J, Walker SR, et al. The JAK2/STAT3 signaling pathway is required for growth of CD44(+)CD24(−) stem cell-like breast cancer cells in human tumors. J Clin Invest. 2011;121(7):2723–35.
79. Britschgi A, Andraos R, Brinkhaus H, Klebba I, Romanet V, Muller U, et al. JAK2/STAT5 inhibition circumvents resistance to PI3K/mTOR blockade: a rationale for cotargeting these pathways in metastatic breast cancer. Cancer Cell. 2012;22(6):796–811.
80. Overmoyer B, Regan M, Schlosnagle E, Bunnell CA, Freedman R, Tolaney SM, et al., editors. Phase I study of the JAK 1/2 inhibitor ruxolitinib with weekly paclitaxel for the treatment of HER2 negative metastatic breast cancer (MBC). 39th Annual San Antonio Breast Cancer Symposium; Dec 6–10. San Antonio, TX (USA); 2016.
81. Bergers G, Benjamin LE. Tumorigenesis and the angiogenic switch. Nat Rev Cancer. 2003;3(6):401–10.
82. Robert NJ, Dieras V, Glaspy J, Brufsky AM, Bondarenko I, Lipatov ON, et al. RIBBON-1: randomized, double-blind, placebo-controlled, phase III trial of chemotherapy with or without bevacizumab for first-line treatment of human epidermal growth factor receptor 2-negative, locally recurrent or metastatic breast cancer. J Clin Oncol. 2011;29(10):1252–60.
83. Gray R, Bhattacharya S, Bowden C, Miller K, Comis RL. Independent review of E2100: a phase III trial of bevacizumab plus paclitaxel versus paclitaxel in women with metastatic breast cancer. J Clin Oncol. 2009;27(30):4966–72.
84. Miles DW, Chan A, Dirix LY, Cortes J, Pivot X, Tomczak P, et al. Phase III study of bevacizumab plus docetaxel compared with placebo plus docetaxel for the first-line treatment of human epidermal growth factor receptor 2-negative metastatic breast cancer. J Clin Oncol. 2010;28(20):3239–47.
85. Tolaney SM, Nechushtan H, Ron IG, Schoffski P, Awada A, Yasenchak CA, et al. Cabozantinib for metastatic breast carcinoma: results of a phase II placebo-controlled randomized discontinuation study. Breast Cancer Res Treat. 2016;160(2):305–12.
86. Soria JC, DeBraud F, Bahleda R, Adamo B, Andre F, Dienstmann R, et al. Phase I/IIa study evaluating the safety, efficacy, pharmacokinetics, and pharmacodynamics of lucitanib in advanced solid tumors. Ann Oncol. 2014;25(11):2244–51.
87. Bergh J, Bondarenko IM, Lichinitser MR, Liljegren A, Greil R, Voytko NL, et al. First-line treatment of advanced breast cancer with sunitinib in combination with docetaxel versus docetaxel alone: results of a prospective, randomized phase III study. J Clin Oncol. 2012;30(9):921–9.
88. Gradishar WJ, Kaklamani V, Sahoo TP, Lokanatha D, Raina V, Bondarde S, et al. A double-blind, randomised, placebo-controlled, phase 2b study evaluating sorafenib in combination with paclitaxel as a first-line therapy in patients with HER2-negative advanced breast cancer. Eur J Cancer. 2013;49(2):312–22.
89. Rugo HS, Stopeck AT, Joy AA, Chan S, Verma S, Lluch A, et al. Randomized, placebo-controlled, double-blind, phase II study of axitinib plus docetaxel versus docetaxel plus placebo in patients with metastatic breast cancer. J Clin Oncol. 2011;29(18):2459–65.
90. Diamantis N, Banerji U. Antibody-drug conjugates – an emerging class of cancer treatment. Br J Cancer. 2016;114(4):362–7.

91. Bardia A, Diamond JR, Mayer IA, Isakoff S, Abramson V, Starodub AN, et al., editors. Sacituzumab govitecan (IMMU-132), an anti-Trop-2-SN-38 antibody-drug conjugate (ADC) for the treatment of relapsed/refractory, metastatic triple-negative breast cancer (mTNBC): updated results. 39th Annual San Antonio Breast Cancer Symposium; Dec 6–10. San Antonio, TX (USA); 2016.
92. Ogitani Y, Aida T, Hagihara K, Yamaguchi J, Ishii C, Harada N, et al. DS-8201a, a novel HER2-targeting ADC with a novel DNA topoisomerase I inhibitor, demonstrates a promising antitumor efficacy with differentiation from T-DM1. Clin Cancer Res. 2016;22(20):5097–108.
93. Glozak MA, Seto E. Histone deacetylases and cancer. Oncogene. 2007;26(37):5420–32.
94. Hodges-Gallagher L, Valentine CD, Bader SE, Kushner PJ. Inhibition of histone deacetylase enhances the anti-proliferative action of antiestrogens on breast cancer cells and blocks tamoxifen-induced proliferation of uterine cells. Breast Cancer Res Treat. 2007;105(3):297–309.
95. Sabnis GJ, Goloubeva OG, Kazi AA, Shah P, Brodie AH. HDAC inhibitor entinostat restores responsiveness of letrozole-resistant MCF-7Ca xenografts to aromatase inhibitors through modulation of Her-2. Mol Cancer Ther. 2013;12(12):2804–16.
96. Yardley DA, Ismail-Khan RR, Melichar B, Lichinitser M, Munster PN, Klein PM, et al. Randomized phase II, double-blind, placebo-controlled study of exemestane with or without entinostat in postmenopausal women with locally recurrent or metastatic estrogen receptor-positive breast cancer progressing on treatment with a nonsteroidal aromatase inhibitor. J Clin Oncol. 2013;31(17):2128–35.
97. Woods DM, Sodre AL, Villagra A, Sarnaik A, Sotomayor EM, Weber J. HDAC inhibition upregulates PD-1 ligands in melanoma and augments Immunotherapy with PD-1 blockade. Cancer Immunol Res. 2015;3(12):1375–85.
98. Schultz N, Lopez E, Saleh-Gohari N, Helleday T. Poly(ADP-ribose) polymerase (PARP-1) has a controlling role in homologous recombination. Nucleic Acids Res. 2003;31(17):4959–64.
99. Turner N, Tutt A, Ashworth A. Hallmarks of 'BRCAness' in sporadic cancers. Nat Rev Cancer. 2004;4(10):814–9.
100. Puhalla S, Beumer JH, Pahuja S, Appleman LJ, Abdul-Hassan Tawbi H, Stoller RG, et al., editors. Final results of a phase 1 study of single-agent veliparib (V) in patients (pts) with either BRCA1/2-mutated cancer (BRCA+), platinum-refractory ovarian, or basal-like breast cancer (BRCA-wt). 2014 American Society of Clinical Oncology (ASCO) Annual Meeting; May 30-June 3, 2014; Chicago, IL (USA): J Clin Oncol. 2014;32:5s. (suppl; abstr 2570).
101. Sandhu SK, Schelman WR, Wilding G, Moreno V, Baird RD, Miranda S, et al. The poly(ADP-ribose) polymerase inhibitor niraparib (MK4827) in BRCA mutation carriers and patients with sporadic cancer: a phase 1 dose-escalation trial. Lancet Oncol. 2013;14(9):882–92.
102. de Bono JS, Mina LA, Gonzalez M, Curtin NJ, Wang E, Henshaw JW, et al., editors. First-in-human trial of novel oral PARP inhibitor BMN 673 in patients with solid tumors. 2013 American Society of Clinical Oncology (ASCO) Annual Meeting; May 31 – June 4, 2013; Chicago, IL (USA): J Clin Oncol. 2013;31(suppl; abstr 2580).
103. Tutt A, Robson M, Garber JE, Domchek SM, Audeh MW, Weitzel JN, et al. Oral poly(ADP-ribose) polymerase inhibitor olaparib in patients with BRCA1 or BRCA2 mutations and advanced breast cancer: a proof-of-concept trial. Lancet. 2010;376(9737):235–44.
104. Donawho CK, Luo Y, Luo Y, Penning TD, Bauch JL, Bouska JJ, et al. ABT-888, an orally active poly(ADP-ribose) polymerase inhibitor that potentiates DNA-damaging agents in preclinical tumor models. Clin Cancer Res. 2007;13(9):2728–37.
105. Isakoff S, Overmoyer B, Tung N, Gelman R, Habin K, Qian J, et al. P3-16-05: a phase II trial expansion cohort of the PARP inhibitor veliparib (ABT888) and temozolomide in BRCA1/2 associated metastatic breast cancer. Cancer Res. 2011;71(24 Suppl):P3-16-05-P3-16-05.
106. Rodler ET, Kurland BF, Griffin M, Gralow JR, Porter P, Yeh RF, et al. Phase I study of veliparib (ABT-888) combined with cisplatin and vinorelbine in advanced triple-negative breast cancer and/or BRCA mutation-associated breast cancer. Clin Cancer Res. 2016;22(12):2855–64.
107. Pahuja S, Beumer JH, Appleman LJ, Abdul-Hassan Tawbi H, Stoller RG, Lee JJ, et al., editors. A phase I study of veliparib (ABT-888) in combination with weekly carboplatin

and paclitaxel in advanced solid malignancies and enriched for triple-negative breast cancer (TNBC). 2015 American Society of Clinical Oncology (ASCO) Annual Meeting; May 29-June 2, 2015; Chicago, IL (USA): J Clin Oncol. 2015;33(suppl; abstr 1015).
108. Jiang T, Safonov A, Bianchini G, Shi W, Wali V, Pusztai L, et al. Abstract P4-07-01: DNA repair deficiency enhances immune response and correlates with excellent clinical outcome in triple negative breast cancer. Cancer Res. 2016;76(4 Suppl):P4-07-1-P4--1.
109. Beliakoff J, Whitesell L. Hsp90: an emerging target for breast cancer therapy. Anti-Cancer Drugs. 2004;15(7):651–62.
110. Zagouri F, Sergentanis TN, Nonni A, Papadimitriou CA, Michalopoulos NV, Domeyer P, et al. Hsp90 in the continuum of breast ductal carcinogenesis: evaluation in precursors, preinvasive and ductal carcinoma lesions. BMC Cancer. 2010;10:353.
111. Modi S, Stopeck A, Linden H, Solit D, Chandarlapaty S, Rosen N, et al. HSP90 inhibition is effective in breast cancer: a phase II trial of tanespimycin (17-AAG) plus trastuzumab in patients with HER2-positive metastatic breast cancer progressing on trastuzumab. Clin Cancer Res. 2011;17(15):5132–9.
112. Jhaveri K, Chandarlapaty S, Lake D, Gilewski T, Robson M, Goldfarb S, et al. A phase II open-label study of ganetespib, a novel heat shock protein 90 inhibitor for patients with metastatic breast cancer. Clin Breast Cancer. 2014;14(3):154–60.
113. Lin NU. Breast cancer brain metastases: new directions in systemic therapy. Ecancermedicalscience. 2013;7:307.
114. Freedman RA, Gelman RS, Wefel JS, Melisko ME, Hess KR, Connolly RM, et al. Translational Breast Cancer Research Consortium (TBCRC) 022: a phase II trial of neratinib for patients with human epidermal growth factor receptor 2-positive breast cancer and brain metastases. J Clin Oncol. 2016;34(9):945–52.
115. Lin NU, Dieras V, Paul D, Lossignol D, Christodoulou C, Stemmler HJ, et al. Multicenter phase II study of lapatinib in patients with brain metastases from HER2-positive breast cancer. Clin Cancer Res. 2009;15(4):1452–9.
116. Borges VF, Ferrario C, Aucoin N, Falkson CI, Khan QJ, Krop I, et al., editors. Efficacy results of a phase 1b study of ont 380, a CNS-penetrant TKI, in combination with T-DM1 in HER2+ metastatic breast cancer (MBC), including patients (pts) with brain metastases. 2016 American Society of Clinical Oncology (ASCO) Annual Meeting; June 3–7, 2016; Chicago, IL (USA): J Clin Oncol. 2016;34(suppl; abstr 513).
117. DeMichele A, Clark AS, Tan KS, Heitjan DF, Gramlich K, Gallagher M, et al. CDK 4/6 inhibitor palbociclib (PD0332991) in Rb+ advanced breast cancer: phase II activity, safety, and predictive biomarker assessment. Clin Cancer Res. 2015;21(5):995–1001.
118. Finn R, Jiang Y, Rugo H, Moulder SL, Im SA, Gelmon KA, et al. Biomarker analyses from the phase 3 PALOMA-2 trial of palbociclib (P) with letrozole (L) compared with placebo (PLB) plus L in postmenopausal women with ER + /HER2– advanced breast cancer (ABC). Ann Oncol. 2016;27(suppl_6):LBA15–LBA.
119. Fribbens C, O'Leary B, Kilburn L, Hrebien S, Garcia-Murillas I, Beaney M, et al. Plasma ESR1 mutations and the treatment of estrogen receptor-positive advanced breast cancer. J Clin Oncol. 2016;34:2961–8.

Breast Cancer Treatment in Elderly Patients

13

Akiko Chiba and Marissa Howard-McNatt

Introduction

Breast cancer remains a substantial health issue in the elderly population. Breast cancer risk increases with age, and the incidence of breast cancer peaks between 70 and 84 years of age [1]. Forty-two percent of all breast cancers occur in women over 65 years of age and 20% in those over 75 years of age [2]. In addition, the population in the USA is expected to become older, thereby increasing the number of patients at risk for breast cancer. By 2030, more than 20% of US residents are projected to be over 65 compared with 13% in 2010. An increase in life expectancy plays a major role in these demographic shifts. Life expectancy at age 65 was 15.2 years in 1992 and increased to 19.1 years by 2010 [3]. The life expectancy for white, black, and Hispanics from 2010 is showed in Table 13.1 [4]. Based on trends in mortality, it is projected that life expectancy will continue to improve. This article addresses treatment of breast cancer in the elderly, discussing age-appropriate screening, variations in treatment choice compared to the standard of care, quality of life, and survival compared to their younger counterparts.

A. Chiba, MD (✉)
Department of Surgical Oncology, Wake Forest Baptist Health, Medical Center Boulevard, Winston-Salem, NC 27157, USA
e-mail: achiba@wakehealth.edu

M. Howard-McNatt, MD
Associate Professor of Surgery, Department of Surgery, Wake Forest Baptist Health, Medical Center Boulevard, Winston-Salem, NC 27157, USA
e-mail: mmcnatt@wakehealth.edu

M. Howard-McNatt (ed.), *Changing Paradigms in the Management of Breast Cancer*, DOI 10.1007/978-3-319-60336-0_13

Table 13.1 Life expectancy at selected ages by race: United States, 2010

Age (years)	White female (years)	Black female (years)	Hispanic female (years)
60	24.5	23	26.3
65	20.3	19.3	22.0
70	16.4	15.8	18.0
75	12.8	9.6	14.0
80	9.6	7.1	10.7
85	6.9	5.2	7.7
90	4.8	3.8	5.4

National Vital Statistics Reports, Vol. 61, No. 4, May 8, 2013

Treatment Pattern

Despite breast cancer being a disease of the elderly, this age group has historically been excluded from clinical trials [5]. Given this lack of data, physicians are left to decide their treatment plan based on extrapolated data and experience. This has led to deviations from the standard of care in treating elderly women with breast cancer. When standard of care was applied, such as mastectomy and axillary dissection, these women were thought to be overtreated. However, those patients who underwent breast-conserving surgery and had omission of axillary dissection and/or radiation therapy might be considered to be under treated. Older women with breast cancer are less likely to receive standard treatments, such as axillary lymph node dissection or radiation therapy, after breast-conserving surgery compared to younger patients [6]. Possible explanations of under treatment include shorter life expectancy, increasing medical comorbidities, and less aggressive biologic behavior of breast cancer [7–10].

Screening

The risk of developing breast cancer increases with age, making screening older women valuable. A quarter of breast cancer deaths each year are attributed to breast cancer diagnosed after the age of 74 [11]. Screening methods include mammograms, clinical breast examination, and breast self-awareness. Sensitivity and specificity of mammography increase as patient gets older due to decrease in glandular breast tissues and replacement with fatty tissue. This decreases unnecessary biopsies and intuitively provides a substantial opportunity to reduce breast cancer death in older populations. Unfortunately, none of the randomized prospective trials of screening mammography included women over the age of 75 making continued use of screening mammography clinical decision in this population difficult [12]. There have been a few observational studies demonstrating a reduction in breast cancer mortality associated with mammographic screening in women 75 years and older; however, the benefits were limited to those without severe comorbidities, and no benefit was observed in women with severe comorbidities [13, 14]. These results must be interpreted with caution given the limitations of study design. It has been

Table 13.2 Variations in current mammography screening guidelines for average-risk women

	Screening frequency	Age to start screening	Age to stop screening
US Preventative Services Task Force [39]	Biennial	50	75
American Cancer Society [40]	Annual	45–54	Continue as long as healthy and life expectancy ≥10 years
	Biennial	≥55	
American College of Radiology [41]	Annual	40	Stop when life expectancy is <5–7 based on comorbidities and when abnormal result would not be acted on because of comorbidity

suggested that older women with comorbidities, such as those with Charleston Comorbidity Index of two or more, may not benefit from screening mammography due to competing causes of mortality [15].

Another issue with older women and breast screening is determining when to stop screening. The United States Preventive Service Task Force recommends stopping at age 75, whereas the American Cancer Society recommends continuing as long as a patient is healthy and has a life expectancy of more than 10 years. The American College of Radiology also recommends continued screening if the patient is healthy and willing to undergo additional testing (including biopsy). Variations in screening recommendations are shown in Table 13.2. Overscreening in elderly women is a health-care concern as well, with recent studies demonstrating that many elderly women with multiple comorbidities and advanced cancer are still undergoing screening mammography [16, 17]. It is important to evaluate individual patients to determine if mammographic screening is of benefit as patients with multiple comorbidities will not experience reduction in breast cancer mortality from screening.

Tumor Biology

Breast cancer in the elderly patient is less aggressive. Older women tend to have more favorable tumors at diagnosis that are likely small, have less nodal involvement, express both estrogen and progesterone receptors, are more low grade, and are HER-2 negative [32]. Molecular genetics shows that more favorable luminal A and luminal B subtypes are found in older women. However, older women can present with triple negative or HER-2 amplified cancers. Treatment needs to be based on these phenotypes as well as tumor size and nodal involvement.

Treatment

Surgical resection remains the mainstay of treatment in elderly women with breast cancer. Treatment should be based on staging of the cancer, and patients should receive standard of care if possible. Surgery and anesthesia carry some risks independent of age, however, the main factor influencing morbidity and mortality from breast surgery is comorbidity rather than age alone [18]. A recent retrospective study of SEER analysis evaluated outcomes of 1784 breast cancer patients over the age of 70 undergoing mastectomy and lumpectomy [19]. Of these, 596 (33%) underwent mastectomy, 918 (51%) underwent lumpectomy with radiation, and 270 (15.4%) underwent lumpectomy alone. The type of surgery was not an independent factor in determining overall survival. The SEER study showed worse breast cancer-specific survival that was associated with an inability to perform more than two activities of daily living, two or more comorbidities, larger tumor size, and positive lymph nodes. On multivariate analysis, larger tumor size and positive lymph nodes were identified as independent determinants for worse survival [19]. This suggests that even in elderly patients, nodal staging remains an important part of breast cancer treatment. In contrast, another study of 140 women over the age of 70 who did not undergo sentinel lymph node biopsy demonstrated a low axillary recurrence and low mortality for patients with clinical T1–2 N0 breast cancer [20].

Surgical staging of the axilla may be omitted in elderly patients with clinically node-negative disease as information from axillary surgery may not alter treatment decisions in many cases. This is especially true in the frail patient who is not a candidate to receive chemotherapy regardless of their nodal status. In elderly women with clinically node-negative, hormone receptor-positive disease, adjuvant therapy will likely be limited to endocrine therapy. The rate of axillary recurrence following lumpectomy and endocrine therapy in patients without radiation therapy or axillary surgery was 1% at 5 years as demonstrated in CALGB 9343 [20, 21]. This is a small enough risk that axillary staging may be omitted in selected patients.

Radiation Therapy

There have been two recent prospective randomized trials to determine whether there is a benefit of adjuvant radiation therapy after breast-conserving surgery in elderly patients with early breast cancer. CALGB-9343 randomized 636 stage I, estrogen receptor-positive breast cancer patient's age ≥70 to lumpectomy with tamoxifen only or lumpectomy with tamoxifen and radiation therapy [21]. This study showed there were no significant differences in time to distant metastasis, breast cancer-specific survival, or overall survival between the two groups. Ten-year overall survival was 67% (95% CI, 62–72%) and 66% (95% CI, 61–71%) in the tamoxifen and radiation therapy and tamoxifen only groups, respectively [20].The PRIME II study was another study evaluating the effect of omitting whole-breast irradiation on local control in women aged 65 years or older undergoing lumpectomy and endocrine treatment for early stage breast cancer. After a median follow-up of 5 years, local recurrence was 1.3% (95% CI 0·2–2·3; $n = 5$) in the whole-breast irradiation group and 4.1% (2•4–5•7; $n = 26$) in the group without radiation therapy. Whole-breast irradiation after breast-conserving surgery and adjuvant endocrine therapy resulted in a small, but statistical significant reduction in local recurrence; however, there was no difference in 5-year overall survival between the two groups 93.9% (95% CI 91.8–96.0) [22]. Especially in in early stage estrogen receptor-positive breast cancer in the elderly, radiation therapy may be omitted without significant consequence. Despite these data, the omission of radiation therapy in selected older population has not been widely applied [23, 24].

Chemotherapy

Chemotherapy is underutilized in older women, and there are few prospective randomized clinical trials in this population. For the older patient, their comorbidities, functional status, social support, and life expectancy must all be taken into account before selecting patients for treatment [32]. Standard-of-care treatments should be used in those healthy older adults whose life expectancy is equal to or greater than 10 years.

Adjuvant chemotherapy is generally recommended for women with ER-negative or Her-2/neu amplified tumors that are larger than 1 cm or any subtype in which lymph node involvement is found. A retrospective review of four randomized studies has shown that the administration of intensive chemotherapy regimens in older patients results in a reduction in breast cancer recurrence and morality, regardless of age [25]. Furthermore, a consensus panel as part of the NCCN's published recommendations in 2008 suggested that the use of adjuvant chemotherapy in older patients should be guided by a well-balanced consideration of benefit-fit risk ratio. No specific chemotherapy regimen is recommended for older patients, but caution should be given for anthrocyclines and consideration for hepatic and renal function [32]. ER-negative breast cancer can be particularly aggressive and tend to recur in the first 5 years. For older women with ER-negative breast cancer, several retrospective analyses also support the use of adjuvant chemotherapy. Two analyses using the Surveillance, Epidemiology, and End Results database have demonstrated that adjuvant chemotherapy in the treatment of node-positive, ER-negative breast cancer is associated with a reduction in mortality [26, 27].

The use of trastuzumab in Her-2-positive breast cancer in the elderly also needs special attention. Trastuzumab is associated with improvement in disease-free and overall survival; however, the scope of the benefit in older patients is hard to determine given that few older women enrolled in the randomized trials [28, 29]. Older age is a recognized risk factor for trastuzumab-related cardiotoxicity [30]. Significant associations with CHF and trastuzumab exposure include use of hypertensive medications, lower baseline left ventricular ejection fraction (LVEF), and lower LVEF following treatment with doxorubicin/cyclophosphamide. In conclusion, consensus opinion issued by the NCCN is that the small numbers of cardiac-related deaths and added valued and therapeutic index of adjuvant trastuzumab should not preclude trastuzumab's use in the treatment of healthy elderly women [31, 32].

Table 13.3 Summary of management

Screening	Reasonable to continue annual mammography in patients with:
	Life expectancy $\geq$10 years
	Less than 2 comorbidities
	No terminal illness, such as other cancer
Surgical options	Axillary lymph node status remains to be an important prognostic factors in elderly and may change adjuvant treatment based on result. Consider perofrming lymph node staging.
Local adjuvant therapy	Radiation therapy may be omitted in patients >70 years old.
Systemic adjuvant therapy	Risk/benefit discusson of chemotherapy and endocrine therapy with medical oncologist.

Endocrine Therapy

All women with hormone receptor-positive breast cancer need to be considered as candidates for endocrine therapy with tamoxifen or an aromatase inhibitor (AI). Tamoxifen belongs to a class of drugs recognized as selective estrogen receptor (ER) modulators. It acts as an antagonist of the ER in breast tissue but an agonist in others. AIs decrease the levels of circulating estrogen by inhibiting aromatase, the enzyme that converts androgens to estrogens in tissues like adipose and the adrenal glands. AIs only work in postmenopausal women. Tamoxifen is comparable to AIs in term of survival, but AIs have a decreased risk of relapse [33]. Thus, 5 years of an AI is more effective than tamoxifen for the same duration and results in fewer recurrences in women older than 60 [33].

Elderly patients with estrogen receptor-positive breast cancer who are considered unsuitable to undergo surgical resection are often treated with primary endocrine monotherapy. This type of treatment has been more commonly applied in Europe. Tamoxifen has been initially used as the first-line agent for this treatment, which has now been replaced by aromatase inhibitors. However, aromatase inhibitors must be used with caution in elderly population as the Arimidex, Tamoxifen, Alone or in Combination (ATAC) trial showed that when used in the adjuvant setting, there were significantly more incidence of fractures in the Arimidex group when compared with tamoxifen [34].

Several randomized controlled trials comparing tamoxifen as a sole therapy vs. surgery have demonstrated improved local control with surgery versus tamoxifen alone; however most of these studies have failed to demonstrate improvement in overall survival [35–37]. The study reported by Fennessy et al. was the only randomized trial which demonstrated reduction in survival in patients undergoing surgical resection [38].

For a general summary of the management of breast cancer treatment, see Table 13.3.

Conclusion

Treating breast cancer in the older patient is very complex. Each patient must be evaluated on an individual basis as to their functional reserve, comorbidities, personal wishes, and estimated life expectancy. More studies need to be done on this rapidly rising population.

References

1. Howlader N, Noone A, Krapcho M, et al. SEER Cancer Statistics Review, 1975–2012, National Cancer Institute. Bethesda, MD, http://seer.cancer.gov/csr/1975_2012/, based on November 2014 SEER data submission, posted to the SEER web site, April 2015. Http://SeerCancerGov/Csr/1975_2012/. 2015:1–101. http://seer.cancer.gov/csr/1975_2012/sections.html.
2. Howlader N, Noone AM, Krapcho M, et al. SEER Cancer Statistics Review, 1975–2013, National Cancer Institute. Bethesda, MD, http://seer.Cancer.Gov/csr/1975_2013/, based on November 2015 SEER data submission, posted to the SEER web site, Apr 2016.
3. U. S. Census Bureau. An Aging Nation: The Older Population in the United States Retrieved November 5, 2016, from https://www.census.gov/prod/2014pubs/p25-1140.pdf. 2014.
4. Murphy SL, Xu JQ, Kochanek KD. Deaths: final data for 2010. National vital statistics reports; vol 61 no 4. Hyattsville: National Center for Health Statistics; 2013.
5. Hutchins LF, Unger JM, Crowley JJ, Coltman CA, Albain KS. Underrepresentation of patients 65 years of age or older in cancer-treatment trials. N Engl J Med. 1999;341(27):2061–7. doi:10.1056/NEJM199912303412706.
6. Wyld L, Garg DK, Kumar ID, Brown H, Reed MWR. Stage and treatment variation with age in postmenopausal women with breast cancer: compliance with guidelines. Br J Cancer. 2004;90(8):1486–91. doi:10.1038/sj.bjc.6601742.
7. Diab SG, Elledge RM, Clark GM. Tumor characteristics and clinical outcome of elderly women with breast cancer. J Natl Cancer Inst. 2000;92(7):550–6. http://www.ncbi.nlm.nih.gov/pubmed/10749910%5Cn; http://jnci.oxfordjournals.org/content/92/7/550.full.pdf
8. Pierga JY, Girre V, Laurence V, et al. Characteristics and outcome of 1755 operable breast cancers in women over 70 years of age. Breast. 2004;13(5):369–75. doi:10.1016/j.breast.2004.04.012.
9. Bouchardy C, Rapiti E, Blagojevic S, Vlastos AT, Vlastos G. Older female cancer patients: importance, causes, and consequences of undertreatment. J Clin Oncol. 2007;25(14):1858–69. doi:10.1200/JCO.2006.10.4208.
10. Velanovich V, Gabel M, Walker EM, et al. Causes for the undertreatment of elderly breast cancer patients: tailoring treatments to individual patients. J Am Coll Surg. 2002;194(1):8–13. doi:10.1016/S1072-7515(01)01132-2.
11. Howlander N, Noone A, Krapcho M, Garshell J, Miller D, Altekruse S, et al. SEER cancer statistics review, 1975–2012. Bethesda: National Cancer Institute; 2015.
12. Gøtzsche PC, Nielsen M. Screening for breast cancer with mammography. Cochrane Database Syst Rev. 2011;1:CD001877. doi:10.1002/14651858.CD001877.pub4.
13. Jonsson H, Bordás P, Wallin H, Nyström L, Lenner P. Service screening with mammography in northern Sweden: effects on breast cancer mortality – an update. J Med Screen. 2007;14(2):87–93. doi:10.1258/096914107781261918.
14. Roder D, Houssami N, Farshid G, et al. Population screening and intensity of screening are associated with reduced breast cancer mortality: evidence of efficacy of mammography screening in Australia. Breast Cancer Res Treat. 2008;108(3):409–16. doi:10.1007/s10549-007-9609-5.

15. Braithwaite D, Zhu W, Hubbard RA, et al. Screening outcomes in older US women undergoing multiple mammograms in community practice: does interval, age, or comorbidity score affect tumor characteristics or false positive rates? J Natl Cancer Inst. 2013;105(5):334–41. doi:10.1093/jnci/djs645.
16. Tan A, Kuo YF, Goodwin JS. Potential overuse of screening mammography and its association with access to primary care. Med Care. 2014;52(6):490–5. doi:10.1097/MLR.0000000000000115.
17. Sima CS, Panageas KS, Schrag D. Cancer screening among patients with advanced cancer. JAMA. 2010;304(14):1584–91. doi:10.1001/jama.2010.1449.
18. Bergman L, Kluck HM, van Leeuwen FE, et al. The influence of age on treatment choice and survival of elderly breast cancer patients in south-eastern Netherlands: a population-based study. Eur J Cancer. 1992;28(8–9):1475–80. doi:10.1016/0959-8049(92)90547-F.
19. Mogal HD, Clark C, Dodson R, Fino NF, Howard-McNatt M. Outcomes after mastectomy and lumpectomy in elderly patients with early-stage breast cancer. Ann Surg Oncol. 2017;4(1):100–107. doi:10.1245/s10434–016–5582-8.
20. Chung A, Gangi A, Amersi F, et al. Not performing a sentinel node biopsy for older patients with early-stage invasive breast cancer. JAMA Surg. 2015;150(7):683–4.
21. Hughes KS, Schnaper LA, Bellon JR, et al. Lumpectomy plus tamoxifen with or without irradiation in women age 70 years or older with early breast cancer: long-term follow-up of CALGB 9343. J Clin Oncol. 2013;31(19):2382–7. doi:10.1200/JCO.2012.45.2615.
22. Kunkler IH, Williams LJ, Jack WJL, Cameron DA, Dixon JM. Articles breast-conserving surgery with or without irradiation in women aged 65 years or older with early breast cancer (PRIME II): a randomised controlled trial. Lancet Oncol. 2015;16:266–73. doi:10.1016/S1470-2045(14)71221-5.
23. Soulos PR, Yu JB, Roberts KB, et al. Assessing the impact of a cooperative group trial on breast cancer care in the medicare population. J Clin Oncol. 2012;30(14):1601–7. doi:10.1200/JCO.2011.39.4890.
24. McCormick B, Ottesen RA, Hughes ME, et al. Impact of guideline changes on use or omission of radiation in the elderly with early breast cancer: practice patterns at national comprehensive cancer network institutions. J Am Coll Surg. 2014;219(4):796–802. doi:10.1016/j.jamcollsurg.2014.05.013.
25. Muss HB, Woolf S, Berry D, et al. Adjuvant chemotherapy in older and younger women with lymph node-positive breast cancer. JAMA. 2005;293:1073–81.
26. Giordano SH, Duan Z, Kuo YF, et al. Use and outcomes of adjuvant chemotherapy in older women with breast cancer. J Clin Oncol. 2006;24:2750–6.
27. Elkin EB, Hurria A, Mitra N, et al. Adjuvant chemotherapy and survival in older women with hormone receptor-negative breast cancer: assessing outcome in a population-based, observational cohort. J Clin Oncol. 2006;24:2757–64.
28. Piccart-Gebhart MJ, Procter M, Leyland-Jones B, et al. Trastuzumab after adjuvant chemotherapy in HER2-positive breast cancer. N Engl J Med. 2005;353:1659–72.
29. Smith I, Procter M, Gelber RD, et al. 2-year follow-up of trastuzumab after adjuvant chemotherapy in HER2-positive breast cancer: a randomised controlled trial. Lancet. 2007;369:29–36.
30. Tan-Chiu E, Yothers G, Romond E, et al. Assessment of cardiac dysfunction in a randomized trial comparing doxorubicin and cyclophosphamide followed by paclitaxel, with or without trastuzumab as adjuvant therapy in node-positive, human epidermal growth factor receptor 2-overexpressing breast cancer: NSABP B-31. J Clin Oncol. 2005;23:7811–9.
31. Carlson RW, Moench S, Hurria A, et al. NCCN task force report: breast cancer in the older woman. J Natl Compr Cancer Netw. 2008;6:S1–S25.
32. Karuturi M, VanderWalde N, Muss H. Approach and management of breast cancer in the elderly. Clin Geriatr Med. 2016;32(1):133–53.
33. Dowsett M, Cuzick J, Ingle J, et al. Meta-analysis of breast cancer outcomes in adjuvant trials of aromatase inhibitors versus tamoxifen. J Clin Oncol. 2010;28:509–18.

34. Howell PA. Results of the ATAC (Arimidex, tamoxifen, alone or in combination) trial after completion of 5 years' adjuvant treatment for breast cancer. Lancet. 2005;365(9453):60–2. doi:10.1016/S0140-6736(04)17666-6.
35. Robertson JF, Ellis IO, Elston CW, Blamey RW. Mastectomy or tamoxifen as initial therapy for operable breast cancer in elderly patients: 5-year follow-up. Eur J Cancer. 1992;28A(4–5):908–10.
36. Gazet JC, Ford HT, Coombes RC, et al. Prospective randomized trial of tamoxifen vs surgery in elderly patients with breast cancer. Eur J Surg Oncol.1994;20(3):207–14.
37. Fentiman IS, Christiaens MR, Paridaens R, et al. Treatment of operable breast cancer in the elderly: a randomised clinical trial EORTC 10851 comparing tamoxifcn alone with modified radical mastectomy. Eur J Cancer. 2003;39(3):309–16. doi:10.1016/S0959-8049(02)00673-1.
38. Fennessy M, Bates T, MacRae K, Riley D, Houghton J, Baum M. Late follow-up of a randomized trial of surgery plus tamoxifen versus tamoxifen alone in women aged over 70 years with operable breast cancer. Br J Surg. 2004;91(6):699–704. doi:10.1002/bjs.4603.
39. U.S. Preventive Services Task Force. Final update summary: breast cancer: screening. Sept 2016. https://www.uspreventiveservicestaskforce.org/Page/Document/UpdateSummaryFinal/breast-cancer-screening1.
40. Oeffinger KC, Fontham ET, Etzioni R, et al. Breast cancer screening for women at average risk: 2015 guideline update from the American Cancer Society. JAMA. 2015;314(15):1599–614. doi:10.1001/jama.2015.12783.
41. Lee CH, Dershaw DD, Kopans D, et al. Breast cancer screening with imaging: recommendations from the Society of Breast Imaging and the ACR on the use of mammography, breast MRI, breast ultrasound, and other Technologies for the Detection of clinically occult breast cancer. J Am Coll Radiol. 2010;7(1):18–27. doi:10.1016/j.jacr.2009.09.022.

Breast Cancer Treatment in Young Women

14

Susan K. Boolbol and Sarah Cate

Introduction

Breast cancer affects one in eight women. Of the women who are diagnosed with breast cancer, 25% are premenopausal, and 15% are under the age of 45 [1]. Premenopausal women face different issues than postmenopausal women. All women under the age of 50 who are diagnosed with breast cancer may have a genetic mutation and should undergo genetic testing according to the NCCN guidelines. This is a complex psychosocial issue, in the era of panel testing. Patients may have a low penetrance cancer mutation, which does not mandate prophylactic contralateral surgery, but this may be difficult to explain to patients in the midst of a breast cancer diagnosis. Additionally, as women delay childbearing, many premenopausal breast cancer patients may not have had children. Patients should be offered fertility preservation, which in turn can be expensive and can delay treatment. Finally, there are many psychosocial issues that younger breast cancer patients face, which are unique to younger patients.

Younger women may have more aggressive subtypes of breast cancer. Some of these subtypes, including triple-negative breast cancer, are more prevalent in young women, especially BRCA 1 carriers, African-Americans, and Latino women [2]. African-American women have been shown to be diagnosed at earlier ages [2]. All of these factors contribute to adjuvant treatment, which usually involves chemotherapy in triple-negative breast cancers.

S.K. Boolbol, MD (✉) • S. Cate, MD
Mount Sinai Beth Israel Hospital, 10 Union Square East,
Suite 4E, New York, NY 10003, USA
e-mail: susan.boolbol@mountsinai.org

M. Howard-McNatt (ed.), *Changing Paradigms in the Management of Breast Cancer*, DOI 10.1007/978-3-319-60336-0_14

Fertility

Fertility preservation is a crucial factor for many patients to consider while undergoing treatment during their childbearing years. One of the many side effects of chemotherapy in young women is an increased risk of infertility. Chemotherapy leads to follicle loss in the ovaries due to apoptosis. Since women are born with all of their follicles, once follicles are damaged or lost, there is no way to regenerate new ones. In addition, certain hormonal treatment modalities, such as tamoxifen, have been shown to delay pregnancy for an average of 5 years due to risk of teratogenicity. As many as 73% of women aged 36–40 undergoing certain chemotherapy regimens face amenorrhea, and even if menstruation returns, fertility does not. There are many methods of fertility preservation for women who are undergoing breast cancer treatments.

The primary method of fertility preservation is embryo cryopreservation, which must take place prior to chemotherapy treatment [3]. Embryo cryopreservation is a three-step process. Initially, hormones are taken to mature the follicles, followed by in vitro fertilization (IVF), and finally the embryo is frozen for implantation at a later time. A second viable option for patients is oocyte cryopreservation, in which the oocyte, or egg, is frozen as an alternative to the embryo. This method of fertility preservation may be a more plausible option for women without a male partner to fertilize the oocyte. In 2012, oocyte cryopreservation became a standard recognized treatment by the American Society of Reproductive Medicine, in addition to embryo cryopreservation. However, there are some risks associated with undergoing these cryopreservation procedures. Primarily, chemotherapy must be delayed for an average of 2–6 weeks, until the follicles have matured. Delaying the initiation of chemotherapy may allow more aggressive cancers to progress. In addition, for patients with estrogen receptor-positive (ER+) cancers, the supplementation of additional hormones that increase estrogen levels can lead to progression of the cancer.

Recently, additional methods of fertility preservation have been investigated. One method that requires no hormonal stimulation, no male partner, and a shorter treatment delay is ovarian tissue cryopreservation for reimplantation. Women undergo an oophorectomy, and the removed ovarian tissue is preserved through cryopreservation, until it is later implanted back into the patient. While many of the previous risks are not a threat with this type of procedure, there is a chance that cancerous cells may be reintroduced into the body through ovarian tissue. This method is still under investigation and is not yet considered a standard treatment. Similarly, there is another investigational option, in which the cryopreserved ovarian tissue is matured in vitro, followed by IVF, and a subsequent uterine transfer (IUI). This option may be beneficial as it limits the risk of cancer cell reintroduction. This method is not yet considered standard treatment.

A less invasive method of fertility preservation, gonadotropin-releasing hormone (GnRH) agonist, has been shown to help some patients; however the supporting data is controversial. This hormone agonist acts as a competitive inhibitor and is thought to prevent follicles from undergoing apoptosis, while minimizing ovarian and uterine perfusion, and protecting germline stem cells, therefore reducing the infertility itself from occurring. Unfortunately, despite various research trials, there is no consensus on the benefits of this treatment [3].

Due to the time-sensitive nature of cancer treatment, it is important for women to be aware of their fertility preservation options in order to make a prompt decision on which method if any to proceed with. With such a large number of young women facing breast cancer and chemotherapy, fertility preservation is becoming a substantial aspect of cancer treatment for many.

Genetic Testing

Genetic counseling and testing is standard of care in premenopausal breast cancer patients. Diagnosis at a young age, specifically below 50 years old, should raise concern for a genetic mutation, in addition to a strong family history of the same or similar cancers and multiple affected family members in multiple generations. In fact, 6.2% of screening mammography populations are considered to be at high risk for a hereditary breast cancer gene, significantly elevating their lifetime cancer risk [4].

BRCA 1 (17q21) and BRCA 2 (13q12.3) are two genetic mutations most indicative of elevated breast cancer risk. These normally function as tumor suppressor genes likely involved in DNA repair and regulation of the cell cycle. When mutated, the genes fail to properly function and lose the ability to appropriately control cell division and tumor growth. To date, over 1000 mutations have been discovered. Since the BRCA genes are inherited in an autosomal dominant fashion, only one copy of the mutated gene is necessary to cause an increased cancer risk. Approximately 1/500–1/800 individuals in the general population have either the BRCA 1 or BRCA 2 mutation, which has an associated increased risk of not only breast cancer but also ovarian, pancreatic, prostate, and colon cancers and melanoma [5]. Furthermore, within the Ashkenazi Jewish population, the prevalence rate of BRCA mutations is as high as 1/40. Compared to the average population which has an 8% risk of developing breast cancer and less than a 1% risk of developing ovarian cancer by age 70, BRCA-positive patients have up to an 87% risk of developing breast cancer and a 44% risk of ovarian cancer [5].

Due to the heightened cancer risk, it is crucial for premenopausal breast cancer patients, who have a greater risk of having a gene mutation, to undergo testing in order to determine the best course of treatment for not only their future but for their family's as well. According to the National Comprehensive Cancer Network (NCCN) guidelines, BRCA-positive patients should begin self-breast examinations by age 18. Beginning at age 25, patients should receive biannual clinical breast examinations and annual mammography and breast MRI. Additionally, screening for ovarian cancer is indicated with transvaginal ultrasound and CA-125 biannually, starting at age 30–35 or 5–10 years earlier than the earliest ovarian cancer diagnosis in the family. Alternatively, some patients may opt for prophylactic surgery in order to reduce the chance of developing a cancer. In the management of BRCA carriers with breast cancer, most patients will elect to undergo bilateral mastectomies, to reduce their risk of a future breast cancer. Additionally, some clinical trials, such as those with PARP inhibitors, are only available to BRCA mutation carriers.

More recently, additional genes have been found that contribute to increased cancer risks. Other than BRCA 1 and BRCA 2, genes including CDH1, STK11, and TP53 have been found to increase the risk of developing breast cancer, and genes such as AR, ATM, BARD1, BRIP1, CHEK2, DIRAS3, ERBB2, NBN, PALB2, RAD50, and RAD51 are associated with breast cancer. Consequentially, panel testing, which screens for an array of genes associated with various cancers, has been highly beneficial for patients, especially those with extensive family histories of cancer, patients with more than one primary cancer, or patients with early-onset cancers. NCCN guidelines state that women under the age of 35 should receive not only BRCA testing but also p53 testing as standard of care. Currently, seven different labs offer panel testing for Hereditary Breast and Ovarian Cancer Syndrome (HBOC) and other high-risk genes. The panel includes high-penetrance genes, which have a high lifetime risk of manifesting a cancer (70–100%), and moderate penetrance genes, with a modest-moderate lifetime risk (30–60%) [6].

NCCN guidelines for panel testing state that testing should be offered by a genetic counselor due to test variants and the need for pre- and posttesting counseling. Testing should be offered on the basis of clinically actionable information. Therefore, they should be performed only if a positive or negative result would influence the management of the patient. Several companies offer various panel options that the genetic counselor and patients may choose from depending on the patient's specific history. Ambry Genetics, for example, offers both the BRCAplus, which screens for BRCA1, BRCA2, CDH1 (hereditary diffuse gastric cancer and lobular breast cancer), PTEN (Cowden syndrome), and TP53 (Li-Fraumeni syndrome) and the BreastNext panel, which screens for ATM, BARD1, BRCA1, BRCA2, BRIP1, CDH1, CHEK2, MRE11A, MUTYH, NBN, NF1, PALB2, PTEN, RAD50, RAD51C, RAD51D, STK11, and TP53. Myriad Genetics, on the other hand, offers myRisk, which is a 28-gene panels that looks at risk of eight cancer sites including breast, ovarian, gastric, colorectal, pancreatic, melanoma, prostate, and endometrial cancers. Testing should be performed before any surgery, so that patients can decide whether or not they want to undergo prophylactic contralateral mastectomy in the event of a positive result or bilateral mastectomies. For women deciding to do so, some reconstruction options including DIEP flap reconstruction are one-time procedures that can take place simultaneously during the mastectomies. Consequently, patients should have the maximal information available to them prior to a definitive surgery. For non-BRCA mutations on the panel, prophylactic surgery is not recommended. However patients would receive increased screening with both annual mammograms and breast MRIs.

Some of the considerations that should be used to determine which panel best suits the patient include variant of uncertain significance (VUS) rate and ability to reclassify VUS, test affordability and financial assistance programs, time from testing to results, screening methodology, insurance preauthorization policies, and specimen types. It is important to note that although positive results for carrying recessive gene mutations such as ATM, NBN, and PALB2 are insignificant to the patient's health, they may influence management of the patients' children as there is a possibility of disease risk if the other parent also carries a mutation in the same gene. Having two copies of a mutated gene that follow autosomal recessive dominance can indicate diseases such as ataxia-telangiectasia, Nijmegen breakage syndrome, and Fanconi anemia, among others.

Several studies have been conducted to determine the prevalence of positive findings in panel testing. In one study, 1951 participants referred to a diagnostic laboratory for BRCA1/BRCA2 testing underwent panel screening [7]. Two-hundred seventy-five (14.1%) patients were mutation carriers in at least of the 25 genes that were screened. Furthermore, 182 (9.3%) of patients had a BRCA mutation, and 93 (4.8%) patients had a mutation in a non-BRCA gene. In a separate study, 390 BRCA-negative patients underwent panel testing, and 4.4% were found to have a mutation in at least 1 of the 23 non-BRCA genes. The most common non-BRCA mutations included CHEK2, NBN, ATM, and PALB2. This data indicates the importance of panel testing over simply BRCA1/BRCA2 gene testing since compared with BRCA1/BRCA2 testing alone, using the 25-gene panel increased the identification of mutations in cancer susceptibility genes by 4.76% (95% CI: 2.71–6.81%).

Though panel testing can create more uncertainty for patients, the benefits of capturing more genetic mutations for cancer often outweigh the harms. Mutation carriers may need doctors' additional preventative measures and closer surveillance in order to increase early detection of cancers. Further research is necessary to determine the exact implications of various gene mutations on cancer risk as well as to discover more genes associated with elevated risk.

Psychosocial Issues

Significant psychosocial issues face young women undergoing breast cancer treatment. These include sexual side effects from treatment, loss of financial independence, and nonadherence to treatment regimens. Young patients have been shown to have greater benefit from 10 years of adjuvant treatment with tamoxifen versus 5 years of treatment, as a result of the ATLAS Trial [8]. These patients in turn tend to have a higher incidence of side effects from tamoxifen [9]. This affects patient compliance and adherence to tamoxifen. There is evidence to suggest that these women are less likely to comply with treatment, due to these side effects and psychosocial issues [10]. In study by Cluze et al., a prospective cohort of women under age 40 diagnosed with breast cancer was analyzed, to examine the incidence of tamoxifen interruption. They found that 42% of women interrupt their treatment for two or more consecutive months. A lack of support was identified as one factor, while treatment side effects were noted to be a cause of interruption after 16–28 months of treatment. Additionally, they identified that those patients who had taken tamoxifen for 16–28 months were less apprehensive about breast cancer relapse and, therefore, stopped taking the medication.

Additionally, quality of life in younger women diagnosed with breast cancer is lower than that of older women diagnosed with breast cancer [11]. These women experience higher levels of clinical depression, anxiety, and stress perceptions.

Factors thought to contribute to higher levels of depression and distress include fear of infertility and menopause. Additionally, weight gain and lack of physical activity were observed in the premenopausal women with breast cancer.

Another area of complex management in young women with breast cancer is sexuality. In a study by Charif et al., 623 women were analyzed who were diagnosed with breast cancer between the ages of 18 and 40 [12]. A significant number of these patients were dissatisfied with their sexual health and fertility. In this study, 319 patients participated in telephone interviews, at 10, 16, 28, and 48 months after their breast cancer diagnosis. At 4 years post-breast cancer diagnosis, 53% of women were satisfied with their fertility, and 42.6% were satisfied with their sexuality. This suggests that a significant percentage of breast cancer patients face sexuality issues. These can vary from vasomotor symptoms to vaginal atrophy [9]. Patients who have been treated for breast cancer need to be integrated into a survivorship program, which addresses such issues [13].

Local recurrence rates due to a long lifespan are an additional concern for young women. This has been thought to affect the choice of mastectomy over breast conservation therapy (BCT). The EORTC trials 10,804, 10,854, and 10,902 found that young age and BCT were independent risk factors for local regional recurrence [14]. These trials included almost 1200 young patients and demonstrated that women under 35 had a 2.8 times risk of LRR compared with older patients.

References

1. Sonmezer M, Oktay K. Fertility preservation in young women undergoing breast cancer therapy. The Oncologist. 2006;11(5):422–34.
2. Brinton LA, Sherman ME, Carreon JD, Anderson WF. Recent trends in breast cancer among younger women in the United States. J Natl Cancer Inst. 2008;100:1643.
3. Waks AG, Partridge AH. Fertility preservation in patients with breast cancer: necessity, methods, and safety. J Natl Compr Cancer Netw. 2016;14(3):355–63.
4. Bellcross CA, et al. Evaluation of a breast/ovarian cancer genetics referral screening tool in a mammography population. Genet Med. 2009;11.11:783–9.
5. Antoniou A, et al. Average risks of breast and ovarian cancer associated with BRCA1 or BRCA2 mutations detected in case series unselected for family history: a combined analysis of 22 studies. Am J Hum Genet. 2003;72(5):1117–30.
6. Hall MJ, et al. Gene panel testing for inherited cancer risk. J Natl Cancer Netw. 2014;12(9):1339–46.
7. Tung, Nadine, Battelli, Chiara, Allen, Brian, et al.. Prevalence of gene mutations among hereditary breast and ovarian cancer patients using a 25 gene panel. Beth Israel Deaconess Medical Center. Presented at San Antonio Breast Cancer Symposium, December 2013.
8. Davies C, Pan H, Godwin J, Gray R, Arriagada R, Raina V, et al. Long-term effects of continuing adjuvant tamoxifen to 10 years versus stopping at 5 years after diagnosis of oestrogen receptor-positive breast cancer: ATLAS, a randomised trial. Lancet. 2013;381(9869):805–16.
9. Ganz PA, Greendale GA, Petersen L, Kahn B, Bower JE. Breast cancer in younger women: reproductive and late health effects of treatment. J Clin Oncol. 2003;21:4184–93.
10. Cluze C, Rey D, Huiart L, Bendiane MK, Bouhnik AD, Berenger C, Carrieri MP, Giorgi R. Adjuvant endocrine therapy with tamoxifen in young women with breast cancer: determinants of interruptions vary over time. Ann Oncol. 2012;23:882–90.

11. Howard-Anderson J, Ganz PA, Bower JE, Stanton AL. Quality of life, fertility concerns, and behavioral health outcomes in younger breast cancer survivors: a systematic review. J Natl Cancer Inst. 2012;104:386–405.
12. Ben Charif A, Bouhnik AD, Rey D, Provansal M, Courbiere B, Spire B, Mancini J. Satisfaction with fertility- and sexuality-related information in young women with breast cancer – ELIPPSE40 cohort. BMC Cancer. 2015;15:572. doi:10.1186/s12885-015-1542-0.
13. Patricia Ganz, Julienne Bower, Annette Stanton. Special issues in younger women with breast cancer. Improving Outcomes for Breast Cancer Survivors. Volume 862 of the series Advances in Experimental Medicine and Biology, pp 9–21 (n.d.).
14. de Bock GH, van der Hage JA, Putter H, et al. Isolated loco-regional recurrence of breast cancer is more common in young patients and following breast conserving therapy: long-term results of European Organisation for Research and Treatment of Cancer studies. Eur J Cancer. 2006;42:351–6.

Genetic Risk Prediction in Breast Cancer 15

Anvy Nguyen, Jennifer K. Plichta, Jessica Cintolo-Gonzalez, Kinyas Kartal, Molly Elizabeth Griffin, and Kevin Hughes

Introduction

The expansion of knowledge related to genetic susceptibility in breast cancer, in particular the identification of *BRCA1* and *BRCA2* genes, has greatly enhanced the accuracy of breast cancer prediction for the subset of individuals with heritable disorders. Genetic testing for hereditary breast cancer makes early detection and cancer prevention feasible through screening, surgical prophylaxis, and chemoprevention. Genetic risk prediction, combined with prevention or early detection and targeted therapy, can greatly improve survival rates of breast cancer patients [2]. The health care system falls short when women with BRCA mutations are not identified and notified of their status. Ideally, all mutation carriers should be identified through testing before they develop disease, and subsequent management should be aimed at preventing or minimizing the stage of cancer once it occurs. Unfortunately, most patients who carry a genetic mutation for hereditary breast cancer have not been identified [1].

A. Nguyen, MD (✉)
Department of Breast Oncology, Susan F. Smith Center for Women's Cancers, Dana-Farber Cancer Institute, Boston, MA 02115, USA
e-mail: anvy_nguyen@dfci.harvard.edu

J.K. Plichta, MD, MS
Department of Surgery, Duke University Medical Center, DUMC 3513, Durham, NC 27710, USA
e-mail: jennifer.plichta@duke.edu

J. Cintolo-Gonzalez, MD
Brigham and Women's Hospital, 75 Francis St., Boston, MA 02115, USA
e-mail: jcintolo-gonzalez@partners.org

K. Kartal, MD • M.E. Griffin, BA • K. Hughes, MD
Division of Surgical Oncology, Massachusetts General Hospital, 55 Fruit St., Boston, MA 02114, USA
e-mail: kkartal@mgh.harvard.edu; megriff@post.harvard.edu; kshughes@partners.org

M. Howard-McNatt (ed.), *Changing Paradigms in the Management of Breast Cancer*, DOI 10.1007/978-3-319-60336-0_15

As recently stated by Mary Claire King, "Identifying a woman's high risk of cancer only after she is diagnosed with it is an obvious failure of cancer prevention" [3]. Even more egregious is the failure to identify a mutation carrier *after* she develops cancer. Women identified as mutation carriers after a breast cancer develops can still garner benefits from this knowledge. These include, but are not limited to, directing surgical management, selecting systemic therapy, managing other at-risk organs, determining a follow-up approach, and managing recurrent disease. In addition, identifying a mutation carrier may lead to the identification of mutation carriers in other family members, ideally before they develop cancer.

For those mutation carriers who are not identified at the time of cancer diagnosis, it is important to minimize the negative impact of this failure by supporting a program of genetic testing in the large cadre of women who are currently being followed for breast cancer. Identifying the mutation status in patients with previous breast cancers can still influence how the patient is being followed, how in-breast and/or distant recurrences are managed, and if family members need to be tested. Patients found to be mutation carriers through genetic testing are suddenly empowered to make decisions about further cancer prevention, reproduction, and treatment not just for their breast cancer but for looming cancers that may arise in other organs. Patients and family members who participate in genetic screening can be appropriately counseled, and those individuals who test negative for mutation can avoid unnecessary interventions.

The initial step and cornerstone of assessing genetic risk in breast cancer is to perform an evaluation of the patient's personal and family history. The evaluation should include the construction of a detailed three-generation pedigree that includes ethnicity, cancer history of each family member, current ages, ages at diagnosis/death, and causes of death [4]. Based on the results of the personal and/or family history, their risk of carrying a mutation and/or their eligibility under the National Comprehensive Cancer Network (NCCN) guidelines [5] may render them good candidates for genetic testing.

Hereditary Breast Cancers

High-Penetrance Genes

Hereditary cancer syndromes are characterized by germline gene mutations, which are associated with a high risk for cancer development. These mutations are usually inherited in an autosomal dominant pattern and often have an early age of onset. Hereditary cancer syndromes are rare, accounting for only approximately 5–10% of all breast cancers [6]. Genetic predispositions that confer a high risk for breast cancer include hereditary breast and ovarian cancer syndrome (HBOC, *BRCA1*/*BRCA2*), Li-Fraumeni syndrome (*TP53*), Peutz-Jeghers syndrome (*STK11*), Cowden syndrome (*PTEN*), and hereditary diffuse gastric cancer syndrome (*CDH1*). Breast cancer risk is higher in individuals diagnosed with these syndromes, and there is a risk for developing tumors in other organs [7–10]. These high-penetrance genes can be tested in clinical practice, and patients and other family members can derive significant benefit from knowing whether or not they have mutations in these genes.

Most hereditary breast cancers are caused by deleterious mutations in *BRCA1* and *BRCA2*. Mutation carriers have a 50–85% risk of developing breast cancer and a 15–60% risk of developing ovarian cancer by age 70. The risk of bilateral breast cancers has been estimated to be as high as 64% in *BRCA1* mutation carriers diagnosed with breast cancer by age 60. Male *BRCA2* mutation carriers have an increased risk of developing breast cancer, and male carriers of *BRCA1/BRCA2* mutations are at increased risk for developing prostate cancer [11, 12]. *BRCA1/BRCA2* mutation carriers have also been found to have an increased risk of developing pancreatic cancer [13, 14].

Low- and Moderate-Penetrance Genes

Deleterious mutations in low and moderately penetrant genes, such as *CHEK2*, *ATM*, *PALB2*, *BRIP1*, *BARD1*, *NBN*, and *RAD50*, have also been shown to confer an increased breast cancer risk, although to a lesser degree than *BRCA1* or *BRCA2*.

Truncating mutations in *CHEK2* have been associated with a clinically meaningful risk of breast cancer, ranging from 20% in mutation carriers with no affected relative to 44% in mutation carriers with either a first- or second-degree relative affected [15]. Biallelic mutations in *ATM*, a gene encoding a protein involved in DNA repair, were originally associated with ataxia-telangiectasia, a recessive early-onset progressive neurological disorder. More recently, monoallelic *ATM* mutations have been shown to play a role in breast cancer susceptibility, conferring an estimated relative risk of 2.23 in all carriers and 4.94 in patients younger than 50 years [16]. Biallelic mutations in *PALB2* have been linked with Fanconi anemia, whereas monoallelic mutations are associated with a predisposition to breast as well as pancreatic cancer. *PALB2* mutations have been shown to confer an absolute breast cancer risk of 33–58% by 70 years of age [17]. Monoallelic mutations in *BRIP1*, a gene encoding the BRCA1-interacting helicase, confer a relative risk of 2.0 for developing breast cancer [18]. Breast cancer penetrance of low-risk genes including *BARD1*, *NBN*, and *RAD50* is not well defined; however, laboratories are now including them as a component of panel testing.

The Breast Cancer Patient

Breast cancer patients can be classified as (1) patients diagnosed in the past who are being followed (currently cancer-free), (2) patients who have developed a local recurrence, (3) patients who have developed distant metastases, and (4) patients with a newly diagnosed breast cancer. Identifying the mutation status for women in each of these groups has common benefits, as well as specific benefits for certain groups.

Previously Diagnosed Breast Cancer Patients

In those patients being followed for a history of breast cancer, one might expect that they should have already been tested if they were at risk. Unfortunately, as mentioned previously, this seldom occurs. Even today, many patients who are at high risk never undergo genetic testing.

However, genetic testing rates have increased for younger women. One study reported an increase from 76.9% in 2006 to 95.3% in 2013 [19]. The study participants included 897 women with breast cancer aged 40 years or younger from academic and community medical centers. This is in contrast to a 2005 study, where the genetic testing rate was 16.7% based on a survey conducted of 551 women under age 45 who had been diagnosed with breast cancer between 1993 and 2002 [20]. There is a strong likelihood that genetic testing in younger women with breast cancer has increased given the prevalence of mutation carriers in this group [21].

Patients who were previously ineligible for genetic testing at the time of their diagnosis may now be eligible under the new expanded criteria for genetic testing. The statement on Genetic Testing for Cancer Susceptibility from the American Society of Clinical Oncology (ASCO) issued in 2003 recommended genetic counseling/testing if (i) there was a personal or family history suggesting genetic cancer susceptibility, (ii) the test could be adequately interpreted, and (iii) the results would aid in the diagnosis or influence the medical or surgical management of the patient or family members at hereditary risk of cancer [22]. In 2010, the Hereditary Breast and Ovarian Cancer (HBOC) testing criteria for breast cancer patients as set forth by the NCCN included multiple criteria, including:

(a) Individuals from a family with a known BRCA1/BRCA2 gene mutation
(b) Personal history of epithelial ovarian/fallopian tube/primary peritoneal cancer
(c) Personal history of male breast cancer
(d) An individual of ethnicity associated with higher mutation frequency (Ashkenazi Jewish)

In 2016, the NCCN expanded their criteria for genetic testing of individuals at risk, to include individuals:

(a) Diagnosed at age ≤60 with a triple-negative breast cancer
(b) Diagnosed at any age with a family history of pancreatic and/or prostate cancer (≥2 close blood relatives)
(c) With a personal history of pancreatic and/or prostate cancer and a family history of breast, ovarian, pancreatic, and/or prostate cancer

The current guidelines highlight the importance of recognizing pancreatic cancer and prostate cancer risk related to *BRCA1/BRCA2* mutations. It has been shown that there is a two- to threefold and two- to sevenfold higher risk of developing pancreatic cancer in patients with *BRCA1* and *BRCA2* mutations, respectively [14, 23–25]. Mutations in *ATM*, *PALB2*, *STK11*, and *TP53* are also associated with both breast cancer and pancreatic cancer risk [26]. These expanded criteria now make genetic testing applicable in patients who were previously not eligible.

Performing patient follow-up and updating family histories are also critical as an individual's family history can change over time. Relatives who were previously unaffected may have developed a cancer, and this might make the patient eligible for genetic testing when she previously was not. It is difficult to understate the importance of updating the family history for patients in follow-up to avoid a missed opportunity for genetic testing.

Some patients may have undergone testing with an outmoded instrument resulting in a false-negative finding. For example, traditional methods fail to detect very large rearrangement mutations which account for 6–10% of all HBOC mutations identified [27]. Prior to 2006, standard genetic testing for mutations in the *BRCA1* and *BRCA2* genes failed to identify mutations in 12% of 300 breast cancer patients from high-risk families [28]. These subjects had genomic rearrangements of *BRCA1* and *BRCA2* that were too large to be detected by conventional sequencing. At that time, genetic testing of *BRCA1* and *BRCA2* was carried out by a single commercial firm whose protocol was to sequence the exons and flanking regulatory regions of each gene, which can miss many mutations. A more comprehensive testing strategy now includes detection of large rearrangements in *BRCA1* and *BRCA2* [29]. The NCCN has updated their guidelines to support the inclusion of large rearrangement testing for all patients undergoing genetic testing for *BRCA1* and *BRCA2* mutations [5].

The NCCN also now acknowledges that multigene panel testing for hereditary forms of cancer may be more efficient and cost-effective. Multigene panel testing utilizes next-generation sequencing technology to interrogate multiple genes simultaneously and is recommended when more than one gene might explain an inherited cancer syndrome or when a patient with a personal or family history suggestive of an inherited predisposition to cancer previously tested negative.

Most patients who have undergone even recent genetic testing have been tested only for *BRCA1* and *BRCA2*, leaving many other mutation carriers unidentified. There are over 25 breast cancer susceptibility genes in addition to *BRCA1* and *BRCA2*. As described above, the six genes with high-penetrance mutations associated with a significantly elevated cancer risk include *BRCA1*, *BRCA2*, *TP53*, *PTEN*, *STK11*, and *CDH1* [30]. *ATM*, *CHEK2*, and *PALB2* are moderate-penetrance genes conferring a lower but significant breast cancer risk [31]. It has been shown that 7% of patients who previously underwent non-informative genetic testing were found to have a pathogenic mutation with multigene panel testing [32]. In a study of 1046 *BRCA1-/BRCA2*-negative individuals who underwent multi-panel gene testing, 3.8% were found to harbor mutations in breast and ovarian cancer genes (*CHEK2*, *ATM*, and *PALB2*) and Lynch syndrome genes [33], suggesting that patients who were only tested for *BRCA1/BRCA2* mutations should be tested for mutations in other breast cancer susceptibility genes.

In *BRCA1-/BRCA2*-negative individuals, further testing of other breast cancer susceptible genes should be considered in those who have a suggestive personal and/or family history. As such, a thorough family history should not be limited to breast cancer and should include the identification of cancers of other organs that may be part of a breast cancer syndrome or other hereditary cancer syndromes. In patients whose personal or family histories suggest more than one hereditary cancer syndrome or in patients with such histories who tested negative, the NCCN suggests that multigene panel testing should be offered [5].

As multigene panels are being increasingly used for genetic testing, it is important to note that there will be a resultant increase in variants of uncertain significance (VUS) for which there is insufficient evidence to determine their clinical relevance. Thus patients must be counseled prior to testing regarding the higher percentages of these results.

The largest benefit of identifying mutation carrier status in breast cancer patients is to help determine optimal surgical management, which may include completion mastectomy with or without contralateral prophylactic mastectomy. Patients who underwent breast-conserving surgery without knowledge of their mutation status may reconsider mastectomy with or without contralateral prophylactic mastectomy after receiving a positive BRCA mutation result. The risk for contralateral breast cancer is 36.1% and 28.5% at 15 years after diagnosis in *BRCA1*- and *BRCA2*-positive breast cancer patients, respectively, with women younger than 50 years of age more at risk than those older than 50 years [34]. In *BRCA1/BRCA2* mutation carriers previously treated for unilateral breast cancer, contralateral prophylactic mastectomy was found to reduce the risk of contralateral breast cancer by 91% [35]. The potential benefit of prophylactic mastectomy on the contralateral side would be greatest in these patients, and the Society of Surgical Oncology (SSO) recommends mastectomy in the contralateral breast for women with a previous diagnosis of breast cancer at high risk for contralateral breast cancer [36]. This recommendation must be tempered by the age of the patient. Prophylactic removal of the contralateral breast will be of far more benefit to a 35-year-old carrier than a 70-year-old carrier newly diagnosed with her first breast cancer. Posttreatment surveillance with breast MRI may be considered for patients who do not elect to undergo mastectomy.

Breast cancer patients with a *BRCA1/BRCA2* mutation must also consider undergoing a risk-reducing salpingo-oophorectomy (RRSO), which is recommended between the ages of 35 and 40 years or at completion of childbearing. In addition to reducing the risk of ovarian cancer, RRSO has been associated with a reduced risk of contralateral breast cancer and ipsilateral breast recurrence in *BRCA1/BRCA2* patients with a history of breast cancer [37, 38].

Tamoxifen has also been shown to be protective against cancers arising in the contralateral breast for carriers of *BRCA1/BRCA2* mutations. This finding suggests that tamoxifen should be strongly considered in patients with ER+ cancers [39, 40]. In an observational study of 2464 *BRCA1/BRCA2* mutation carriers with a history of breast cancer, patients who received tamoxifen following unilateral mastectomy experienced a lower incidence of cancer in the contralateral breast [41].

A positive result on susceptibility testing in breast cancer patients does not necessarily alter clinical management. First, one must assess the clinical actionability of each test result, defined as clinically prescribed interventions based on results of genetic testing. Desmond's study found that 31.7% of patients who harbored mutations in high-risk genes would have had a change in pretest recommendations for screening and/or preventive surgery. In contrast, a management change would have been recommended in 25% of patients who harbored mutations in genes associated with low or moderately increased cancer risk. The identification of low- and moderate-risk genes was found to benefit family members who also harbored mutations, as family members with mutations in low- or moderate-risk genes would be recommended for enhanced screening. Desmond's study also found that in total, 52% of mutation-positive patients would receive additional recommendations for screening and/or prevention based on NCCN guidelines [33]. Both the NCCN and Tung et al. have established screening guidelines and management approaches for patients with moderate-penetrance mutations in an effort to provide assistance to clinicians caring for these patients (Table 15.1) [5, 42].

Patients with high-penetrance mutations in *TP53*, *PTEN*, *STK11*, and *CDH1* can be managed according to established guidelines for each associated hereditary cancer syndrome. For instance, it has been shown that patients with a *TP53* mutation are at higher risk of secondary radiation-induced malignancies [43]. In these patients, avoidance of radiotherapy is recommended, and a bilateral mastectomy is favored. It is important to note that *TP53* mutation carriers tend to have an earlier age of breast cancer diagnosis with an average age of 30 at the time of diagnosis. Thus, multigene panel testing should be considered in young breast cancer patients who test negative for BRCA1/BRCA2 mutations. Early identification of *CDH1* mutation carriers is also critical, as these patients have a higher lifetime risk of developing diffuse gastric cancer and lobular breast cancer. Given the high mortality associated with diffuse gastric cancer, prophylactic total gastrectomy is recommended in these patients [44].

When a mutation carrier is identified, one of the most important things to do is cascade testing of as many at-risk relatives as possible. The identification of family members will markedly improve outcomes by identifying patients who are at extremely high risk and managing them in a way that will detect cancer earlier or prevent cancer altogether.

Cascade genetic screening is a methodology for identifying and testing family members at increased risk for a heritable disease. Cascade screening follows a systematic process of family tracing which minimizes costs and the number of family members who need to be tested. In 2012, the Center for Disease Control (CDC) developed an evidence-based classification schema for genomic applications in public health and clinical settings. Cascade screening was included as a Tier 1 application. Tier 1 genomic applications are defined as those having "significant potential for positive impact on public health" and include applications for HBOC and Lynch syndrome, as well as familial hypercholesterolemia [45]. The CDC recommends a two-phase approach for HBOC with the Phase 1 approach including (1) enhancing cancer registry reporting, (2) informing evidence-based policy-making by partner payers to enhance coverage, (3) developing and tracking surveillance indicators, and (4) instituting outreach programs. The Phase 2 approach uses cascade screening to identify at-risk family members who may benefit from preventive strategies [46].

Table 15.1 Comparison of proposed management strategies from Tung et al. [42] and the NCCN [5] for moderate-penetrance breast cancer predisposition

Gene	Mammography[a]		RRM		RRSO		Colonoscopy		RR proctocolectomy		Pancreatic screening		RR gastrectomy	
	Tung	NCCN	Tung	NCCN	Tung	NCCN	Tung	NCCN	Tung	NCCN	Tung	NCCN	Tung	NCCN
ATM	Annually starting at age 40	Annually starting at age 40	NA	IE	FH	NC	NC	NA	NC	NC	Clinical trial	NC	NC	NC
CHEK2 (truncating)	Annually starting at age 40	Annually starting at age 40	NA	IE	FH	NC	**Discuss at age 40**	**Every 5 years, starting at age 40**	NC	NC	NC	NC	NC	NC
NBN	Annually starting at age 40	Annually starting at age 40	NA	NA	FH	NC	NC	NC	NC	NC	NC	NC	NC	NC
PALB2 BRIP1 RAD51C	**Annually starting at age 30**	**Annually starting at age 40**	NA	**DO**	FH	IE	NC	NC	NC	NC	Clinical trial	NC	NC	NC
RAD51D	FH	FH	NA	NC	**R/C at age 50–55**	**R/C at age 45–50**	NC	NC	NC	NC	NC	NC	NC	NC
APC	NC	NC	NC	NC	NC	NC	**FH**[b]	**Annually starting at age 10–15**	NC	**R/C at age 20**	NC	Clinical trial	NC	NC
CDH1	NC	**Annually starting at age 30**	NA	**DO**	NA	NA	NC	NC	NC	NC	NC	NC	NC	FH

RRM risk-reducing mastectomy, *RRSO* risk-reducing salpingo-oophorectomy, *RR* risk-reducing, *NCCN* National Comprehensive Cancer Network, *FH* family history, *NC* no comment, *NA* no available data, *IE* insufficient evidence for any recommendation, *DO* discuss option, *R/C* recommend/consider

[a]Clinical breast examination and/or breast MRI

[b]For individuals without a family history of colorectal cancer or adenomatous polyps, population screening guidelines should be followed

Previously Diagnosed Patients Who Develop Local Recurrence

BRCA1-/BRCA2-positive patients with stage I/II breast cancer have a 12.9% 10-year risk of developing an ipsilateral breast recurrence [47]. These patients may elect to undergo completion mastectomy with or without contralateral prophylactic mastectomy. After undergoing treatment, these patients require close follow-up in the same manner as all breast cancer patients.

Previously Diagnosed Patients Who Develop Distant Metastasis

Mutation status can potentially help guide systemic therapy decisions in BRCA mutation carriers who develop distant metastases. While still under study, it appears that cisplatin chemotherapy and PARP inhibitors (small molecular inhibitors of the enzyme poly ADP-ribose polymerase) may be more effective in BRCA mutation carriers [48]. Developing data shows that *BRCA1*-associated cancers are more sensitive to platinum therapy and less sensitive to taxanes [49, 50]. *BRCA1*-positive patients with breast cancer who are treated with cisplatin in both the neoadjuvant and metastatic setting have been shown to respond well to treatment [51]. Preclinical studies in breast cancer models show that the combination of a PARP1 inhibitor with cisplatin induces a larger response in *BRCA2*-deficient tumors than either compound alone [52]. Currently, clinical trials with several PARP inhibitors are being conducted to assess the toxicities, efficacies, and benefits of the drugs in *BRCA1-/BRCA2*-related breast cancer [53, 54]. *PTEN*-deficient tumors have also been shown to be sensitive to PARP inhibitors both in vitro and in vivo suggesting that treatment with PARP inhibitors may be considered for those with *PTEN*-positive breast cancer in the near future [55]. A similar result has been shown in *ATM*-deficient cells indicating that *ATM* depletion sensitizes breast cancer cells to PARP inhibitors [56].

Newly Diagnosed Breast Cancer Patients

Most newly diagnosed patients accept genetic counseling and testing when offered [57]. Newly diagnosed breast cancer patients identified as mutation carriers have the option of breast-conserving therapy versus mastectomy with or without contralateral prophylactic mastectomy. In a prospective study of 194 newly diagnosed breast cancer patients, 48% of patients found to carry a *BRCA1/BRCA2* mutation chose bilateral mastectomy as their definitive breast cancer surgery compared to 24% of patients in whom no mutation was detected, highlighting the significance of genetic testing in newly diagnosed patients in surgical decision-making [58]. It has been shown that women found to have a mutation would have opted for bilateral mastectomy if they had been identified as mutation carriers at the time of diagnosis [59]. Knowledge of one's mutation status prior to definitive surgery may help women avoid a second surgery for those who would have chosen bilateral mastectomy over breast-conserving therapy. Patients with knowledge of their mutation status at the time of diagnosis may also avoid radiation therapy after breast-conserving surgery, which may negatively affect the cosmetic outcome of reconstructive surgery. As mentioned above, platinum-based chemotherapy may be preferentially considered as systemic therapy for *BRCA1* mutation carriers, and PARP inhibitors have thus far shown great potential in clinical trials.

Breast Cancer Risk Prediction Models

Numerous risk models have been developed that use mathematical strategies to predict the risk of having a mutation in a cancer susceptibility gene such as *BRCA1/BRCA2*. These models, used in conjunction with clinical guidelines and judgment, can assist in determining the need for a genetic counseling referral and genetic testing. While many models focus on predicting BRCA mutation carrier status, the top three in terms of validation and common use in clinical practice are Myriad, BRCAPRO, and BOADICEA.

The Myriad model (Myriad I, also known as the Shattuck-Eidens model) predicts the risk of having a deleterious *BRCA1* mutation based on logistic regression analysis of a group of 798 women who underwent genetic sequencing by Myriad laboratories [60]. The risk factors incorporated into this prediction model are age of first diagnosis of breast or ovarian cancer, Ashkenazi Jewish ethnicity, diagnosis of bilateral breast cancers, number of relatives (any degree) affected by breast cancer, number of relatives (any degree) affected by ovarian cancer, and number of relatives (any degree) affected by both breast and ovarian cancer. The Myriad II model, sometimes referred to as the Frank model [61], also uses logistic regression to refine its correlations between similar risk factors and mutation status albeit in a larger cohort of 10,000 women. Risk factors incorporated into the Myriad II tables include personal breast cancer history, with age of onset of breast cancer categorized as ≥50 or <50, history of ovarian cancer, history of male breast cancer, and the combination of both breast and ovarian cancer. The family history assessment includes breast cancer accounting for age (≥50 or <50) and ovarian cancer at any age in first- or second-degree relatives. In contrast to Myriad I, this updated version predicts the risk of carrying a *BRCA1* or *BRCA2* mutation [62]. In comparison with other models that predict *BRCA1/BRCA2* mutation status, including BRCAPRO and BOADICEA, the Myriad II model has comparable sensitivities and specificities for predicting BRCA carrier status [63–65, 66]. The Myriad model can be applied in the clinical setting either by using an online risk calculator [67] or by using tables, which are also accessible online and routinely updated [68]. Separate tables exist for those with or without Ashkenazi Jewish ancestry. However, there are some drawbacks. The Myriad model is limited in that it can only incorporate risk from two relatives and it attributes the same degree of risk to all breast cancer patients under age 50, rather than looking at various age intervals for further risk stratification, such that a diagnosis of breast cancer in one's early 20s is treated the same as a diagnosis in one's late 40s.

BRCAPRO, like the Myriad model, initially was developed to predict the risk of carrying a deleterious *BRCA1* mutation [69] but was subsequently updated to predict the probability of a *BRCA2* mutation as well [70]. In addition to predicting the likelihood of carrying a deleterious *BRCA1/BRCA2* germline mutation, BRCAPRO also predicts the likelihood of developing breast or ovarian cancer within a set time period and more recently also predicts the risk of contralateral breast cancer in those already diagnosed with breast cancer [71]. While Myriad uses logistic regression to analyze risk factors predicting carrier status, BRCAPRO applies Bayes' theorem and calculates risk based on published estimates of the prevalence and penetrance of *BRCA1/BRCA2* and baseline rates of breast cancer in the population. BRCAPRO is thus updated regularly based on these changing rates. Familial factors incorporated into the model for each relative assessed include relation to patient, current age, breast cancer and ovarian cancer status, and age of diagnosis if affected. BRCAPRO also incorporates pathologic markers (ER, PR, HER2, CK14, CK5/CK6) for known breast cancer, race, and ethnicity (Ashkenazi Jewish, non-Ashkenazi Jewish, Italian, Asian, other), as well as information as to whether family members have undergone interventions such as mastectomy (specifying male mastectomy and bilateral mastectomy) or oophorectomy [71]. Additional modifications, such as BRCAPROLyte and BRCAPROLyte-plus, have been made to provide simplified versions to ease the extent of data collection in the clinical setting [72]. For clinical use, BRCAPRO can be accessed via its native R implementation as part of the open source BayesMendel [73] package or via multiple web-based and commercial software packages [74–77].

Both Myriad and BRCAPRO models are most useful for assessing individual as well as familial risk in high-risk populations [78]. However, because they focus on assessing the probability of carrying a *BRCA1/BRCA12* mutation, they do not address lower-penetrance susceptibility genes. In contrast, the Breast and Ovarian Analysis of Disease Incidence and Carrier Estimation Algorithm (BOADICEA) model, first described in 2002 [79] with further description of the refined model published in 2004 [80], predicts the likelihood of carrying a clinically harmful *BRCA1/BRCA2* mutation and also assesses a purported polygenetic component of risk separate from *BRCA1/BRCA2* mutations. Like BRCAPRO, BOADICEA uses Bayes' theorem and additionally predicts the risk of developing breast cancer over time [80]. BOADICEA was developed in an original cohort of women from the Anglian Breast Cancer (ABC) study who were diagnosed with breast cancer under the age of 55 [79], and it was validated in multiple additional cohorts [80]. The model was updated in 2008 by incorporating data from two additional cohorts (the UK National Case-Control Study and the Manchester Study) and by accounting for family history of male breast cancer, prostate cancer, and pancreatic cancer [81].

Further updates in 2014 account for tumor pathology characteristics, including ER status, triple-negative status, and expression of basal markers (CK5/CK6 and CK14), and incorporate updated cancer incidences into the calculations [82]. Although all relatives within a patient's pedigree may be incorporated into the algorithm, permitting more complete data, this also increases the risk of recall bias [80]. When compared with other genetic-based models, including BRCAPRO and Myriad, BOADICEA demonstrates good overall predictive accuracy of carrier incidence within the population, as well as discriminatory accuracy regarding mutation carrier status at the individual level [81, 83–85]. BOADICEA can be accessed via an online web application [86].

Conclusion

Currently, it is recommended that genetic testing should be offered to all eligible breast cancer patients regardless of when they were diagnosed. Patients with a previous diagnosis of breast cancer should have close follow-up and be continually reassessed for their eligibility for genetic testing. Mutation carriers benefit from knowledge of mutation status in terms of definitive management, future risk management, and systemic therapy. Cascade genetic screening of relatives is critical. As multigene panel testing and the identification of actionable mutations is increasing, it is important for health care professionals to identify not only *BRCA1/BRCA2* mutation carriers but also patients who are mutation carriers of other heritable syndromes. Tools that are designed only to identify BRCA mutation carriers can potentially miss carriers of other gene mutations. Any patient at risk for a mutation in a cancer-causing gene should undergo genetic testing, and a comprehensive family history should include cancers of all other organ systems to evaluate for heritable syndromes.

Rapid advances in genomic sequencing technology have led to increasingly personalized surgical and medical treatment options. It is likely that mutation-specific treatments for cancer-causing genes will become the standard in the future by providing accurate genetic diagnoses, comprehensive risk assessment, informed counseling, therapeutic profiling, and early prevention.

References

1. Drohan B, Roche CA, Cusack JC Jr, Hughes KS. Hereditary breast and ovarian cancer and other hereditary syndromes: using technology to identify carriers. Ann Surg Oncol. 2012;19(6):1732–7.
2. Ingham SL, Sperrin M, Baildam A, Ross GL, Clayton R, Lalloo F, et al. Risk-reducing surgery increases survival in BRCA1/2 mutation carriers unaffected at time of family referral. Breast Cancer Res Treat. 2013;142(3):611–8.
3. Levy-Lahad E, Lahad A, King MC. Precision medicine meets public health: population screening for BRCA1 and BRCA2. J Natl Cancer Inst. 2015;107(1):420.
4. Srivastava A, McKinnon W, Wood ME. Risk of breast and ovarian cancer in women with strong family histories. Oncology (Williston Park). 2001;15(7):889–902. discussion, 5–7, 11–13
5. NCCN Clinical practice guidelines in oncology: genetic/familial high risk assessment: breast and ovarian. https://www.nccn.org. Accessed 27 Aug 2016
6. Schwartz GF, Hughes KS, Lynch HT, Fabian CJ, Fentiman IS, Robson ME, et al. Proceedings of the international consensus conference on breast cancer risk, genetics, & risk management, April, 2007. Cancer. 2008;113(10):2627–37.

7. Guenard F, Labrie Y, Ouellette G, Beauparlant CJ, Bessette P, Chiquette J, et al. Germline mutations in the breast cancer susceptibility gene PTEN are rare in high-risk non-BRCA1/2 French Canadian breast cancer families. Familial Cancer. 2007;6(4):483–90.
8. Bradbury AR, Olopade OI. Genetic susceptibility to breast cancer. Rev Endocr Metab Disord. 2007;8(3):255–67.
9. Hearle N, Schumacher V, Menko FH, Olschwang S, Boardman LA, Gille JJ, et al. Frequency and spectrum of cancers in the Peutz-Jeghers syndrome. Clin Cancer Res. 2006;12(10):3209–15.
10. Kaurah P, MacMillan A, Boyd N, Senz J, De Luca A, Chun N, et al. Founder and recurrent CDH1 mutations in families with hereditary diffuse gastric cancer. JAMA. 2007;297(21):2360–72.
11. Thompson D, Easton D, Breast Cancer Linkage C. Variation in cancer risks, by mutation position, in BRCA2 mutation carriers. Am J Hum Genet. 2001;68(2):410–9.
12. Ford D, Easton DF, Bishop DT, Narod SA, Goldgar DE. Risks of cancer in BRCA1-mutation carriers. Breast Cancer Linkage Consortium. Lancet. 1994;343(8899):692–5.
13. Breast Cancer Linkage C. Cancer risks in BRCA2 mutation carriers. J Natl Cancer Inst. 1999;91(15):1310–6.
14. Thompson D, Easton DF, Breast Cancer Linkage C. Cancer incidence in BRCA1 mutation carriers. J Natl Cancer Inst. 2002;94(18):1358–65.
15. Cybulski C, Wokolorczyk D, Jakubowska A, Huzarski T, Byrski T, Gronwald J, et al. Risk of breast cancer in women with a CHEK2 mutation with and without a family history of breast cancer. J Clin Oncol. 2011;29(28):3747–52.
16. Thompson D, Duedal S, Kirner J, McGuffog L, Last J, Reiman A, et al. Cancer risks and mortality in heterozygous ATM mutation carriers. J Natl Cancer Inst. 2005;97(11):813–22.
17. Antoniou AC, Casadei S, Heikkinen T, Barrowdale D, Pylkas K, Roberts J, et al. Breast-cancer risk in families with mutations in PALB2. N Engl J Med. 2014;371(6):497–506.
18. Seal S, Thompson D, Renwick A, Elliott A, Kelly P, Barfoot R, et al. Truncating mutations in the Fanconi anemia J gene BRIP1 are low-penetrance breast cancer susceptibility alleles. Nat Genet. 2006;38(11):1239–41.
19. Rosenberg SM, Ruddy KJ, Tamimi RM, Gelber S, Schapira L, Come S, et al. BRCA1 and BRCA2 mutation testing in young women with breast cancer. JAMA Oncol. 2016;2(6):730–6.
20. Brown KL, Hutchison R, Zinberg RE, McGovern MM. Referral and experience with genetic testing among women with early onset breast cancer. Genet Test. 2005;9(4):301–5.
21. Loman N, Johannsson O, Kristoffersson U, Olsson H, Borg A. Family history of breast and ovarian cancers and BRCA1 and BRCA2 mutations in a population-based series of early-onset breast cancer. J Natl Cancer Inst. 2001;93(16):1215–23.
22. American Society of Clinical O. American Society of Clinical Oncology policy statement update: genetic testing for cancer susceptibility. J Clin Oncol. 2003;21(12):2397–406.
23. Brose MS, Rebbeck TR, Calzone KA, Stopfer JE, Nathanson KL, Weber BL. Cancer risk estimates for BRCA1 mutation carriers identified in a risk evaluation program. J Natl Cancer Inst. 2002;94(18):1365–72.
24. Risch HA, McLaughlin JR, Cole DE, Rosen B, Bradley L, Fan I, et al. Population BRCA1 and BRCA2 mutation frequencies and cancer penetrances: a kin-cohort study in Ontario, Canada. J Natl Cancer Inst. 2006;98(23):1694–706.
25. Iqbal J, Ragone A, Lubinski J, Lynch HT, Moller P, Ghadirian P, et al. The incidence of pancreatic cancer in BRCA1 and BRCA2 mutation carriers. Br J Cancer. 2012;107(12):2005–9.
26. Grant RC, Selander I, Connor AA, Selvarajah S, Borgida A, Briollais L, et al. Prevalence of germline mutations in cancer predisposition genes in patients with pancreatic cancer. Gastroenterology. 2015;148(3):556–64.
27. Judkins T, Rosenthal E, Arnell C, Burbidge LA, Geary W, Barrus T, et al. Clinical significance of large rearrangements in BRCA1 and BRCA2. Cancer. 2012;118(21):5210–6.
28. Walsh T, Casadei S, Coats KH, Swisher E, Stray SM, Higgins J, et al. Spectrum of mutations in BRCA1, BRCA2, CHEK2, and TP53 in families at high risk of breast cancer. JAMA. 2006;295(12):1379–88.
29. Hendrickson BC, Judkins T, Ward BD, Eliason K, Deffenbaugh AE, Burbidge LA, et al. Prevalence of five previously reported and recurrent BRCA1 genetic rearrangement mutations

in 20,000 patients from hereditary breast/ovarian cancer families. Genes Chromosom Cancer. 2005;43(3):309–13.
30. Campeau PM, Foulkes WD, Tischkowitz MD. Hereditary breast cancer: new genetic developments, new therapeutic avenues. Hum Genet. 2008;124(1):31–42.
31. Li J, Meeks H, Feng BJ, Healey S, Thorne H, Makunin I, et al. Targeted massively parallel sequencing of a panel of putative breast cancer susceptibility genes in a large cohort of multiple-case breast and ovarian cancer families. J Med Genet. 2016;53(1):34–42.
32. Frey MK, Kim SH, Bassett RY, Martineau J, Dalton E, Chern JY, et al. Rescreening for genetic mutations using multi-gene panel testing in patients who previously underwent non-informative genetic screening. Gynecol Oncol. 2015;139(2):211–5.
33. Desmond A, Kurian AW, Gabree M, Mills MA, Anderson MJ, Kobayashi Y, et al. Clinical actionability of multigene panel testing for hereditary breast and ovarian cancer risk assessment. JAMA Oncol. 2015;1(7):943–51.
34. Metcalfe K, Gershman S, Lynch HT, Ghadirian P, Tung N, Kim-Sing C, et al. Predictors of contralateral breast cancer in BRCA1 and BRCA2 mutation carriers. Br J Cancer. 2011; 104(9):1384–92.
35. van Sprundel TC, Schmidt MK, Rookus MA, Brohet R, van Asperen CJ, Rutgers EJ, et al. Risk reduction of contralateral breast cancer and survival after contralateral prophylactic mastectomy in BRCA1 or BRCA2 mutation carriers. Br J Cancer. 2005;93(3):287–92.
36. Giuliano AE, Boolbol S, Degnim A, Kuerer H, Leitch AM, Morrow M. Society of Surgical Oncology: position statement on prophylactic mastectomy. Approved by the Society of Surgical Oncology Executive Council, March 2007. Ann Surg Oncol. 2007;14(9):2425–7.
37. Valachis A, Nearchou AD, Lind P. Surgical management of breast cancer in BRCA-mutation carriers: a systematic review and meta-analysis. Breast Cancer Res Treat. 2014;144(3):443–55.
38. Metcalfe K, Lynch HT, Ghadirian P, Tung N, Olivotto I, Warner E, et al. Contralateral breast cancer in BRCA1 and BRCA2 mutation carriers. J Clin Oncol. 2004;22(12):2328–35.
39. Narod SA, Brunet JS, Ghadirian P, Robson M, Heimdal K, Neuhausen SL, et al. Tamoxifen and risk of contralateral breast cancer in BRCA1 and BRCA2 mutation carriers: a case-control study. Hereditary Breast Cancer Clinical Study Group. Lancet. 2000;356(9245):1876–81.
40. Gronwald J, Tung N, Foulkes WD, Offit K, Gershoni R, Daly M, et al. Tamoxifen and contralateral breast cancer in BRCA1 and BRCA2 carriers: an update. Int J Cancer. 2006;118(9):2281–4.
41. Phillips KA, Milne RL, Rookus MA, Daly MB, Antoniou AC, Peock S, et al. Tamoxifen and risk of contralateral breast cancer for BRCA1 and BRCA2 mutation carriers. J Clin Oncol. 2013;31(25):3091–9.
42. Tung N, Domchek SM, Stadler Z, Nathanson KL, Couch F, Garber JE, et al. Counselling framework for moderate-penetrance cancer-susceptibility mutations. Nat Rev Clin Oncol. 2016;13(9):581–8.
43. Heymann S, Delaloge S, Rahal A, Caron O, Frebourg T, Barreau L, et al. Radio-induced malignancies after breast cancer postoperative radiotherapy in patients with Li-Fraumeni syndrome. Radiat Oncol. 2010;5:104.
44. van der Post RS, Vogelaar IP, Carneiro F, Guilford P, Huntsman D, Hoogerbrugge N, et al. Hereditary diffuse gastric cancer: updated clinical guidelines with an emphasis on germline CDH1 mutation carriers. J Med Genet. 2015;52(6):361–74.
45. Prevention CfDCa. Tier 1 genomics applications and their importance to public health.
46. Prevention CfDCa. Hereditary Breast and Ovarian Cancer (HBOC) Phase 1.
47. Metcalfe K, Lynch HT, Ghadirian P, Tung N, Kim-Sing C, Olopade OI, et al. Risk of ipsilateral breast cancer in BRCA1 and BRCA2 mutation carriers. Breast Cancer Res Treat. 2011;127(1):287–96.
48. Farmer H, McCabe N, Lord CJ, Tutt AN, Johnson DA, Richardson TB, et al. Targeting the DNA repair defect in BRCA mutant cells as a therapeutic strategy. Nature. 2005;434(7035):917–21.
49. Quinn JE, James CR, Stewart GE, Mulligan JM, White P, Chang GK, et al. BRCA1 mRNA expression levels predict for overall survival in ovarian cancer after chemotherapy. Clin Cancer Res. 2007;13(24):7413–20.

50. Rottenberg S, Nygren AO, Pajic M, van Leeuwen FW, van der Heijden I, van de Wetering K, et al. Selective induction of chemotherapy resistance of mammary tumors in a conditional mouse model for hereditary breast cancer. Proc Natl Acad Sci U S A. 2007;104(29):12117–22.
51. Clergue O, Jones N, Sevenet N, Quenel-Tueux N, Debled M. Should knowledge of BRCA1 status impact the choice of chemotherapy in metastatic breast cancer: a review. Bull Cancer. 2015;102(3):245–55.
52. Bryant HE, Schultz N, Thomas HD, Parker KM, Flower D, Lopez E, et al. Specific killing of BRCA2-deficient tumours with inhibitors of poly(ADP-ribose) polymerase. Nature. 2005;434(7035):913–7.
53. Fong PC, Boss DS, Yap TA, Tutt A, Wu P, Mergui-Roelvink M, et al. Inhibition of poly(ADP-ribose) polymerase in tumors from BRCA mutation carriers. N Engl J Med. 2009;361(2):123–34.
54. PARP inhibitors. https://www.breastcancertrials.org/bct_nation/browse_trials.seam%3Bjsessionid=13FBD071E8DF7F064AF70D8C262EE2EF?categoryString=PARP&Search_Operator=OR.Accessed 27 Aug 2016.
55. Mendes-Pereira AM, Martin SA, Brough R, McCarthy A, Taylor JR, Kim JS, et al. Synthetic lethal targeting of PTEN mutant cells with PARP inhibitors. EMBO Mol Med. 2009;1(6–7):315–22.
56. Gilardini Montani MS, Prodosmo A, Stagni V, Merli D, Monteonofrio L, Gatti V, et al. ATM-depletion in breast cancer cells confers sensitivity to PARP inhibition. J Exp Clin Cancer Res. 2013;32:95.
57. Schwartz MD, Lerman C, Brogan B, Peshkin BN, Isaacs C, DeMarco T, et al. Utilization of BRCA1/BRCA2 mutation testing in newly diagnosed breast cancer patients. Cancer Epidemiol Biomark Prev. 2005;14(4):1003–7.
58. Schwartz MD, Lerman C, Brogan B, Peshkin BN, Halbert CH, DeMarco T, et al. Impact of BRCA1/BRCA2 counseling and testing on newly diagnosed breast cancer patients. J Clin Oncol. 2004;22(10):1823–9.
59. Meijers-Heijboer H, Brekelmans CT, Menke-Pluymers M, Seynaeve C, Baalbergen A, Burger C, et al. Use of genetic testing and prophylactic mastectomy and oophorectomy in women with breast or ovarian cancer from families with a BRCA1 or BRCA2 mutation. J Clin Oncol. 2003;21(9):1675–81.
60. Shattuck-Eidens D, Oliphant A, McClure M, McBride C, Gupte J, Rubano T, et al. BRCA1 sequence analysis in women at high risk for susceptibility mutations. Risk factor analysis and implications for genetic testing. JAMA. 1997;278(15):1242–50.
61. Frank TS, Manley SA, Olopade OI, Cummings S, Garber JE, Bernhardt B, et al. Sequence analysis of BRCA1 and BRCA2: correlation of mutations with family history and ovarian cancer risk. J Clin Oncol. 1998;16(7):2417–25.
62. Frank TS, Deffenbaugh AM, Reid JE, Hulick M, Ward BE, Lingenfelter B, et al. Clinical characteristics of individuals with germline mutations in BRCA1 and BRCA2: analysis of 10,000 individuals. J Clin Oncol: Off J Am Soc Clin Oncol. 2002;20(6):1480–90.
63. Barcenas CH, Hosain GM, Arun B, Zong J, Zhou X, Chen J, et al. Assessing BRCA carrier probabilities in extended families. J Clin Oncol. 2006;24(3):354–60.
64. Bodmer D, Ligtenberg MJ, van der Hout AH, Gloudemans S, Ansink K, Oosterwijk JC, et al. Optimal selection for BRCA1 and BRCA2 mutation testing using a combination of 'easy to apply' probability models. Br J Cancer. 2006;95(6):757–62.
65. Parmigiani G, Chen S, Iversen ES Jr, Friebel TM, Finkelstein DM, Anton-Culver H, et al. Validity of models for predicting BRCA1 and BRCA2 mutations. Ann Intern Med. 2007;147(7):441–50.
66. Panchal SM, Ennis M, Canon S, Bordeleau LJ. Selecting a BRCA risk assessment model for use in a familial cancer clinic. BMC Med Genet. 2008;9:116.
67. MYRIAD PRO: BRCA risk calculator. https://www.myriadpro.com/hereditary-cancer-testing/hereditary-breast-and-ovarian-cancer-hboc-syndrome/brca-risk-calculator/.Accessed 27 Aug 2016.

68. MYRIAD PRO: prevalence tables. https://www.myriadpro.com/hereditary-cancer-testing/hereditary-breast-and-ovarian-cancer-hboc-syndrome/prevalence-tables/. Accessed 27 Aug 2016.
69. Berry DA, Parmigiani G, Sanchez J, Schildkraut J, Winer E. Probability of carrying a mutation of breast-ovarian cancer gene BRCA1 based on family history. J Natl Cancer Inst. 1997;89(3):227–38.
70. Parmigiani G, Berry D, Aguilar O. Determining carrier probabilities for breast cancer-susceptibility genes BRCA1 and BRCA2. Am J Hum Genet. 1998;62(1):145–58.
71. Mazzola E, Blackford A, Parmigiani G, Biswas S. Recent enhancements to the genetic risk prediction model BRCAPRO. Cancer Informat. 2015;14(Suppl 2):147–57.
72. Biswas S, Atienza P, Chipman J, Hughes K, Barrera AM, Amos CI, et al. Simplifying clinical use of the genetic risk prediction model BRCAPRO. Breast Cancer Res Treat. 2013; 139(2):571–9.
73. Recent enhancements to the genetic risk prediction model BRCAPRO. http://www.la-press.com/recent-enhancements-to-the-genetic-risk-prediction-model-brcapro-article-a4822. Accessed 27 Aug 2016.
74. Online Risk Service. http://bayesmendel.dfci.harvard.edu/risk/. Accessed 27 Aug 2016.
75. Progeny: cancer risk assessment. http://www.progenygenetics.com/clinical/risk. Accessed 27 Aug 2016.
76. CancerGene. https://www4.utsouthwestern.edu/breasthealth/cagene/. Accessed 27 Aug 2016.
77. CRA health: risk assessment. Accessed 27 Aug 2016.
78. Rao NY, Hu Z, Yu JM, Li WF, Zhang B, Su FX, et al. Evaluating the performance of models for predicting the BRCA germline mutations in Han Chinese familial breast cancer patients. Breast Cancer Res Treat. 2009;116(3):563–70.
79. Antoniou AC, Pharoah PD, McMullan G, Day NE, Stratton MR, Peto J, et al. A comprehensive model for familial breast cancer incorporating BRCA1, BRCA2 and other genes. Br J Cancer. 2002;86(1):76–83.
80. Antoniou AC, Pharoah PP, Smith P, Easton DF. The BOADICEA model of genetic susceptibility to breast and ovarian cancer. Br J Cancer. 2004;91(8):1580–90.
81. Antoniou AC, Hardy R, Walker L, Evans DG, Shenton A, Eeles R, et al. Predicting the likelihood of carrying a BRCA1 or BRCA2 mutation: validation of BOADICEA, BRCAPRO, IBIS, Myriad and the Manchester scoring system using data from UK genetics clinics. J Med Genet. 2008;45(7):425–31.
82. Lee AJ, Cunningham AP, Kuchenbaecker KB, Mavaddat N, Easton DF, Antoniou AC. BOADICEA breast cancer risk prediction model: updates to cancer incidences, tumour pathology and web interface. Br J Cancer. 2014;110(2):535–45.
83. Antoniou AC, Durocher F, Smith P, Simard J, Easton DF. BRCA1 and BRCA2 mutation predictions using the BOADICEA and BRCAPRO models and penetrance estimation in high-risk French-Canadian families. Breast cancer research : BCR. 2006;8(1):R3.
84. Schneegans SM, Rosenberger A, Engel U, Sander M, Emons G, Shoukier M. Validation of three BRCA1/2 mutation-carrier probability models Myriad, BRCAPRO and BOADICEA in a population-based series of 183 German families. Familial Cancer. 2012;11(2):181–8.
85. Fischer C, Kuchenbacker K, Engel C, Zachariae S, Rhiem K, Meindl A, et al. Evaluating the performance of the breast cancer genetic risk models BOADICEA, IBIS, BRCAPRO and Claus for predicting BRCA1/2 mutation carrier probabilities: a study based on 7352 families from the German Hereditary Breast and Ovarian Cancer Consortium. J Med Genet. 2013;50(6):360–7.
86. BOADICEA web application. http://ccge.medschl.cam.ac.uk/boadicea/boadicea-web-application/. Accessed 27 Aug 2016.

Correction to: Percutaneous Ablation in the Treatment of Breast Cancer

Vivian J. Bea, Dalliah Black, and Kelly Hunt

Correction to:
Chapter 6: M. Howard-McNatt (ed.), *Changing Paradigms in the Management of Breast Cancer*,
https://doi.org/10.1007/978-3-319-60336-0_6

After publication of this chapter it has come to the authors' attention that Fig. 6.5 needs changes to better protect the privacy of the patient. A modified Fig. 6.5 is included in this Erratum. The original Fig. 6.5 has been removed to protect the patient's privacy.

The updated original version of this chapter can be found at
https://doi.org/10.1007/978-3-319-60336-0_6

M. Howard-McNatt (ed.), *Changing Paradigms in the Management of Breast Cancer*, https://doi.org/10.1007/978-3-319-60336-0_16

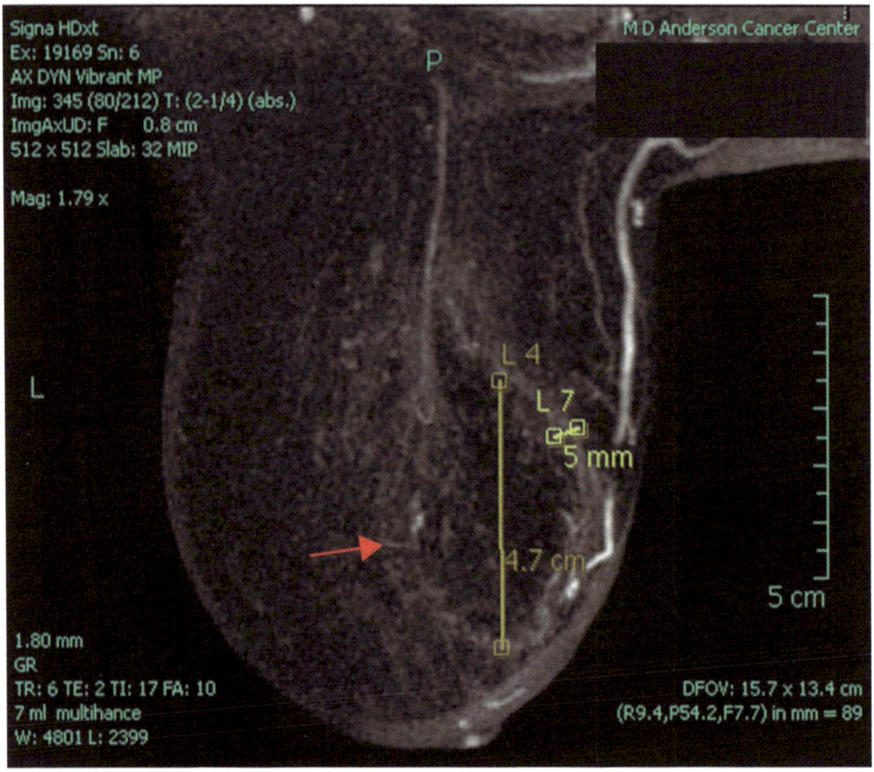

Fig. 6.5 Post-cryoablation breast MRI. *Red arrow* marks cryoablation halo cavity; no residual enhancing mass is seen

Index

A
Abemaciclib, 175, 177
ACOSOG Z0011, 53
ACOSOG Z1072, 80
Adipose-derived regenerative cells (ADRC), 108
Adjuvant chemoradiation therapy, 146
Adjuvant systemic therapy, 141
Alpelisib (BYL719), 183
American College of Chest Physicians (ACCP), 89
American College of Surgeons Oncology Group (ACOSOG), 49, 141
American Society of Clinical Oncology (ASCO), 220
American Society of Plastic Surgeons (ASPS), 90
Antibody-drug conjugates (ADC), 177, 186, 187
Arimidex, Tamoxifen, Alone or in Combination (ATAC), 204
Atezolizumab, 163
Atypical ductal hyperplasia (ADH), 117, 118, 120, 122–124
Atypical lobular hyperplasia (ALH), 120–124
Axilla
  ACOSOG Z1071 trial, 51
  ALND, 55
  cN0, 48
  DCIS, 54
  levels, 48
  management, 55
  multi-institutional trials, 52
  NCCN Guidelines, 53
  node-positive disease, 51
  radiation therapy, 52
  SLN, 47
  SN FNAC study, 52
  ultrasound, 50
Axillary lymph node (ALN), 147
Axillary lymph node dissection (ALND), 47, 127–133, 135, 139–145, 147, 151
Axillary ultrasound, 48, 50

B
Bayes' theorem, 227
Bevacizumab, 158, 186
Body mass index (BMI), 89, 156
Brain metastases, 188, 189
BRCA, 209, 211–213
BRCAPRO models, 227
Breast and Ovarian Analysis of Disease Incidence and Carrier Estimation Algorithm (BOADICEA), 227
Breast atypias, 117
Breast cancer, 17–21, 28, 54, 59
  margins and (*see* Margins and breast cancer)
  and radiation therapy, 127
Breast cancer patients
  BRCA mutation, 225
  BRCA1/BRCA2 mutation, 222
  BRCA1-/BRCA2-negative individuals, 221
  genetic testing rates, 220
  multigene panels, 222
  NCCN, 220, 221
  newly diagnosed patients, 225
  previously diagnosed patients, 220–223, 225
  TP53 mutation, 223
Breast cancer treatment in elderly patients, 199, 200
  chemotherapy, 203
  endocrine therapy, 204, 205
  radiation therapy, 202, 203
  screening, 200, 201
  treatment, 201, 202
  treatment pattern, 200
  tumor biology, 201

M. Howard-McNatt (ed.), *Changing Paradigms in the Management of Breast Cancer*, DOI 10.1007/978-3-319-60336-0

Breast cancer treatment in young women
fertility, 210, 211
genetic testing, 211–213
psychosocial issues, 213, 214
Breast conservation surgery (BCS), 33
Breast conservation therapy (BCT), 214
Breast imaging, 1
abbreviated (Fast) MRI, 12
CEM, 11, 12
digital mammography and breast tomosynthesis, 2–4, 6
magnetic resonance imaging, 8–11
ultrasound and elastography, 7, 8
Breast Imaging Reporting and Data System (BIRADS), 2, 3
Breast implant technology, 96–99
Breast MRI and Atypias, 123, 124
Breast nodal volumes, 148
Breast prosthetic placement, 87
Breast reconstruction
ADMs, 86
autologous tissue, 86
BCS, 94
BRAVA technique, 109
breast prosthesis, 98
CTA, 90
dermal grafts, 101
fTRAM, 104
ICGFA, 92
MRA, 90
neoadjuvant and adjuvant therapies, 87
NSM, 95
patient education, 88
round-shaped implants, 99
saline implants, 98
SIEAV, 104
SSM, 94
timing and technique, 86
Breast screening programs, 71
Breast volume replacement, 104
Breast-conserving surgery (BCS), 127, 129, 131–135
Buparlisib (BKM120), 183

C
Cabozantinib, 186
Cascade genetic screening, 223
CDK4/CDK6 inhibitors, 178–179
Cell-cycle machinery, 176
Center for Disease Control (CDC), 223
Central nervous system disease, 188–189
Charleston Comorbidity Index, 201
Chemotherapy, 203
Clinically node negative (cN0), 48
Coleman technique, 108
Computed tomography angiogram (CTA), 91
Contralateral breast cancer (CBC), 35
characteristics, 37
rates, 38
risk, 37
Contralateral prophylactic mastectomy (CPM), 33, 39, 40
CBC characteristics, 37
CBC rates, 38
CBC risk, 37
counseling patients on, 41
patient perspectives on
patient knowledge, 40
patient motivations for choosing CPM, 39
patient satisfaction and quality of life, 39, 40
pros and cons, 42
reasons to consider or not consider, 42
surgeon perspectives, 40, 41
and survival, 35–37
trends in, 34, 35
Contrast-enhanced mammography (CEM), 11, 12
Cook-Swartz implantable Doppler system, 92
Core biopsy, 117, 119–124
Cryoablation, 73
ACOSOG Z1072, 76–77
concept, 74
fibroadenomas, 73
retrospective study, 75
skin damage, 73
surgical excision, 75
ultrasound-guided, 74
Cyclin D1, 175

D
Diffusion-weighted imaging (DWI), 10
Digital breast tomosynthesis (DBT), 2–6
Digital mammography, 2–4, 6
Dinaciclib, 177
Doppler/duplex ultrasonography, 90
Ductal carcinoma in situ (DCIS), 2, 54, 60, 118–120, 122, 124

E
EBCTCG meta-analysis data, 147
Elastography, 7, 8
Embryo cryopreservation, 210
Endocrine Therapy, 204

Entinostat, 187
ER-negative breast cancer, 203
Extra-nodal extension (ECE), 140

F
False-negative rate (FNR), 48, 51
Fat grafting, 107
Fat harvest, 108
Fertility preservation, 210, 211
FibroAdenoma Cryoablation Treatment (FACT) registry, 73
First-generation prosthesis, 99
Flap innervation, 105–107
Flap-Based Breast Reconstruction, 103–109
Flat epithelial atypia (FEA), 117–120, 123, 124
Fluorescent Angiography (FA), 92
Free Tissue Transfer Assessment, 90–93

G
Genetic risk prediction
  BRCA1 and *BRCA2* genes, 217
  health care system, 217
  hereditary cancer syndromes, 218
  mutation, 218
Gonadotropin-releasing hormone (GnRH) agonist, 210
Graft survival, 108

H
Heat shock proteins, 188
HER2-positive disease, 177
Hereditary Breast and Ovarian Cancer Syndrome (HBOC), 212, 220
Hereditary cancer syndromes, 218
  mutations, 219
  penetrant genes, 219
High-intensity focused ultrasound (HIFU), 79
Histone deacetylases (HDAC), 187
Hormone agonist, 210

I
Immunotherapy clinical trials, 181–182
Implantable Doppler Monitoring, 92–93
Implant-based breast reconstruction, 89
Indocyanine green fluorescent angiography (ICGFA), 91
Inferolateral approach, 24
Inflammatory breast cancer (IBC), 54
Internal mammary nodes (IMN), 129, 132
The International Breast Cancer Study Group (IBCSG), 49
Intraoperative specimen imaging, 62, 63
Intraoperative ultrasound, 63

J
Janus kinase 2 (JAK2), 185

L
Laser ablation, 79
Latissimus dorsi myocutaneous (LDMC) flap, 86
Left ventricular ejection fraction (LVEF), 203
Liposculpting, 107
Lobular carcinoma in situ (LCIS), 119–124
Lobular neoplasia, 117, 120–124
Local recurrence rates, 214
Local-regional recurrence (LRR), 147
Locoregional failure (LRF), 129
Locoregional recurrence (LRR), 127, 128, 131, 134
Luminal androgen receptor (LAR) type, 161
Lumpectomy, 85, 140–144, 151, 202
Lumpectomy cavity, 64
Lynch syndrome, 223

M
Magnetic resonance angiography, 90
Magnetic resonance imaging (MRI), 1, 2, 8–11, 60
Mammogram, 2–4, 6, 19
Margins and breast cancer, 60–65
  DCIS, 60
  intraoperative ultrasound, 63
  invasive cancer, 59
  recurrence rates, 60, 65
  techniques to improve clearance, 60
    intraoperative pathologic evaluation, 65
    intraoperative specimen imaging, 62, 63
    localization techniques for non-palpable tumors, 61, 62
    novel technology, 63, 64
    preoperative imaging, 60, 61
    routine cavity shave margins, 64
Mastectomy, 202
Maximum intensity projection image (MIP), 12
Metastatic breast cancer (MBC)
  abemaciclib, 188
  ADC, 186
  AKT and mTOR, 180
  CD28, 177

Metastatic breast cancer (MBC) (*cont.*)
CDK4/CDK6 inhibitors, 175
cell cycle, 175
checkpoints, 175
CNS, 188
drugs, 168–174
ER-positive breast cancer, 175
FGFR genes, 185
growth factor receptor, 185, 186
HDAC inhibitors, 187
IGF-1R, 185
immune checkpoint, 177–180
leptomeningeal metastases, 189
ligand binding, 180
monotherapy, 189
mTOR inhibitor, 183
oncogenic signaling pathways, 167, 175
ORR, 180
PARP inhibition, 187
PI3 kinases, 180
PI3K inhibitors, 183
PI3K/AKT/mTOR, 183
PIK3CA mutations, 183, 185
Meticulous surgical technique, 28
Modified radical mastectomy (MRM), 94
Multidisciplinary approach, 52
Myriad model, 226

N
National Cancer Data Base (NCDB), 34
National Comprehensive Cancer Network (NCCN) guidelines, 53, 60, 211, 218, 224
National Surgical Adjuvant Breast and Bowel Project (NSABP), 49
Neoadjuvant chemotherapy (NACT), 50–52, 133–135, 147–151, 157
Neratinib, 160, 161
Neurotization, 107
Nipple areola complex (NAC), 110
Nipple reconstruction, 109–110
Nipple-sparing mastectomy (NSM), 18, 19, 23–28, 94
for breast cancer, 28
complications, 27
for cancer, 22
oncologic outcome of therapeutic, 21–23
oncologic safety occult nipple involvement, 18, 19
patient satisfaction, cosmetic outcome, 27, 28
patient selection, 19, 20
prophylactic, 21
for risk reduction, 20, 21
surgical technique
incision placement, 23, 24
nipple margin assessment, 25–27
overview of technique, 24, 25
Non-skin-sparing mastectomy (NSSM), 94
NSQIP registry, 89

O
Oncoplastic breast surgery, 102
Overall response rates (ORR), 180

P
Palbociclib, 175
Pathologic complete response (pCR) rate, 133
Pathologic-radiologic concordance, 122, 123
Pedicle transverse rectus abdominis myocutaneous (pTRAM) flap, 86
Percutaneous ablation
advantages, 71
cryoablation, 72
HIFU's, 79
laser ablation, 79
mammogram and ultrasound, 80
MRI, 81
PMC, 79
RFA, 77
Percutaneous microwave coagulation (PMC), 79
PI3K inhibitors, 184
Poly-ADP-ribose polymerase (PARP), 159, 187
Post-mastectomy radiation therapy (PMRT), 127–129, 132, 134, 144–147, 149, 151
Profunda artery perforator (PAP) flap, 105
Progression-free survival (PFS) rates, 158
Prophylactic NSM, 21
Prosthesis location modifications, 97

R
Radiation therapy and breast cancer, 127
Radioactive seed localization (RSL), 61
Radiofrequency ablation (RFA)
hepatocellular carcinoma, 77
limitations, 78
temperature, 77
two-center pilot study, 77
Radio-occult lesion localization (ROLL), 61
Radiotherapy and regional nodes
axillary management, 139–142
neoadjuvant chemotherapy and adjuvant radiation, 147–151
post-mastectomy radiation therapy, 144–147
supraclavicular and internal mammary management, 142–144

Regional nodal irradiation (RNI), 49, 128, 129
after breast-conserving surgery, 129, 130
by extent of axillary surgery, 130–132
and neoadjuvant chemotherapy, 133–135
Rosen triad, 117

S
Screening mammography, 117
SENTINA trial, 51
Sentinel lymph node biopsy (SLNB), 139–142, 151
Silicone gel polymers, 98
Single-stage implant-based breast reconstruction, 99, 100
Skin-sparing mastectomy (SSM), 94
Society of Surgical Oncology (SSO), 222
Soft tissue flaps, 107
SOUND trial, 55
Stacked flaps, 107
Subcutaneous mastectomy, 18, 20
Surgical decision making, 41
Surveillance Epidemiology End Results (SEER), 34

T
Tamoxifen, 139, 145, 146, 204
Therapeutic nipple-sparing mastectomy, 21–23
Tissue Oximetry, 93
Total skin-sparing mastectomy, 18
Trastuzumab, 203
Triple-negative breast cancer (TNBC), 155
epidemiology and risk factors, 156, 157
immunotherapy, 162, 163
targeted therapies, 159–161
targeted therapies by subtype, 161, 162
treatment, 157, 158
Tumor-infiltrating lymphocytes (TILs), 162, 163
Two-stage implant-based breast reconstruction, 96

U
Ultrasound, 7–9, 72

V
Variant of uncertain significance (VUS) rate, 212, 222
Venous thromboembolism (VTE), 89

W
Whole breast irradiation (WBI), 53, 139

MIX
Papier aus verantwortungsvollen Quellen
Paper from responsible sources
FSC® C105338

If you have any concerns about our products,
you can contact us on
ProductSafety@springernature.com

In case Publisher is established outside the EU,
the EU authorized representative is:
Springer Nature Customer Service Center GmbH
Europaplatz 3, 69115 Heidelberg, Germany

Printed by Libri Plureos GmbH
in Hamburg, Germany